INSTRUCTOR'S GUIDE

to accompany

Psychiatric/Mental Health Nursing: Concepts of Care

Third Edition

Mary C. Townsend
Clinical Nurse Specialist
Adult Psychiatric/Mental Health Nursing
Private Practice
Oklahoma City, OK

Formerly Assistant Professor and
Coordinator, Mental Health Nursing
Kramer School of Nursing
Oklahoma City University
Oklahoma City, OK

 F. A. DAVIS COMPANY • Philadelphia

F. A. Davis Company
1915 Arch Street
Philadelphia, PA 19103

Last digit indicates print number: 10 9 8 7 6 5 4 3 2 1

Printed in the United States of America

ISBN 0-8036-0484-X

CONTENTS

UNIT FOUR   SPECIAL TOPICS IN PSYCHIATRIC/MENTAL HEALTH NURSING

CHAPTER 1. AN INTRODUCTION TO THE CONCEPT OF STRESS

CHAPTER FOCUS

The focus of this chapter is to describe the concept of stress using various definitions that have been identified in the literature. The relationship between stress and illness is discussed.

LEARNING OBJECTIVES

After reading this chapter, the student will be able to:

1. Define *adaptation* and *maladaptation*.
2. Identify physiological responses to stress.
3. Explain the relationship between stress and "diseases of adaptation."
4. Describe the concept of stress as an environmental event.
5. Explain the concept of stress as a transaction between the individual and the environment.
6. Discuss adaptive coping strategies in the management of stress.

KEY TERMS

stress	"fight-or-flight syndrome"
adaptation	precipitating event
maladaptation	predisposing factors

CHAPTER OUTLINE/LECTURE NOTES

I. Introduction
   A. The word *stress* lacks a definitive definition.
   B. Adaptation as a healthy response to stress has been defined as restoration of homeostasis to the internal environmental system. This includes responses directed at stabilizing internal biological processes and psychological preservation of self-identity and self-esteem.
   C. Maladaptive responses are perceived as negative or unhealthy and occur when the integrity of the individual is disrupted.
II. Stress as a Biological Response
   A. This definition of stress is a result of research by Hans Selye. He defined stress as a "nonspecific response by the body to any stressor placed upon it." This syndrome of physical symptoms has come to be known as the "fight-or-flight syndrome."
   B. Selye called this general reaction of the body to stress the *general adaptation syndrome (GAS)*. He described the reaction in three distinct stages.
      1. Alarm reaction stage. During this stage, the physiological responses of the fight-or-flight syndrome are initiated.

2. Stage of resistance. The individual uses the physiological responses of the first stage as a defense in the attempt to adapt to the stressor. If adaptation occurs, the third stage is prevented or delayed. Physiological symptoms may disappear.
3. Stage of exhaustion. Exhaustion occurs when there is a prolonged exposure to the stressor to which the body has become adjusted. The adaptive energy is depleted, and the individual can no longer draw from the resources for adaptation described in the first two stages. Disease of adaptation may occur, and without intervention for reversal, exhaustion and even death can ensue.

C. The fight-or-flight syndrome
  1. The initial stress response
     a. The hypothalamus stimulates the sympathetic nervous system, which in turn stimulates the adrenal medulla. The adrenal medulla releases epinephrine and norepinephrine into the bloodstream.
     b. Changes in the eye include pupil dilation and increased secretion from the lacrimal glands.
     c. In the respiratory system, the bronchioles and pulmonary blood vessels are dilated and the respiration rate is increased.
     d. Changes in the cardiovascular system result in increases in force of contraction, cardiac output, heart rate, and blood pressure.
     e. The gastrointestinal (GI) system undergoes decreases in motility and secretions. Sphincters are contracted.
     f. Effects on the liver result in increased glycogenolysis and gluconeogenesis and decreased glycogen synthesis.
     g. Ureter motility increases. In the bladder, the muscle itself contracts, while the sphincter relaxes.
     h. There is increased secretion from the sweat glands.
     i. The fat cells undergo lipolysis.
  2. The sustained stress response
     a. The hypothalamus stimulates the pituitary gland.
     b. The pituitary gland releases adrenocorticotropic hormone (ACTH), which stimulates the adrenal cortex.
        (1) The adrenal cortex releases glucocorticoids, resulting in increased gluconeogenesis, immunosuppression, and an anti-inflammatory response.
        (2) The adrenal cortex also releases mineralocorticoids, resulting in increased retention of sodium and water.
     c. The pituitary gland releases vasopressin (antidiuretic hormone [ADH]), which results in increases in blood pressure and fluid retention.
     d. The pituitary gland releases growth hormone, which produces a direct effect on protein, carbohydrate, and lipid metabolism, resulting in increased serum glucose and free fatty acids.
     e. The pituitary gland releases thyrotropic hormone (TTH), which stimulates the thyroid gland, resulting in an increase in the basal metabolic rate.
     f. The pituitary gland releases gonadotropins, the initial response of which is an increase in secretion of sex hormones. Later, with sustained stress, secretion is suppressed, resulting in decreased libido or impotence.

III. Stress as an Environmental Event
  A. This concept defines stress as a "thing" or "event" that triggers the adaptive physiological and psychological responses in an individual. The event is one that creates change in the life pattern of the individual, requires significant adjustment in lifestyle, and taxes available personal resources. The change can be either positive or negative.
  B. Easily measured by the Holmes and Rahe Social Readjustment Rating Scale (SRRS).
  C. It is not known for certain whether stress overload merely predisposes a person to illness or actually precipitates it, but there does appear to be a clear causal link.

4. A weakness in the Holmes and Rahe tool is that it does not take into consideration the individual's personal perception of the event or their coping strategies and available support systems at the time of the life change.

IV. Stress as a Transaction between the Individual and the Environment

   A This definition of stress emphasizes the *relationship* between the individual and the environment that is appraised by the individual as taxing or exceeding his or her resources and endangering his or her well-being.

   B. Precipitating event. A stimulus arising from the internal or external environment and perceived by the individual in a specific manner

   C. Individual's perception of the event. When an event occurs, an individual undergoes a primary appraisal and a secondary appraisal of the situation

      1. Primary appraisal. The individual makes a judgment about the situation in one of the following ways.

         a. Irrelevant. When an event is judged irrelevant, the outcome holds no significance for the person.

         b. Benign-positive. This type of event is perceived as producing pleasure for the individual.

         c. Stress appraisal. These types of events include harm/loss, threat, and challenge.

            (1) Harm/loss. This refers to damage or loss already experienced by the individual.

            (2) Threatening. These types are perceived as anticipated harm or loss.

            (3) Challenges. With these types of events, the individual focuses on potential for gain or growth, rather than on risks associated with the event.

      2. Secondary appraisal. This type of appraisal is an assessment of skills, resources, and knowledge that the person possesses to deal with the situation.

      3. The interaction between the primary appraisal of the event that has occurred and the secondary appraisal of available coping strategies determines the individual's quality of adaptation response to stress.

      4. Predisposing factors. These elements influence how an individual perceives and responds to a stressful event. They include genetic influences, past experiences, and existing conditions.

         a. Genetic influences. Circumstances of an individual's life acquired by heredity (e.g., family history of physical and psychological conditions).

         b. Past experiences. Occurrences that result in learned patterns that can influence an individual's adaptation response (e.g., previous exposure to the stressor, learned coping responses, and degree of adaptation to previous stressors).

         c. Existing conditions. Vulnerabilities that influence the adequacy of the individual's physical, psychological, and social resources for dealing with adaptive demands (e.g., current health status, motivation, developmental maturity, severity and duration of the stressor, financial and educational resources, age, existing coping strategies, and a support system of caring others).

V. Stress Management

   A. Stress management is the utilization of coping strategies in the response to stressful situations.

   B. Adaptive coping strategies protect the individual from harm and restore physical and psychological homeostasis.

   C. Coping strategies are considered maladaptive when the conflict being experienced goes unresolved or intensifies.

   D. Some adaptive coping strategies include awareness, relaxation, meditation, interpersonal communication with caring other, problem solving, pets, music, and many others.

VI. Summary

VII. Review Questions

LEARNING ACTIVITIES

When the body encounters a stressor, it prepares itself for fight or flight. Identify the adaptation responses that occur in the initial stress response in each of the physical components listed.

Physical Component	Adaptation Response
Adrenal medulla	
Eye	
Respiratory system	
Cardiovascular system	
GI system	
Liver	
Urinary system	
Sweat glands	
Fat cells	

When the stress response is sustained for an extended period of time, the pituitary gland is stimulated by the hypothalamus to release a number of hormones. Match the ultimate physical effects listed below with the appropriate hormone that triggers the response.

_____ 1. ACTH

_____ 2. Vasopressin (ADH)

_____ 3. Growth hormone

_____ 4. TTH

_____ 5. Gonadotropins

a.. Increased serum glucose and free fatty acids.

b. Suppression of sex hormones resulting in decreased libido and impotence

c. Increased gluconeogenesis; immunosuppression; anti-inflammatory response; increased sodium and water retention

d. Increased basal metabolic rate

e. Increased blood pressure (through constriction of blood vessels) and increased fluid retention.

List the value (in parentheses) for each event that you have experienced in the past 12 months in the column on the right. Add your total value to determine your risk of physical illness due to stress

Holmes and Rahe Social Readjustment Rating Scale

Life Event	Value
Death of spouse (100)	_____
Divorce (73)	_____
Marital separation (65)	_____
Jail term (63)	_____
Death of close family member (63)	_____
Personal illness or injury (53)	_____
Marriage (50)	_____
Fired from work (47)	_____
Marital reconciliation (45)	_____
Retirement (45)	_____
Change in family member's health (44)	_____
Pregnancy (40)	_____
Sex difficulties (39)	_____
Addition to family (39)	_____
Business readjustment (39)	_____
Change in financial status (38)	_____
Death of close friend (37)	_____
Change to different line of work (36)	_____
Change in number of marital arguments (35)	_____
Mortgage or loan over $10,000 (31)	_____
Foreclosure of mortgage or loan (30)	_____
Change in work responsibilities (29)	_____
Son or daughter leaving home (29)	_____
Trouble with in-laws (29)	_____
Outstanding personal achievement (28)	_____
Spouse begins or stops work (26)	_____
Starting or finishing school (26)	_____
Change in living conditions (25)	_____
Revision of personal habits (24)	_____
Trouble with boss (23)	_____
Change in work hours, conditions (20)	_____
Change in residence (20)	_____
Change in schools (20)	_____
Change in recreational habits (19)	_____
Change in church activities (19)	_____
Change in social activities (18)	_____
Mortgage or loan under $10,000 (17)	_____
Change in sleeping habits (16)	_____
Change in number of family gatherings (15)	_____
Change in eating habits (15)	_____
Vacation (13)	_____
Christmas season (12)	_____
Minor violation of the law (11)	_____

Total score

_____

Scoring:
	1–150	No significant possibility of stress-related illness
	150–199	Mild life crisis level—35% chance of illness
	200–299	Moderate life crisis level—50% chance of illness
	300 or over	Major life crisis level—80% chance of illness

From the following case study, identify the predisposing factors (genetic influences, past experiences, and existing conditions) that influence Robert's adaptation response. What is the precipitating stressor in this situation?

Robert, age 56, was admitted to the emergency department of a large hospital at 2 A.M. after vomiting a large amount of blood. In doing the admitting assessment, the nurse learned the following about Robert:

His father and brother are both recovering alcoholics.

Robert had his first drink at age 12 and has been continually increasing the amount and frequency since that time.

His mother died of lung cancer when Robert was age 23. She was a heavy smoker. Robert smokes three packages of cigarettes a day.

He has been hospitalized only once before, about 3 months ago, and diagnosed with an ulcer. The doctor told him at that time he must stop drinking and smoking in order for the ulcer to heal.

Robert is married and has three children. He has a long history of moving from one job to another, staying only until his drinking interferes with his work performance and attendance. He was fired from his job yesterday and spent the evening and nighttime hours drinking two fifths of bourbon. He was engaged in this activity at the time the hematemesis began.

Because of the erratic job history, Robert and his wife experience severe financial difficulties. His wife shows much concern for Robert's condition and stays by his side during the emergency admission. She states to the nurse, "I want so much for our marriage to work, but he is drinking more and more all the time and still doesn't see his drinking as a problem. Every time he gets fired, he blames his boss."

CHAPTER 1. TEST QUESTIONS

1. When an individual's stress response is sustained over a long time, the endocrine system involvement results in:
    - • a. Decreased resistance to disease
      - b. Increased libido
      - c. Decreased blood pressure
      - d. Increased inflammatory response

2. Which of the following symptoms would the nurse identify as typical of the fight or flight response?
      - a. Pupillary constriction
    - • b. Increased heart rate
      - c. Increased salivation
      - d. Increased peristalsis

3. Research undertaken by Holmes and Rahe in 1967 demonstrated a correlation between the effects of life change and illness. In the development of the SRRS, which of the following concepts limits its effectiveness?
      - a. Stress overload always precipitates illness.
      - b. Individual abilities are activated.
      - c. Stress is viewed as a physiological response.
    - • d. Personal perception of the event is excluded.

4. In the transactional model of stress/adaptation, secondary appraisal takes place if the individual judges an event to be:
      - a. Benign
      - b. Irrelevant
      - c. Challenging
      - d. Pleasurable

5. Diseases of adaptation occur when:
      - a. Individuals have not had to face stress in the past
      - b. Individuals inherit maladaptive genes
      - c. Predisposing factors fail
    - • d. Physiological and psychological resources become depleted

6. Meditation has been shown to be an effective stress-management technique. Meditation works by:
    - • a. Producing a state of relaxation
      - b. Providing insight into one's feelings
      - c. Promoting more appropriate role behaviors
      - d. Facilitating problem-solving ability

CHAPTER 2. MENTAL HEALTH AND MENTAL ILLNESS

CHAPTER FOCUS

The focus of this chapter is to differentiate between mental health and mental illness. The history of psychiatric care is explored, various psychological responses to stress are discussed, and cultural components that influence individual attitudes and behaviors toward mental illness are identified.

LEARNING OBJECTIVES

After reading this chapter, the student will be able to:

1. Discuss the history of psychiatric care.
2. Define *mental health* and *mental illness*.
3. Discuss cultural elements that influence attitudes toward mental health and mental illness.
4. Describe psychological adaptation responses to stress.
5. Identify correlation of adaptive/maladaptive behaviors to the mental health/mental illness continuum.

KEY TERMS

anxiety
defense mechanisms

compensation	*rationalization*
denial	*reaction formation*
displacement	*regression*
identification	*repression*
intellectualization	*sublimation*
introjection	*suppression*
isolation	*undoing*
projection	

neurosis	bereavement overload
psychosis	humors
grief	"ship of fools"
anticipatory grief	mental health
	mental illness

CHAPTER OUTLINE/LECTURE NOTES

I. Historical Overview of Psychiatric Care
   1. Early beliefs centered on mental illness in terms of evil spirits or supernatural or magical powers that had entered the body.
   2. The mentally ill were beaten, starved, and otherwise tortured to "purge" the body of these "evil spirits."
   3. Some correlated mental illness with witchcraft, and mentally ill individuals were burned at the stake.
   4. Hippocrates (about 400 B.C.) associated mental Illness with an irregularity in the interaction among the four humors: blood, black bile, yellow bile, and phlegm. Treatment often consisted of induced vomiting and diarrhea with potent cathartic drugs.
   5. During the Middle Ages (A.D. 500 to 1500), the mentally ill were sent out to sea on sailing boats with little guidance and in search of their lost rationality. This practice originated the term "ship of fools."

9

6. During this same period, the Middle Eastern Islamic countries began to establish special units in general hospitals for the mentally ill—creating what were likely the first asylums for the mentally ill.

7. In colonial America, mental illness was equated with witchcraft. Many witches were burned at the stake or put away in places where they could do no harm to others.

8. First hospital in America to admit mentally ill clients was established in Philadelphia in the mid-eighteenth century.

9. Benjamin Rush, often called the father of American psychiatry, was a physician at this hospital and initiated the first humane treatment for mentally ill individuals in the United States.

10. In the nineteenth century, Dorothea Dix was successful in her lobbying for the establishment of state hospitals for the mentally ill. Her goal was to ensure humane treatment for these patients, but the population grew faster than the system of hospitals and the institutions became overcrowded and understaffed.

11. Linda Richards is considered to be the first American psychiatric nurse. She graduated from the New England Hospital for Women and Children.

12. Psychiatric nursing was not included in the curricula of schools of nursing until 1955.

13. The National Mental Health Act was passed by the government in 1946. It provided funds for the education of psychiatrists, psychologists, social workers, and psychiatric nurses. Graduate-level psychiatric nursing was also established during this period.

14. Deinstitutionalization and the community health movement began in the 1960s. (See Chapter 38.)

II. Mental Health

A. Defined as: "The successful adaptation to stressors from the internal or external environment, evidenced by thoughts, feelings, and behaviors that are age-appropriate and congruent with local and cultural norms."

III. Mental Illness

A. Defined as: "Maladaptive responses to stressors from the internal or external environment, evidenced by thoughts, feelings, and behaviors that are incongruent with the local and cultural norms and interfere with the individual's social, occupational, or physical functioning.

B. Horwitz describes cultural influences that affect how individuals view mental illness. These include incomprehensibility (the inability of the general population to understand the motivation behind the behavior) and cultural relativity (the "normality" of behavior is determined by the culture.)

IV. Psychological Adaptation to Stress

A. Anxiety and grief have been described as two major primary psychological response patterns to stress. A variety of thoughts, feelings, and behaviors are associated with each of these response patterns. Adaptation is determined by the degree to which the thoughts, feelings, and behaviors interfere with an individual's functioning.

B. Anxiety

1. Defined: A diffuse apprehension that is vague in nature and is associated with feelings of uncertainty and helplessness.

2. Anxiety is extremely common in our society. Mild anxiety is adaptive and can provide motivation for survival.

3. Peplau identified four levels of anxiety:

a. Mild: seldom a problem. Associated with the tension of day-to-day living. Senses are sharp, motivation is increased, and awareness of the environment is heightened. Learning is enhanced.

b. Moderate: perceptual field diminishes. Less alert to environmental stimuli. Attention span and ability to concentrate decrease, although some learning can still occur. Muscular tension and restlessness may be evident.

c. Severe: perceptual field is so diminished that concentration centers on one detail only or on many extraneous details. Very limited attention span. Physical symptoms may be evident. Virtually all behavior is aimed at relieving the anxiety.

d. Panic: the most intense state. Individual is unable to focus on even one detail. Misperceptions of the environment are common, and there may be a loss of contact with reality. Behavior may be characterized by wild and desperate actions or by extreme withdrawal. Human function and communication with others are ineffective. Prolonged panic anxiety can lead to physical and emotional exhaustion and can be a life-threatening situation.

4. Behavioral adaptation responses to anxiety
   a. At the mild level, individuals employ various coping mechanisms to deal with stress. A few of these include eating, drinking, sleeping, physical exercise, smoking, crying, laughing, and talking to someone with whom they feel comfortable.
   b. At the mild to moderate levels, the ego calls upon defense mechanisms for protection, such as:
      (1) Compensation—covering up a real or perceived weakness by emphasizing a trait one considers more desirable
      (2) Denial—refusal to acknowledge the existence of a real situation or the feelings associated with it
      (3) Displacement—feelings are transferred from one target to another that is considered less threatening or neutral
      (4) Identification—an attempt to increase self-worth by acquiring certain attributes and characteristics of an individual one admires
      (5) Intellectualization—an attempt to avoid expressing actual emotions associated with a stressful situation by using the intellectual processes of logic, reasoning, and analysis
      (6) Introjection—the beliefs and values of another individual are internalized and symbolically become a part of the self, to the extent that the feeling of separateness or distinctness is lost
      (7) Isolation—the separation of a thought or a memory from the feeling, tone, or emotions associated with it
      (8) Projection—feelings or impulses unacceptable to one's self are attributed to another person
      (9) Rationalization—attempting to make excuses or formulate logical reasons to justify unacceptable feelings or behaviors
      (10) Reaction formation—preventing unacceptable or undesirable thoughts or behaviors from being expressed by exaggerating opposite thoughts or types of behaviors
      (11) Regression—a retreat to an earlier level of development and the comfort measures associated with that level of functioning
      (12) Repression—the involuntary blocking of unpleasant feelings and experiences from one's awareness.
      (13) Sublimation—the rechanneling of drives or impulses that are personally or socially unacceptable into activities that are more tolerable and constructive.
      (14) Suppression—the voluntary blocking of unpleasant feelings and experiences from one's awareness.
      (15) Undoing—a mechanism that is used to symbolically negate or cancel out a previous action or experience that one finds intolerable
   c. Anxiety at the moderate to severe levels that remains unresolved over an extended period can contribute to a number of physiological disorders. These may include tension and migraine headaches, angina pectoris, obesity, anorexia nervosa, bulimia nervosa, rheumatoid arthritis, ulcerative colitis, gastric and duodenal ulcers, asthma, irritable bowel syndrome, nausea and vomiting, gastritis, cardiac arrhythmias, premenstrual syndrome, muscle spasms, sexual dysfunction, and cancer. (These disorders are discussed at length in Chapter 33.)
   d. Extended periods of repressed severe anxiety can result in psychoneurotic patterns of behaving. Neuroses are psychiatric disturbances characterized by excessive anxiety or depression, disrupted bodily functions, unsatisfying interpersonal relationships, and behaviors that interfere with routine functioning. Examples of psychoneurotic disorders that are described in the *DSM-IV* include anxiety disorders, somatoform disorders, and dissociative disorders. (These disturbances are discussed at length in Chapters 27 to 29.)
   e. Extended periods of functioning at the panic level of anxiety may result in psychotic behavior. Psychoses are serious psychiatric disturbances characterized by the presence of delusions and/or hallucinations and the impairment of interpersonal functioning and relationship to the external

world. Examples of psychotic responses to anxiety include the schizophrenic, schizoaffective, and delusional disorders. (These disorders are discussed at length in Chapter 25.)

   C. Grief
      1. Defined: The subjective state of emotional, physical, and social responses to the loss of a valued entity. The loss may be real or perceived.
      2. Kubler-Ross has identified five stages of the grief process through which individuals pass as a normal response to loss.
         a. Denial. A stage of shock and disbelief.
         b. Anger, Anger felt for experiencing the loss is displaced upon the environment or turned inward on the self.
         c. Bargaining. Promises are made to God for delaying the loss.
         d. Depression. The full impact of the loss is felt. Disengagement from all association with the lost entity is initiated.
         e. Acceptance. Resignation that the loss has occurred. A feeling of peace regarding the loss is experienced.
      3. Anticipatory grief. The experiencing of the grief process prior to the actual loss.
      4. Resolution. The length of the grief process is entirely individual. It can last from a few weeks to years. It is influenced by a number of factors.
         a. The experience of guilt for having had a "love-hate" relationship with the lost entity. Guilt often lengthens the grieving process.
         b. Anticipatory grieving is thought to shorten the grief response when the loss actually occurs.
         c. The length of the grief response is often extended when an individual has experienced a number of recent losses and when he or she is unable to complete one grieving process before another one begins.
         d. Resolution of the grief response is thought to have occurred when an individual can look back on the relationship with the lost entity and accept both the pleasures and disappointments (both the positive and negative aspects) of the association.
      5. Maladaptive grief responses
         a. Prolonged intense preoccupation with memories of the lost entity for many years after the loss has occurred. Behavior is characterized by disorganization of functioning and intense emotional pain related to the lost entity.
         b. Delayed/inhibited fixation in the denial stage of the grieving process. The loss is not experienced, but there may be evidence of psychophysiological or psychoneurotic disorders.
         c. Distorted fixation in the anger stage of the grieving process. All the normal behaviors associated with grieving are exaggerated out of proportion to the situation. The individual turns the anger inward on the self and is consumed with overwhelming despair. Pathological depression is a distorted grief response. (This response is discussed at length in Chapter 26.)

V. Mental Health/Mental Illness Continuum
   A. In Figure 2–3 of the text, anxiety and grief are presented on a continuum according to degree of symptom severity. Disorders as they appear in the *Diagnostic and Statistical Manual of Mental Disorders* (Edition 4) *(DSM-IV)* are identified at their appropriate placement along the continuum.

VI. The *DSM-IV* Multiaxial Evaluation System
   A. From the psychiatric diagnostic manual, individuals are evaluated on five axes.
      1. Axis I—Clinical disorders and other conditions that may be a focus of clinical attention
      2. Axis II—Personality disorders and mental retardation
      3. Axis III—General medical conditions
      4. Axis IV—Psychosocial and environmental problems
      5. Axis V—Global assessment of functioning rated on the Global Assessment of Functioning (GAF) Scale that measures an individual's psychological, social, and occupational functioning

VII. Summary
VIII. Review Questions

LEARNING ACTIVITIES

On the following Mental Health/Mental Illness continuum, fill in the behavioral experiences or emotional disorders that correspond to the severity of anxiety or grief as it progresses along the continuum.

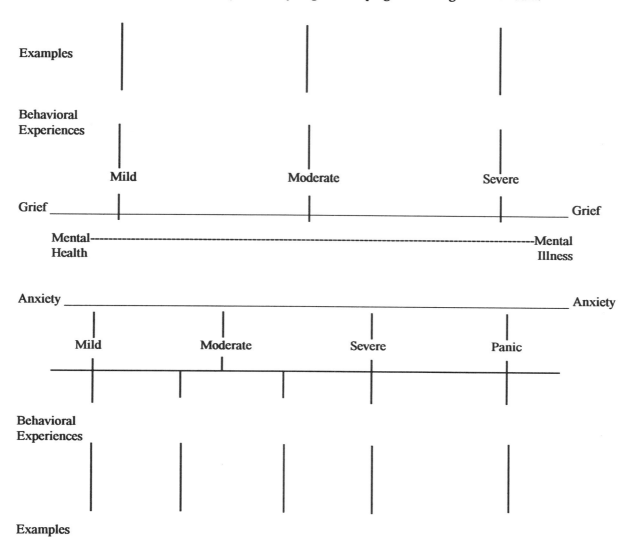

(An explanation of the solution for this activity may be found in Fig. 2–3 of the text.)

EGO DEFENSE MECHANISMS—DEFINITIONS

In the box below, circle the names of the ego defense mechanisms defined as follows. The names may be identified in any direction vertically, horizontally, or diagonally. Number one is completed as an example.

1. Feelings are transferred from one target to another that is considered less threatening or neutral.
2. A mechanism that is used to symbolically negate or cancel out a previous action or experience that one finds intolerable.
3. The separation of a thought or a memory from the feeling, tone, or emotions associated with it.
4. Refusal to acknowledge the existence of a real situation or the feelings associated with it.
5. The beliefs and values of another individual are internalized and symbolically become a part of the self, to the extent that the feeling of separateness or distinctness is lost.
6. An attempt to increase self-worth by acquiring certain attributes and characteristics of an individual one admires.
7. A retreat to an earlier level of development and the comfort measures associated with that level of functioning.
8. Covering up a real or perceived weakness by emphasizing a trait one considers more desirable.
9. The involuntary blocking of unpleasant feelings and experiences from one's awareness.
10. Feelings or impulses unacceptable to one's self are attributed to another person.
11. The voluntary blocking of unpleasant feelings and experiences from one's awareness.
12. Attempting to make excuses or formulate logical reasons to justify unacceptable feelings or behaviors.

THE GRIEF RESPONSE

Kubler-Ross identified five stages of the grief response: denial, anger, bargaining, depression, and acceptance. Fill in the blank with the appropriate stage that describes the verbal or behavioral response. The first one is completed as an example.

1. "I never want to see you again!"   _____Anger_____

2. "Cancer. It can't be! You must have made a mistake!" _____

3. "At last I feel at peace with myself." _____

4. "I'll go to church every Sunday if I can just live till my daughter grows up." _____

5. "I wish I had been a better mother." _____

6. "Why me? I don't deserve this!" _____

7. "I'm feeling much better today. I think I should get a second opinion." _____

8. "I feel as though I'm betraying my family. They depend on me so." _____

9. "If God will only let me live till Christmas. I swear I won't ask for another thing." _____

10. "My family is ready, and so I can rest easy now." _____

CLINICAL EXERCISE

Have students keep a record of ego defense mechanisms they observe being used. These may be identified in the clinical setting, with their classmates, or with families and friends. Have them share these observations in their student group.

CHAPTER 2. TEST QUESTIONS

1. John, a 39-year-old Italian-American, lives in an ethnic community of Italian immigrants. He and most of his peers are of the lower socioeconomic class. Recently John was charged with an act of voyeurism. Which of the following individuals would be most likely to label John's behavior as mental illness?
    a.   John's parents, who are ashamed of his behavior
    b.   John's friends from his "Sons of Italy" social club
    • c.   John's employer who owns the company where he works
    d.   John's wife, who feels she must protect their children

2. Which of the following best describes the characteristics of panic-level anxiety?
    a.   Decreased attention span, hypotension, mild muscle tension
    b.   Frequent body changes, feeling of nervousness, enhanced learning
    c.   Narrow perceptual field, problem solving, mild gastric upset
    • d.   Feeling of losing control, misperceptions of the environment

3. Anne tends to use the defense mechanism of displacement. Her husband, whom she loves very much, yells at her for not having dinner ready when he comes home from work. She is most likely to react by:
    a.   Telling her husband he has no right to yell at her.
    • b.   Yelling at their son for slouching in his chair.
    c.   Burning dinner.
    d.   Saying to her husband, "I'll try to do better tomorrow."

4. Nancy hates her mother, who paid little attention to Nancy when she was growing up. Nancy uses the defense mechanism of reaction formation. Which of the following statements represents this defense mechanism?
    • a.   "I don't like to talk about my relationship with my mother."
    b.   "It's my mother's fault that I feel this way."
    c.   "I have a very wonderful mother whom I love very much."
    d.   "My mom always loved my sister more than she loved me."

5. Jack and Jill were recently divorced. Jill was devastated by the divorce and became very depressed. She sought counseling at the community mental health center. Which of the following statements by Jill would indicate that she has resolved the grief over loss of her marriage?
    a.   "I know things would be different if we could only try again."
    b.   "He will be back. I know he will."
    c.   "I'm sure I did lots of things to provoke his anger."
    • d.   "Yes, it was a difficult relationship, and he abused the children and me."

6. Sarah's husband Frank died 23 years ago. She has not changed a thing in their house since he died. She still has all of Frank's clothing in his closet, and his house slippers are still beside the bed where they were when he died. Sarah talks about Frank unceasingly to anyone who will listen. Which of the following pathological grief responses is Sarah exhibiting?
    a.   Inhibited
    • b.   Prolonged
    c.   Delayed
    d.   Distorted

7. The main difference between neurotic and psychotic behavior is that people experiencing neuroses:
    a.   Are unaware that they are experiencing distress
    b.   Are unaware that their behaviors are maladaptive
    c.   Are aware of possible psychological causes of their behavior
    • d.   Experience no loss of contact with reality

CHAPTER 3. THEORIES OF PERSONALITY DEVELOPMENT

CHAPTER FOCUS

The focus of this chapter is to provide background information for understanding the development of the personality. Major components of seven leading theories are presented.

LEARNING OBJECTIVES

After reading this chapter, the student will be able to:

1. Define *personality*.
2. Identify the relevance of knowledge associated with personality development to nursing in the psychiatric/mental health setting.
3. Discuss the major components of the following developmental theories:
   a. Psychoanalytic theory—Freud
   b. Interpersonal theory—Sullivan
   c. Theory of psychosocial development—Erikson
   d. Theory of object relations development—Mahler
   e. Cognitive development theory—Piaget
   f. Theory of moral development—Kohlberg
   g. A nursing model of interpersonal development—Peplau

KEY TERMS

cognitive development
cognitive maturity
personality
temperament
id
ego
superego
symbiosis
libido
psychodynamic nursing
counselor
technical expert
surrogate

CHAPTER OUTLINE/LECTURE NOTES

I. Introduction
   A. Personality is defined by the *DSM-IV* as "enduring patterns of perceiving, relating to, and thinking about the environment and oneself."
   B. Life-cycle developmentalists believe that people continue to develop and change throughout life, thereby suggesting the possibility for renewal and growth in adults.
   C. Stages are identified by age. However, personality is influenced by temperament (inborn personality characteristics) and the environment.

D. It is possible for behaviors from an unsuccessfully completed stage to be modified and corrected in a later stage.

E. Stages overlap, and individuals may be working on tasks from more than one stage at a time.

F. Individuals may become fixed in a certain stage and remain developmentally delayed.

G. The *DSM-IV* states that personality *disorders* occur when personality traits become inflexible and maladaptive and cause either significant functional impairment or subjective distress.

II. Psychoanalytic Theory—S. Freud

    A. Freud believed basic character was formed by age 5.

    B. He organized the structure of the personality into three major components:

        1. Id. Present at birth, the id serves to satisfy needs and achieve immediate gratification. It has been called the "pleasure principle."

        2. Ego. Development begins at 4 to 6 months. It serves as the rational part of the personality and works to maintain harmony between the external world, the id, and the superego. Also called the "reality principle."

        3. Superego. Development begins at about 3 to 6 years. It is composed of the ego-ideal (the self-esteem that is developed in response to positive feedback) and the conscience (the culturally-influenced sense of right and wrong). It may be referred to as the "perfection principle."

    C. Dynamics of the personality

        1. Freud termed the force required for mental functioning *psychic energy*. It is transferred through all three components of the personality as the individual matures. If an excess of psychic energy is stored in one part of the personality, the behavior reflects that part of the personality.

        2. Freud termed the process by which the id invests energy into an object in an attempt to achieve gratification *cathexis*. Anticathexis is the use of psychic energy by the ego and the superego to control id impulses.

    D. Development of the personality

        1. Freud identified five stages of development and the major developmental tasks of each:

            a. Oral stage (birth to 18 months). Relief from anxiety through oral gratification of needs.

            b. Anal stage (18 months to 3 years). Learning independence and control, with focus on the excretory function.

            c. Phallic stage (3 to 6 years). Identification with parent of same sex; development of sexual identity; focus is on genital organs.

            d. Latency stage (6 to 12 years). Sexuality is repressed; focus is on relationships with same-sex peers.

            e. Genital stage (13 to 20 years). Libido is reawakened as genital organs mature; focus is on relationships with members of the opposite sex.

    E. Relevance to nursing practice. Being able to recognize behaviors associated with the id, ego, and superego will assist in the assessment of developmental level in clients. Understanding the use of ego defense mechanisms is important in making determinations about maladaptive behaviors and in planning care for clients to assist in creating change.

III. Interpersonal Theory—H.S. Sullivan

    A. Based on the belief that individual behavior and personality development are the direct result of interpersonal relationships. The major components of this theory include:

        1. Anxiety. A feeling of emotional discomfort, toward the relief or prevention of which all behavior is aimed.

        2. Satisfaction of needs. Fulfillment of all requirements associated with an individual's physiochemical environment.

        3. Interpersonal security. The feeling associated with relief from anxiety.

        4. Self-system. A collection of experiences, or security measures, adopted by the individual to protect against anxiety. Consists of three components:

            a. The "good me" — the part of the personality that develops in response to positive feedback

            b. The "bad me" —the part of the personality that develops in response to negative feedback

            c. The "not me" — the part of the personality that develops in response to situations that produce intense anxiety in the child.

    B. Stages of development

1. Sullivan identified six developmental stages and the major tasks associated with each.
    a. Infancy (birth to 18 months). Relief from anxiety through oral gratification of needs
    b. Childhood (18 months to 6 years). Learning to experience a delay in personal gratification without undue anxiety
    c. Juvenile (6 to 9 years). Learning to form satisfactory peer relationships
    d. Preadolescence (9 to 12 years). Learning to form satisfactory relationships with persons of the opposite sex; developing a sense of identity
    e. Early adolescence (12 to 14 years). Learning to form satisfactory relationships with persons of the opposite sex; developing a sense of identity
    f. Late adolescence (14 to 21 years). Establishing self-identity; experiencing satisfying relationships; working to develop a lasting, intimate opposite-sex relationship
C. Relevance to nursing practice. Relationship development is a major psychiatric nursing intervention. Knowledge about the behaviors associated with all levels of anxiety and methods for alleviating anxiety helps nurses to assist clients achieve interpersonal security and a sense of well-being.

IV. Theory of Psychosocial Development—E. Erikson
A. Based on the influence of social processes on the development of the personality.
B. Stages of development
    1. Erikson identified eight stages of development and the major tasks associated with each.
        a. Infancy (birth to 18 months): Trust versus mistrust. To develop a trust in the mothering figure and be able to generalize it to others. Failure results in emotional dissatisfaction with self and others, suspiciousness, and difficulty with interpersonal relationships.
        b. Early childhood (18 months to 3 years): Autonomy versus shame and doubt. To gain some self-control and independence within the environment. Failure results in a lack of self-confidence, a lack of pride in the ability to perform, a sense of being controlled by others, and a rage against the self.
        c. Late childhood (3 to 6 years): Initiative versus guilt. To develop a sense of purpose and the ability to initiate and direct own activities. Failure results in feelings of inadequacy and guilt and the accepting of liability in situations for which he or she is not responsible.
        d. School age (6 to 12 years): Industry versus inferiority. To achieve a sense of self-confidence by learning, competing, performing successfully, and receiving recognition from significant others, peers, and acquaintances. Failure results in difficulty in interpersonal relationships because of feelings of inadequacy.
        e. Adolescence (12 to 20 years): Identity versus role confusion. To integrate the tasks mastered in the previous stages into a secure sense of self. Failure results in a sense of self-consciousness, doubt, and confusion about one's role in life.
        f. Young adulthood (20 to 30 years): Intimacy versus isolation. To form an intense, lasting relationship or a commitment to another person, a cause, an institution, or a creative effort. Failure results in withdrawal, social isolation, aloneness, and the inability to form lasting, intimate relationships.
        g. Adulthood (30 to 65 years): Generativity versus stagnation. To achieve the life goals established for oneself, while also considering the welfare of future generations. Failure results in lack of concern for the welfare of others and total preoccupation with the self.
        h. Old age (65 years to death): Ego integrity versus despair. To review one's life and derive meaning from both positive and negative events, while achieving a positive sense of self-worth. Failure results in a sense of self-contempt and disgust with how life has progressed.
C. Relevance to nursing practice. Many individuals with mental health problems are still struggling to achieve tasks from a number of developmental stages. Nurses can plan care to assist these individuals to fulfill these tasks and move on to a higher developmental level.

V. Theory of Object Relations—M. Mahler
A. Based on the separation-individuation process of the infant from the maternal figure (primary caregiver).
B. Stages of development
    1. Mahler identified six phases and subphases through which the individual progresses on the way to object constancy. Major developmental tasks are also described.

a. Phase I: Normal autism (birth to 1 month). Fulfillment of basic needs for survival and comfort. Fixation at this level can predispose to autistic disorder.

b. Phase II: Symbiosis (1 to 5 months). Developing awareness of external source of need fulfillment. Lack of expected nurturing in this phase may lead to symbiotic psychosis.

c. Phase III: Separation-individuation. The process of separating from mothering figure and the strengthening of the sense of self. Divided into four subphases:

    (1) Subphase 1: Differentiation. A primary recognition of separateness from the mother begins.

    (2) Subphase 2: Practicing. Increased independence through locomotor functioning; increased sense of separateness of self.

    (3) Subphase 3: Rapprochement. Acute awareness of separateness of self; learning to seek "emotional refueling" from mothering figure to maintain feeling of security.

    (4) Subphase 4. Consolidation. Sense of separateness established; on the way to object constancy—able to internalize a sustained image of loved object/person when object/person is out of sight; resolution of separation anxiety.

C. Relevance to nursing practice. Understanding the concepts of Mahler's theory of object relations assists the nurse to assess the client's level of individuation from primary caregivers. The emotional problems of many individuals can be traced to lack of fulfillment of the tasks of separation/individuation.

VI. Cognitive Development Theory—J. Piaget

A. Based on the premise that human intelligence is an extension of biological adaptation, or one's ability for psychological adaptation to the environment.

B. Stages of development

  1. Piaget identified four stages of development that are related to age, demonstrating at each successive stage a higher level of logical organization than at the previous stage. Major developmental tasks are also described.

    a. Sensorimotor (birth to 2 years). With increased mobility and awareness develops a sense of self as separate from the external environment; the concept of object permanence emerges as the ability to form mental images evolves.

    b. Preoperational (2 to 6 years). Learning to express self with language; develops understanding of symbolic gestures; achievement of object permanence.

    c. Concrete operations (6 to 12 years). Learning to apply logic to thinking; develops understanding of reversibility and spatiality; learning to differentiate and classify; increased socialization and application of rules.

    d. Formal operations (12 to 15+ years). Learning to think and reason in abstract terms; makes and tests hypotheses; logical thinking and reasoning ability expand and are refined; cognitive maturity achieved.

C. Relevance to nursing practice. Nurses who work in psychiatry may use techniques of cognitive therapy to help clients. Cognitive therapy focuses on changing "automatic thoughts" that occur spontaneously and contribute to negative thinking. Nurses must have knowledge of cognitive development to help clients identify the distorted thought patterns and make the changes required for improvement in affective functioning.

VII. Theory of Moral Development—L. Kohlberg

A. Stages of Development

  1. Not closely tied to specific age groups. More accurately determined by the individual's motivation behind the behavior.

  2. Kohlberg identified three major levels of moral development, each of which is further subdivided into two stages.

    a. Preconventional level (common from ages 4 to 10)

      (1) Punishment and obedience orientation. Behavior is motivated by fear of punishment.

      (2) Instrumental relativist orientation. Behavior is motivated by egocentrism and concern for self.

    b. Conventional level (common from ages 10 to 13 and into adulthood)

      (1) Interpersonal concordance orientation. Behavior is motivated by the expectations of others; strong desire for approval and acceptance.

             (2)   Law and order orientation. Behavior is motivated by respect for authority.
        c.   Postconventional level (can occur from adolescence on)
             (1)   Social contract legalistic orientation. Behavior is motivated by respect for universal laws and moral principles and guided by an internal set of values.
             (2)   Universal ethical principle orientation. Behavior is motivated by internalized principles of honor, justice, and respect for human dignity and guided by the conscience.

    B.   Relevance to nursing practice. Moral development has relevance to psychiatric nursing in that it affects critical thinking about how individuals ought to behave and treat others. Psychiatric nurses must be able to assess the level of moral development of their clients in order to be able to help them in their effort to advance in their progression toward a higher level of developmental maturity.

VIII. A Nursing Model of Interpersonal Development--H. Peplau

    A.   Application of the interpersonal theory to nurse-client relationship development.
    B.   Peplau correlates the stages of personality development in childhood to stages through which clients advance during the progression of an illness.
    C.   Interpersonal experiences are seen as learning situations for nurses to facilitate forward movement in the development of personality.
    D.   Peplau identifies six nursing roles in which nurses function to assist individuals in need of health services:
        1.   Resource person—one who provides specific information
        2.   Counselor—one who listens while the client relates difficulties he or she is experiencing in any aspect of life
        3.   Teacher—one who identifies learning needs and provides information to client or family to fulfill those needs
        4.   Leader—one who guides the interpersonal interactions and ensures the fulfillment of goals
        5.   Technical expert—one who possesses the skills necessary to perform the interventions directed at improvement in the client's condition
        6.   Surrogate--one who serves as a substitute figure for another
    E.   Peplau identifies four stages of personality development:
        1.   Stage 1: Learning to count on others. The infant stage of development. Learning to communicate in various ways with the primary caregiver in order to have comfort needs fulfilled.
        2.   Stage 2: Learning to delay gratification. The toddlerhood stage of development. Learning the satisfaction of pleasing others by delaying self-gratification in small ways.
        3.   Stage 3: Identifying oneself. The early childhood stage of development. Learning appropriate roles and behaviors by acquiring the ability to perceive the expectations of others.
        4.   Stage 4: Developing skills in participation. The late childhood stage of development. Learning the skills of compromise, competition, and cooperation with others; establishment of a more realistic view of the world and a feeling of one's place in it.
    F.   Relevance to nursing practice. Peplau's model provides nurses with a framework to interact with clients, many of whom are fixed in, or because of illness have regressed to, an earlier level of development. Using nursing roles suggested by Peplau, nurses may facilitate client learning of that which has not been learned in earlier experiences.

LEARNING ACTIVITIES

Identify whether each of the behaviors described below is being directed by the id, ego, or superego component of the personality. The first one is completed as an example.

__ID__   1.   Mary stole some makeup off the shelf at the department store.

_____   2.   Mary began to feel very guilty for taking the makeup after she got home with it.

_____   3.   Mary took the makeup back to the store and apologized to the clerk for taking it.

_____   4.   Two-year-old Sandy has a temper tantrum when her Mother takes a dangerous toy away from her.

_____   5.   Sandy sucks on her thumb for comfort.

_____   6.   Frankie wants to do well on the algebra test and stays home to study instead of going out with his friends.

_____   7.   Frankie does not do so well on the algebra test as he had hoped. He becomes despondent and refuses to come out of his room for days.

_____   8.   Jack joins his friends when they invite him to drink beer and smoke marijuana with them.

_____   9.   After having a few beers, Jack decides not to drive his car home.

_____   10.   Jack tells his parents he is sorry for drinking beer and smoking marijuana.

Match the behaviors or statements described on the right with Erikson's stages of development listed on the left. Both achievement and nonachievement are reflected in the choices. The first one is completed as an example.

__e__	1.	Trust
_____	2.	Mistrust
_____	3.	Autonomy
_____	4.	Shame and doubt
_____	5.	Initiative
_____	6.	Guilt
_____	7.	Industry
_____	8.	Inferiority
_____	9.	Identity
_____	10.	Role confusion
_____	11.	Intimacy
_____	12.	Isolation
_____	13.	Generativity
_____	14.	Stagnation
_____	15.	Ego integrity
_____	16.	Despair

a. "I don't like people. I'd rather be alone.

b. "Get away from me with that medicine. I know you are trying to poison me!"

c. "I feel good about my life. I have a lot to be thankful for."

d. Five-year-old girl believes she is the cause of her parents'divorce.

e. "Sure, I'll loan you $10 till your next payday."

f. "I don't know what I want to do with my life. College? Work? What kind of job would I get anyway?"

g. "Mommy! Mommy! I made all A's on my report card!"

h. "I'll have to ask my husband. He's the decision-maker in our family."

i. "When I graduate from college I want to work with handicapped children."

j. "I plan to work as hard as necessary to help women achieve equality. I plan to see this happen before I die."

k. "I hate this place. No one cares what I do anyway. It's just a way to bring home a paycheck."

l. "Look, Mom! I ironed this blouse all by myself!"

m. "If only I could live my life over again. I'd do things so much differently. I feel like a nothing."

n. " I could never be a nurse. I'm not smart enough."

o. "Yes, I will be the chairperson for the cancer drive."

p. "I have been the Girl Scout leader for Troop 259 for 7 years now."

Match the statements/behaviors in the right-hand column to the stages of moral development listed on the left.

_____ 1. Punishment and obedience orientation

_____ 2. Instrumental relativist orientation

_____ 3. Interpersonal concordance orientation

_____ 4. Law and order orientation

_____ 5. Social contract legalistic orientation

_____ 6. Universal ethical principle orientation

a. "I really don't want to take care of this AIDS patient, but he needs care, and it is my moral and legal responsibility."

b. "I'll feed and give water to the pets because if I don't, I won't be allowed to go to the ballgame on Friday night."

c. "I'll wear my seatbelt (even though it is uncomfortable and it wrinkles my dress) because it is the law."

d. "I'll tell him the truth about his prognosis because I would want to be told if it were me."

e. "I only drank the beer because everyone else did. They'd have thought I was a jerk if I didn't!"

f. "Okay, if you pay me $5 I won't tell Mom you skipped school."

CHAPTER 3. TEST QUESTIONS

Please answer the questions based on the following case study.

Mrs. K. is 78-years-old. She has been admitted to the psychiatric unit of a large hospital because she is depressed and told her daughter she no longer had anything to live for. She threatened to swallow her whole bottle of antihypertensive medication.

Mrs. K. lives alone. She has been married and divorced five times. She told the nurse, "Every time I got married, I thought it was for the rest of my life; but every time, we just couldn't get along. I like to be independent. I want to do what I want to do, when I want to do it, and I don't want some man getting in my way! Men are all alike. They think they own their wives. Well, not me!"

On the unit, Mrs. K. is quarrelsome with the other clients. She changes the TV channel to what she wants to watch without consulting the group; she interrupts in group therapy to discuss her own situation when the focus is on another person; and most of the time, she prefers to stay in her room alone, rather than interact with the other clients. She states, "Nobody wants to have anything to do with me, anyway. If I had my life to live over again, I'd sure do a lot of things differently."

1. *Theoretically,* in which level of psychosocial development (according to Erikson) would you place with Mrs. K?
   - a. Trust versus mistrust
   - b. Industry versus inferiority
   - c. Generativity versus stagnation
   - • d. Ego integrity versus despair

2. According to Erikson's theory, where would you place Mrs. K. based on her behavior?
   - a. Trust versus mistrust
   - • b. Industry versus inferiority
   - c. Generativity versus stagnation
   - d. Ego integrity versus despair

3. In what stage of development is Mrs. K. fixed according to Sullivan's interpersonal theory?
   - a. Infancy. She relieves anxiety through oral gratification.
   - • b. Childhood. She has not learned to delay gratification.
   - c. Early adolescence. She is struggling to form an identity.
   - d. Late adolescence. She is working to develop a lasting relationship.

4. Which of the following describes the psychoanalytical structure of Mrs. K.'s personality?
   - a. Weak id, strong ego, weak superego
   - b. Strong id, weak ego, weak superego
   - c. Weak id, weak ego, punitive superego
   - • d. Strong id, weak ego, punitive superego

5. In which of Peplau's stages of development would you assess Mrs. K.?
   - a. Learning to count on others
   - • b. Learning to delay gratification
   - c. Identifying oneself
   - d. Developing skills in participation

CHAPTER 4. CONCEPTS OF PSYCHOBIOLOGY

CHAPTER FOCUS

The focus of this chapter is to explore the role of neurophysiological, neurochemical, genetic, and endocrine influences on psychiatric illness. Various diagnostic procedures used to detect alteration in biological function that may contribute to psychiatric illness are identified, and the implications to psychiatric/mental health nursing are discussed.

LEARNING OBJECTIVES

After reading this chapter, the student will be able to:

1. Identify gross anatomical structures of the brain and describe their functions.
2. Discuss the physiology of neurotransmission within the central nervous system.
3. Describe the role of neurotransmitters in human behavior.
4. Discuss the association of endocrine functioning to the development of psychiatric disorders.
5. Describe the role of genetics in the development of psychiatric disorders.
6. Discuss the correlation of alteration in brain functioning to various psychiatric disorders.
7. Identify various diagnostic procedures used to detect alteration in biological functioning that may be contributing to psychiatric disorders.
8. Discuss the influence of psychological factors on the immune system.
9. Discuss the implications of psychobiological concepts to the practice of psychiatric/mental health nursing.

KEY TERMS

neurotransmitter
synapse
dendrites
axon
neuron
limbic system
receptor sites
neuroendocrinology
circadian rhythms
genotype
phenotype
psychoimmunology
cell body

CHAPTER OUTLINE/LECTURE NOTES

I. Introduction
    A. The 101st Legislature of the United States designated the 1990s as the "decade of the brain," with the challenge being the study of the biological basis of behavior.
    B. In keeping with the "neuroscientific revolution," greater emphasis is placed on the study of the organic basis for psychiatric illness.
II. The Nervous System: An Anatomical Review

A. The brain
   1. The forebrain
      a. The cerebrum
         (1) It consists of a right and left hemisphere connected by a deep groove of neurons (nerve cells) called the corpus callosum.
         (2) The cerebral cortex is identified by numerous folds (called gyri) and deep grooves (called sulci) that extend the surface area of the cortex, thus permitting the presence of millions more neurons than would be possible otherwise.
         (3) Each hemisphere is divided into four lobes, each named for the overlying bones in the cranium: the frontal lobe, parietal lobe, temporal lobe, and occipital lobe.
            (a) Frontal lobes. The frontal lobes are responsible for voluntary body movement, including movements that permit speaking; thinking and judgment formation; and expression of feelings.
            (b) Parietal lobes. The parietal lobes are responsible for perception and interpretation of most sensory information (including touch, pain, taste, and body position).
            (c) Temporal lobes. These are responsible for hearing, short-term memory, and sense of smell; expression of emotions through connection with the limbic system.
            (d) Occipital Lobes. These are responsible for visual reception and interpretation.
      b. The diencephalon. The diencephalon connects the cerebrum with lower brain structures and consists of the thalamus, hypothalamus, and limbic system.
         (1) The thalamus integrates all sensory input (except smell) on the way to the cortex; also has some involvement with emotions and mood.
         (2) The hypothalamus regulates the anterior and posterior lobes of the pituitary gland and exerts control over actions of the autonomic nervous system. Also regulates appetite and temperature.
         (3) The limbic system consists of medially placed cortical and subcortical structures and the fiber tracts connecting them with one another and with the hypothalamus. It is sometimes called the "emotional brain" and is associated with feelings of fear and anxiety; anger and aggression; love, joy, and hope; and with sexuality and social behavior.
   2. The Midbrain
      a. The Mesencephalon. The mesencephalon, or midbrain, is responsible for visual, auditory, and balance ("righting") reflexes.
   3. The Hindbrain
      a. The Pons. The pons is charged with regulation of respiration and skeletal muscle tone; ascending and descending tracts connect brainstem with cerebellum and cortex.
      b. The Medulla. The medulla is a pathway for all ascending and descending fiber tracts. It contains vital centers that regulate heart rate, blood pressure, and respiration; reflex centers for swallowing, sneezing, coughing, and vomiting.
      c. The Cerebellum. The cerebellum regulates muscle tone and coordination and maintains posture and equilibrium.
B. Nerve tissue
   1. The nerve cells of central nervous system (CNS) tissue are called neurons and are composed of three parts: a cell body, an axon, and dendrites.
   2. The cell body contains the nucleus and is essential for the life of the neuron.
   3. The axon transmits impulses away from the cell body.
   4. The dendrites are processes that transmit impulses toward the cell body.
   5. Three classes of neurons exist within the CNS: afferent (sensory), efferent (motor), and interneurons.
      a. Afferent neurons carry impulses from receptors in the internal and external periphery to the CNS, where they are interpreted into various sensations.
      b. Efferent neurons carry impulses from the CNS to muscles (which respond by contracting) and glands (that respond by secreting).

     c.   Interneurons exist entirely within the CNS. They may carry only sensory or motor impulses, or they may serve as integrators in the pathways between afferent and efferent neurons.

    6.   Synapses. The junction between two neurons is called a synapse, and the small space between the two neurons is called a synaptic cleft. Neurons conducting impulses toward the synapse are called presynaptic neurons, and those conducting impulses away are called postsynaptic neurons.

    7.   A chemical neurotransmitter is stored in the axon terminals of the presynaptic neuron. An electrical impulse causes its release into the synaptic cleft, where it combines with receptor sites on the postsynaptic neuron and determines whether another electrical impulse will be generated.

C. Autonomic nervous system (ANS)

    1.   The ANS has two divisions: the sympathetic and the parasympathetic.

        a.   The sympathetic division is dominant in stressful situations and prepares the body for "fight or flight." (See Chapter 1.)

        b.   The parasympathetic division dominates when an individual is in a relaxed, nonstressful condition.

D. Neurotransmitters

    1.   Neurotransmitters play an important role in human emotions and behavior and are the target for the mechanism of action in many psychotropic medications.

    2.   Neurotransmitters are stored in terminal vesicles of neuronal axons. When an electrical impulse reaches this point, the neurotransmitter is released from the vesicles into the synaptic cleft, where it binds with receptor sits on the postsynaptic neuron to determine whether another electrical impulse will be generated. After the neurotransmitter has accomplished this task, it is either inactivated and dissolved by enzymes or returned to the vesicles to be stored and used again.

    3.   Major categories of neurotransmitters include cholinergics, monoamines, amino acids, and neuropeptides.

        a.   Cholinergics

            (1)   Acetylcholine is found in the cerebral cortex, hippocampus, limbic structures, and basal ganglia. It is involved in sleep, arousal, pain perception, movement, and memory.

        b.   Monoamines

            (1)   Norepinephrine is found in the thalamus, hypothalamus, limbic system, hippocampus, cerebellum, and cerebral cortex. It influences mood, cognition, perception, locomotion, cardiovascular functioning, and sleep and arousal.

            (2)   Dopamine is found in the frontal cortex, limbic system, basal ganglia, thalamus, posterior pituitary, and spinal cord. It is involved in movement and coordination, emotions, voluntary judgment, and release of prolactin.

            (3)   Serotonin is found in the hypothalamus, thalamus, limbic system, cerebral cortex, cerebellum, and spinal cord. It influences sleep and arousal, libido, appetite, mood, aggression, pain perception, coordination, and judgment.

            (4)   Histamine is found in the hypothalamus. Its exact function is unclear, but it may have some influence on mood.

        c.   Amino acids

            (1)   Gamma-aminobutyric acid (GABA) is found in the hypothalamus, hippocampus, cortex, cerebellum, basal ganglia, spinal cord, and retina. It is involved in the slowdown of body activity.

            (2)   Glycine is found in the spinal cord and brainstem. It causes recurrent inhibition of motor neurons.

            (3)   Glutamate and aspartate are found in pyramidal cells of the cortex, cerebellum, and the primary sensory afferent systems; also in the hippocampus, thalamus, hypothalamus, and spinal cord. They are involved in the relay of sensory information and in the regulation of various motor and spinal reflexes.

        d.   Neuropeptides

            (1)   Endorphins and enkephalins are found in the hypothalamus, thalamus, limbic structures, midbrain, and brainstem. Enkephalins are also found in the gastrointestinal (GI) tract.

They are involved in the modulation of pain and the reduction of peristalsis (enkephalins).

    (2)   Substance P is found in the hypothalamus, limbic structures, midbrain, brainstem, thalamus, basal ganglia, and spinal cord. It is also found in GI tract and salivary glands. It is involved in the regulation of pain.

    (3)   Somatostatin is found in the cerebral cortex, hippocampus, thalamus, basal ganglia, brainstem, and spinal cord. It inhibits release of serotonin, dopamine, and acetylcholine.

III.   Neuroendocrinology

    A.   Endocrine functioning in the CNS is under the influence of the hypothalamus, which has direct control over the pituitary gland, sometimes called the "master gland."

        1.   The pituitary gland has two major lobes: the posterior lobe (also called the neurohypophysis) and the anterior lobe (also called the adenohypophysis).

           a.   The posterior lobe is under neural control of the hypothalamus. Two hormones—vasopressin and oxytocin—are produced in the hypothalamus and stored in the posterior pituitary. Their release is mediated by neural impulses from the hypothalamus.

              (1)   Vasopressin (antidiuretic hormone) conserves body water and maintains normal blood pressure. Its release is stimulated by pain, emotional stress, dehydration, increased plasma concentration, and decreases in blood volume.

              (2)   Oxytocin stimulates contraction of the uterus at the end of pregnancy and release of milk from the mammary glands. Its role in behavioral functioning is unclear.

           b.   The anterior lobe produces a number of hormones whose release is under the control of releasing hormones that are produced by the hypothalamus. When these pituitary hormones are required by the body, the releasing hormones from the hypothalamus pass through the capillaries and veins of the hypophyseal portal system to capillaries in the anterior pituitary, where they stimulate secretion of these specialized hormones.

              (1)   Growth hormone is responsible for growth in children and for continued protein synthesis throughout life. During prolonged stress, it has a direct effect on protein, carbohydrate, and lipid metabolism, resulting in increased serum glucose and free fatty acids to be used for increased energy.

              (2)   Thyroid-stimulating hormone stimulates the thyroid gland to secrete thyroid hormones necessary for metabolism of food and regulation of temperature.

              (3)   Adrenocorticotropic hormone (ACTH) stimulates the adrenal cortex to secrete cortisol, which plays a role in the response to stress.

              (4)   Prolactin stimulates the breasts to produce milk.

              (5)   Gonadotropic hormones stimulate the ovaries and testes to secrete estrogen, progesterone, and testosterone. Estrogen and progesterone also play a role in ovulation, and testosterone, in sperm production.

              (6)   Melanocyte-stimulating hormone stimulates the pineal gland to secrete melatonin, a hormone that may be implicated in the etiology of seasonal affective disorder.

    B.   Circadian rhythms

        1.   Circadian rhythms follow a near-24-hour cycle in humans and may influence a variety of regulatory functions, including the sleep-wake cycle, body temperature regulation, patterns of activity such as eating and drinking, and hormone secretion.

        2.   The role of circadian rhythms in psychopathology is being studied.

        3.   Some mood disorders have been linked to increased secretion of melatonin during darkness hours.

        4.   Rhythms associated with the menstrual cycle show monthly cycles of progression.

        5.   The sleep-wake cycle is one of the most common biological rhythms that demonstrates circadian influence. Sleep disturbances are common in many individuals.

        6.   Sleep-wake cycle

           a.   The sleep-wake cycle is genetically determined and demonstrates an approximate 24-hour rhythm.

           b.   Sleep is measured by the type of brain-wave activity during various stages of sleep.

               (1)   Stage 0: Alpha rhythm. Relaxed, waking state with eyes closed.

              (2)   Stage 1: Beta rhythm. Transition into sleep; dozing; drift in and out of sleep.

        (3)   Stage 2: Theta rhythm. About half of sleep is spent in this stage. Minimal eye movement and muscular activity occur.

        (4)   Stage 3: Delta rhythm. Deep, restful sleep. Decreased vital signs; no eye movement.

        (5)   Stage 4: Delta rhythm. The age of deepest sleep. Minimal eye movement and muscular activity.

        (6)   REM sleep: Beta rhythm. The dream cycle. Period of rapid eye movement (REM). Vital signs increase.

    7.   Neurochemical influences. A number of neurochemicals have been shown to influence the sleep-wake cycle.

        a.   Serotonin and its precursor, L-tryptophan, have been shown to induce sleep.

        b.   Norepinephrine and dopamine may play a role in REM sleep.

        c.   GABA probably plays a role in sleep facilitation.

        d.   Acetylcholine may induce and prolong REM sleep, whereas histamine may inhibit the effect.

IV.   Genetics

    A.   The goal of behavioral genetics is to clarify the role that genetic factors play in the determination of behavior.

    B.   The term *genotype* refers to the total set of genes present in an individual at the time of conception, coded in the DNA.

    C.   The term *phenotype* refers to the physical manifestations of a particular genotype, such as eye color, height, blood type, language, and hair style. Phenotypes are a combination of genetic and environmental characteristics.

    D.   Various types of studies are conducted to determine etiologic factors associated with psychiatric illness.

        1.   Familial—compare the percentages of family members with the illness to those in the general population or a specific control group. Example of a familial illness: schizophrenia

        2.   Genetic—search for a specific gene that is responsible for the individual having the illness. Example of a genetic illness: Down's syndrome

        3.   Twin studies—examine the frequency of a disorder in monozygotic and dizygotic twins.

        4.   Adoption studies—allow comparisons to be made of the influences of genetic versus environmental factors on the development of a psychiatric disorder. Studies have been conducted with adopted children whose biological parent(s) or relatives had the illness, those whose adoptive parent(s) or relatives had the illness, and with monozygotic twins reared apart by different adoptive parents.

V.   Psychoimmunology

    A.   Normal immune response

        1.   In the cellular immune response, the T4 lymphocytes become sensitized to and specific for the foreign antigen.

        2.   The humoral response is activated when antigen-specific T4 cells communicate with the B cells in the spleen and lymph nodes. The B cells in turn produce the antibodies specific to the foreign antigen.

        3.   The antibodies prevent the foreign antigen from invading body cells.

    B.   Implications for psychiatric illness

        1.   Studies have shown that during times of stress, the immune system is suppressed, resulting in a suppression in lymphocyte proliferation and function.

        2.   Certain neurochemicals may influence the immune system. Growth hormone may enhance immunity, whereas testosterone and increased production of norepinephrine and epinephrine may decrease immunity. Serotonin has demonstrated both enhancing and inhibiting effects.

        3.   Decreased immunity has been associated with grief, bereavement, and depression. Immunological abnormalities have also been associated with alcoholism, autism, and dementia.

        4.   The role of neuroimmunology remains unclear in the relationship to onset and course of schizophrenia.

VI.   Implications for Nursing

    A.   Emphasis in psychiatric nursing is on a smooth transition from a psychosocial approach to one of biopsychosocial focus.

    B.   Psychiatric nurses must have a specialized knowledge about:

        1.   Neuroanatomy and neurophysiology

LEARNING ACTIVITIES

Label the parts indicated.

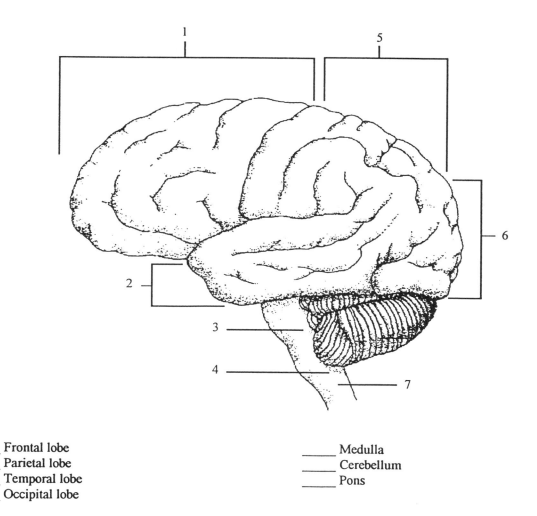

_____ Frontal lobe
_____ Parietal lobe
_____ Temporal lobe
_____ Occipital lobe

_____ Medulla
_____ Cerebellum
_____ Pons

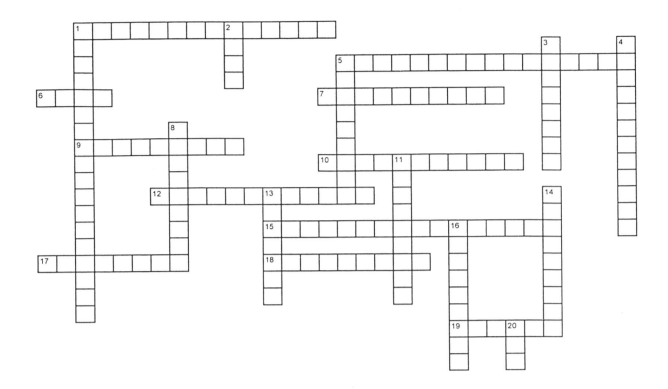

ACROSS

1. Neurotransmitter released in response to stress
5. Study of the implications of the immune system in psychiatry
6. Part of the neuron that carries impulses away from the cell body
7. Structure of the brain associated with muscular coordination and posture
9. Part of the neuron that carries impulses toward the cell body
10. Cells of the immune system
12. Sometimes called the "emotional brain" (two words)
15. Chemical stored in the axon terminals of neurons
17. Part of the neuron that contains the nucleus (two words)
18. Hormone that stimulates breast-milk production and may play a role in depression
19. A nerve cell

DOWN

1. The study of hormones functioning within the neurological system
2. Structure of the brain associated with regulation of respiration
3. Increased levels of this neurotransmitter are implicated in schizophrenia
4. Structure of the brain that controls pituitary function
5. The physical characteristics of a particular genotype
8. Sometimes called the "master gland"
11. Neurotransmitter that mediates allergic and inflammatory reactions
13. The junction between two neurons
14. Neurotransmitter thought to induce sleep and is decreased in depression
16. Hormone secreted by the pineal gland; implicated in the etiology of depression
20. Rapid eye movement; dream-cycle sleep

CHAPTER 4. TEST QUESTIONS

1. Which of the following cerebral structures is sometimes referred to as the "emotional brain"?
   a. The cerebellum
   • b. The limbic system
   c. The cortex
   d. The left temporal lobe

2. Carl's wife of 34 years died unexpectedly 2 months ago. He is very depressed and is being visited at home weekly by a community mental health nurse. The nurse encourages Carl to talk about his wife, their life together, and what he's lost with her death. In addition, at each visit she strongly reinforces the need for Carl to eat properly and get daily exercise and adequate rest. She emphasizes these self-care activities *primarily* because:
   a. The nurse is substituting for Carl's wife.
   b. Carl has developed bad habits since his wife's death.
   c. It is routine to remind patients about nutrition, exercise, and rest.
   • d. Carl is more susceptible to illness because of his depression.

3. The nurse knows that the mechanism responsible for the correct answer in the vignette above is:
   a. Denial
   b. Inhibitory response
   • c. Hypothalamic-pituitary-adrenal axis
   d. Increased secretion of melatonin

Neurotransmitters and hormones may play a significant role in psychiatric illness. In questions 4 to 7, match the neurotransmitters named on the left with the implication for psychiatric illness on the right.

4.	<u>b</u> Increased dopamine	a.	Alzheimer's disease
5.	<u>d</u> Decreased norepinephrine	b.	Schizophrenia
6.	<u>c</u> Decreased GABA	c.	Anxiety disorders
7.	<u>a</u> Decreased acetylcholine	d.	Depression

In questions 8 to 10, match the hormones named on the left with the implication for psychiatric illness on the right.

8.	<u>c</u> Elevated cerebrospinal fluid cortisol	a.	Acute mania
9.	<u>a</u> Elevated thyroid hormone	b.	Schizophrenia
10.	<u>b</u> Decreased prolactin	c.	Anorexia Nervosa

CHAPTER 5. RELATIONSHIP DEVELOPMENT

CHAPTER FOCUS

The focus of this chapter is to describe the role of the psychiatric nurse and the importance of a therapeutic relationship between client and nurse. Steps in the development of a therapeutic relationship are discussed.

LEARNING OBJECTIVES

After reading this chapter, the student will be able to:

1. Describe the relevance of a therapeutic nurse-client relationship.
2. Discuss the dynamics of a therapeutic nurse-client relationship.
3. Discuss the importance of self-awareness in the nurse-client relationship.
4. Identify goals of the nurse-client relationship.
5. Identify and discuss essential conditions for a therapeutic relationship to occur.
6. Describe the phases of relationship development and the tasks associated with each phase.

KEY TERMS

rapport
concrete thinking
confidentiality
unconditional positive regard
genuineness
empathy
sympathy
beliefs
attitudes
values

CHAPTER OUTLINE/LECTURE NOTES

I. Role of the Psychiatric Nurse
   A. Nurses have evolved through various roles from custodial caregivers and physicians' handmaidens to being recognized as unique, independent members of the professional health-care team.
   B. Hildegard Peplau identified six subroles within the role of the nurse.
      1. Mother-surrogate—fulfills needs associated with mothering basic needs, such as bathing, feeding, dressing, toileting, warning, disciplining, and approving
      2. Technician—focuses on the competent, efficient, and correct performance of technical procedures
      3. Manager—manages and manipulates the environment to improve conditions for client recovery
      4. Socializing agent—participates in social activities with the client
      5. Health teacher—identifies learning needs and provides information required by the client or family to improve the health situation
      6. Counselor or psychotherapist—uses "interpersonal techniques" to assist clients in learning to adapt to difficulties or changes in life experiences
   C. Peplau believes the emphasis in psychiatric nursing is on the counseling or psychotherapeutic subrole.

D. Peplau and Sullivan, both interpersonal therapists, emphasize the importance of relationship development in the provision of emotional care.

II. Dynamics of a Therapeutic Nurse-Client Relationship
    A. Therapeutic nurse-client relationship can occur only when each views the other as a unique human being. When this occurs, both participants have needs met by the relationship.
    B. Therapeutic relationships are goal oriented and directed at learning and growth promotion.
    C. Goals are often achieved through use of the problem-solving model.
        1. Identify the client's problem.
        2. Promote discussion of desired changes.
        3. Identify realistic changes.
        4. Discuss aspects that cannot be realistically changed and ways to cope with them more adaptively.
        5. Discuss alternative strategies for creating changes the client desires to make.
        6. Weigh benefits and consequences of each alternative.
        7. Assist client to select an alternative.
        8. Encourage client to implement the change.
        9. Provide positive feedback for client's attempts to create change.
        10. Assist client to evaluate outcomes of the change and make modifications as required.

III. Therapeutic Use of Self
    A. Defined: The ability to use one's personality consciously and with full awareness in an attempt to establish relatedness and to structure nursing interventions.
    B. Nurse must possess self-awareness, self-understanding, and a philosophical belief about life, death, and the overall human condition.

IV. Gaining Self-Awareness
    A. Values clarification is one process by which an individual may gain self-awareness.
        1. Beliefs. Beliefs are ideas that one holds to be true. Beliefs may be:
            a. Rational—objective evidence exists to substantiate their truth
            b. Irrational—an individual holds the idea as true despite the existence of objective, contradictory evidence
            c. Held on faith— ideas that an individual holds as true for which no objective evidence exists
            d. Stereotypical—the belief describes a concept in an oversimplified or undifferentiated manner
        2. Attitudes. Attitudes are frames of reference around which an individual organizes knowledge about his or her world.
            a. Attitudes have an emotional component. They may be judgmental, selective, and biased.
            b. Attitudes may be positive or negative.
        3. Values. Values are abstract standards, positive or negative, that represent an individual's ideal mode of conduct and ideal goals.
            a. Values differ from attitudes and beliefs in that they are action oriented or action producing.
            b. Attitudes and beliefs become values only when they have been acted upon.
            c. Attitudes and beliefs flow out of one's set of values.
    B. The Johari Window
        1. The Johari Window is a representation of the self and a tool that can be used to increase self-awareness. It is divided into four quadrants:
            a. The Open or Public Self. The part of the self that is public; that is, aspects of the self about which both the individual and others are aware.
            b. The Unknowing Self. The part of the self that is known to others but remains hidden from the awareness of the individual.
            c. The Private Self. The part of the self that is known to the individual, but which the individual deliberately and consciously conceals from others.
            d. The Unknown Self. The part of the self that is unknown to both the individual and to others.
        2. The goal of increasing self-awareness by using the Johari Window is to increase the size of the quadrant that represents the Open or Public Self.
        3. Increased self-awareness allows an individual to interact with others comfortably, to accept differences in others, and to observe each person's right to respect and dignity.

V. Conditions Essential to Development of a Therapeutic Relationship

A. Rapport—implies special feelings on the part of both the client and the nurse based on acceptance, warmth, friendliness, common interest, a sense of trust, and a nonjudgmental attitude.

B. Trust—implies a feeling of confidence in another person's presence, reliability, integrity, veracity, and sincere desire to provide assistance when requested. Trust is the basis of a therapeutic relationship.

C. Respect—implies the dignity and worth of an individual regardless of his or her unacceptable behavior. Carl Rogers called this unconditional positive regard.

D. Genuineness—refers to the nurse's ability to be open, honest, and "real" in interactions with the client. Genuineness implies congruence between what is felt and what is being expressed.

E. Empathy—a process wherein an individual is able to see beyond outward behavior, and sense accurately another's inner experience at a given time. With empathy, the nurse's feelings remain on an objective level. It differs from sympathy in that, with sympathy, the nurse actually shares what the client is feeling and experiences a need to alleviate distress.

VI. Phases of a Therapeutic Nurse-Client Relationship
   A. The preinteraction phase
      1. Obtain information about the client from chart, significant others, or other health team members.
      2. Examine one's own feelings, fears, and anxieties about working with a particular client.
   B. The orientation (introductory) phase
      1. Create environment for trust and rapport.
      2. Establish contract for intervention.
      3. Gather assessment data.
      4. Identify client's strengths and weaknesses.
      5. Formulate nursing diagnoses.
      6. Set mutually agreeable goals.
      7. Develop a realistic plan of action.
      8. Explore feelings of both client and nurse.
   C. The working phase
      1. Maintain trust and rapport.
      2. Promote client's insight and perception of reality.
      3. Use problem-solving model to work toward achievement of established goals.
      4. Overcome resistance behaviors.
      5. Continuously evaluate progress toward goal attainment.
   D. Termination Phase
      1. Therapeutic conclusion of the relationship occurs when:
         a. Progress has been made toward attainment of the goals
         b. A plan of action for more adaptive coping with future stressful situations has been established
         c. Feelings about termination of the relationship are recognized and explored

VII. Summary
VIII. Review Questions

LEARNING ACTIVITIES

Situation: Pam comes to the psychiatric clinic for assistance with more adaptive coping. Nurse Jones will be her therapist.

Match the behaviors described on the right with the essential condition for therapeutic relationship development listed on the left.

_____ 1. Rapport

_____ 2. Trust

_____ 3. Respect

_____ 4. Genuineness

_____ 5. Empathy

a. Nurse Jones does not approve of Pam's gay lifestyle but accepts her unconditionally nonetheless.

b. Nurse Jones and Pam develop an immediate mutual regard for each other.

c. Pam knows that Nurse Jones is always honest with her and will tell her the truth even if it is sometimes painful.

d. Pam knows that Nurse Jones will not tell anyone else about what they discuss in therapy.

e. When Pam talks about her problems, Nurse Jones listens objectively and encourages Pam to reflect on her feelings about the situation.

PHASES OF RELATIONSHIP DEVELOPMENT

Identify the appropriate phase of relationship development for each of the following tasks. The four phases include:

a.   Preinteraction phase
b.   Orientation (introductory) phase
c.   Working phase
d.   Termination phase

The first one is completed as an example.

__b__   1.   Pam and Nurse Jones set goals for their time together.

_____   2.   Nurse Jones reads Pam's previous medical records.

_____   3.   Having identified Pam's problem, they discuss aspects for possible change and ways to accomplish them.

_____   4.   They establish a mutual contract for intervention.

_____   5.   The established goals have been met.

_____   6.   Nurse Jones explores her feelings about working with a gay person.

_____   7.   Pam weighs the benefits and consequences of various alternatives for change.

_____   8.   Pam and Nurse Jones discuss a plan of action for Pam to employ in the advent of stressful situations following therapy.

_____   9.   Pam cries and says she cannot stop coming to therapy.

_____   10.   Nurse Jones gives Pam positive feedback for attempting to make adaptive changes in her life.

PERSONAL COAT OF ARMS

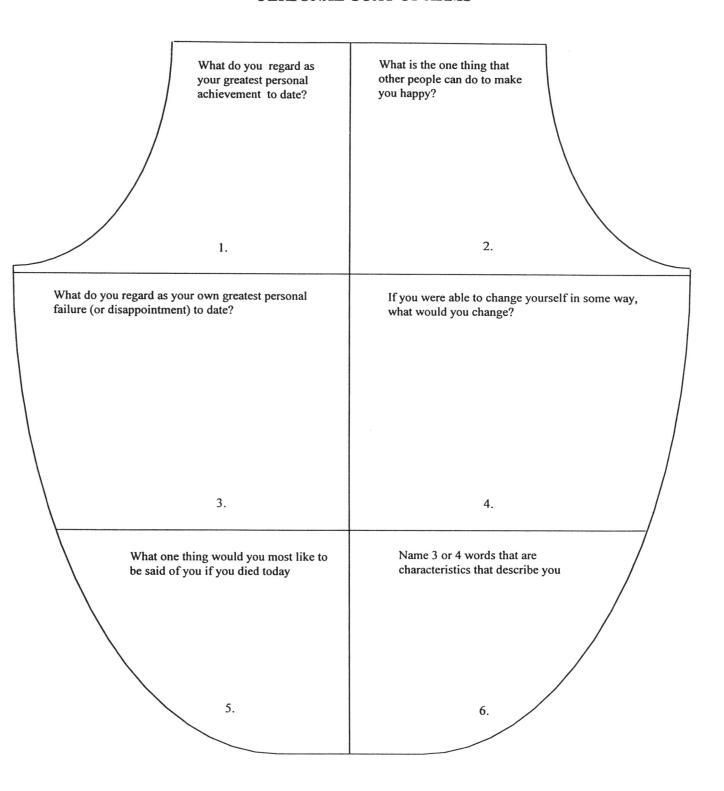

What do you regard as your greatest personal achievement to date?

1.

What is the one thing that other people can do to make you happy?

2.

What do you regard as your own greatest personal failure (or disappointment) to date?

3.

If you were able to change yourself in some way, what would you change?

4.

What one thing would you most like to be said of you if you died today

5.

Name 3 or 4 words that are characteristics that describe you

6.

CHAPTER 5. TEST QUESTIONS

1. When there is congruence between what the nurse is feeling and what is being expressed, the nurse is conveying:
    a. Respect
    • b. Genuineness
    c. Sympathy
    d. Rapport

Situation: Sally has made the decision to leave her alcoholic husband. She is feeling very depressed right now. Which of the following statements by the nurse conveys *empathy* and which conveys *sympathy?*

   a. "I know you are feeling very depressed right now. I felt the same way when I decided to leave my husband. But I can tell you from personal experience, you are doing the right thing."

   b. "I can understand that you are feeling depressed right now. It was a very difficult decision to make. I'll sit here with you for awhile."

2. <u>b</u> Empathy

3. <u>a</u> Sympathy

4. Which of the following tasks takes place during the working phase of relationship development?
    a. Establishing a contract for intervention
    b. Examining feelings about working with a particular client
    c. Establishing a plan for continuing aftercare
    • d. Promoting the client's insight and perception of reality

5. The Johari Window is a representation of the self and a tool that can be used to increase self-awareness. Because Nurse J. suppresses painful memories of an abortion, she would prefer not to discuss these issues with anyone. However, she volunteers her time to counsel potential abortion clients at the women's clinic. In the Johari Window, this is an example of:
    a. The Open or Public Self
    b. The Unknowing Self
    • c. The Private Self
    d. The Unknown Self

CHAPTER 6. THERAPEUTIC COMMUNICATION

CHAPTER FOCUS

The focus of this chapter is to introduce the student to the concept of communication. Both verbal and nonverbal components of expression are discussed, and a description of therapeutic and nontherapeutic techniques is given.

LEARNING OBJECTIVES

After reading this chapter, the student will be able to:

1. Discuss the transactional model of communication.
2. Identify types of preexisting conditions that influence the outcome of the communication process.
3. Define *territoriality, density,* and *distance* as components of the environment.
4. Identify components of nonverbal expression.
5. Describe therapeutic and nontherapeutic verbal communication techniques.
6. Describe active listening.
7. Discuss therapeutic feedback.

KEY TERMS

territoriality
density
intimate distance
personal distance
social distance
public distance
paralanguage

CHAPTER OUTLINE/LECTURE NOTES

I. Introduction
   A. The nurse must be aware of the therapeutic or nontherapeutic value of the communication techniques used with the client, because they are the "tools" of psychosocial intervention.
II. What Is Communication?
   A. Interpersonal communication is a transaction between the sender and the receiver. Both persons participate simultaneously.
   B. In the transactional model, both participants perceive each other, listen to each other, and simultaneously engage in the process of creating meaning in a relationship.
III. The Impact of Preexisting Conditions
   A. Both sender and receiver bring certain preexisting conditions to the exchange that influence both the intended message and the way in which it is interpreted.
      1. Values, attitudes, and beliefs. Examples: Attitudes of prejudice are expressed through negative stereotyping. A person who values youth may dress and behave in a manner that is characteristic of one who is much younger.
      2. Culture or religion. Cultural mores, norms, ideas, and customs provide the basis for our way of thinking. Examples: Men who hug each other on the street give a different message in the Italian culture than they would in the American culture. Some messages about religion are conveyed by wearing crosses around one's neck or hanging crucifixes on the wall.

3. Social status. High-status persons often convey their high-power position with gestures. Examples: less eye contact, more relaxed posture, louder voice pitch, more frequent use of hands on hips, power dressing, greater height, and more distance when communicating with individuals considered to be of lower social status.

4. Gender. Masculine and feminine gestures influence messages conveyed in communication with others. Examples: differences in posture and gender roles within various cultures.

5. Age or developmental level. Examples of the influence of developmental level on communication are especially evident during adolescence, with words such as "cool," "groovy," "awesome," and others. Sign language is a unique system of gestures used by individuals who are deaf or hearing impaired.

6. Environment in which the transaction takes place. Territoriality, density, and distance are aspects of environment that communicate messages.
    a. Territoriality—the innate tendency to own space. All individuals lay claim to certain areas as their own, and feel safer in their own area.
    b. Density—the number of people within a given environmental space. Prolonged exposure to high-density situations elicits certain behaviors, such as aggression, stress, criminal activity, and hostility.
    c. Distance— the means by which various cultures use space to communicate.
        (1) Intimate distance—the closest distance that individuals will allow between themselves and others. In America, it is 0 to 18 inches.
        (2) Personal distance—interactions that are personal in nature, such as close conversations with friends. In America, it is 18 to 40 inches.
        (3) Social distance—conversations with strangers or acquaintances (e.g., at a cocktail party). In America, it is 4 to 12 feet.
        (4) Public distance—speaking in public or yelling to someone some distance away. In America, the distance exceeds 12 feet.

IV. Nonverbal Communication
    A. Physical appearance and dress. Ways in which individuals dress or wear their hair conveys a message to all who observe their appearance. Example: Unkempt appearance may give an impression to some people that the individual is sloppy and irresponsible.
    B. Body movement and posture. The way in which an individual positions his or her body communicates messages regarding self-esteem, gender identity, status, and interpersonal warmth or coldness. Examples:
        1. Slumped posture, head and eyes pointed downward conveys a message of low self-esteem.
        2. Sitting with legs crossed at the thighs sometimes depicts feminine identity.
        3. Standing tall with head high and hands on hips indicates a superior status over the person being addressed.
        4. Warmth is conveyed by a smile, direct eye contact, and keeping the hands still.
    C. Touch. Can elicit both negative and positive reactions, depending upon cultural interpretation. Types of touch:
        1. Functional-professional—impersonal, businesslike touch. Example: a tailor fitting a suit.
        2. Social-polite—impersonal, but affirming. Example: a handshake.
        3. Friendship-warmth—indicates a strong liking for another person. Example: laying one's hand upon the shoulder of another.
        4. Love-intimacy—conveys an emotional attachment or attraction for another person. Example: to engage in a strong, mutual embrace.
        5. Sexual arousal—an expression of physical attraction. Example: touching another in the genital region.
    D. Facial expressions. Next to human speech, facial expression is the primary source of communication. The face can give multiple messages, such as happiness, sadness, anger, surprise, doubt, fear, disgust.
    E. Eye behavior. Eyes have been called the "windows of the soul." Social and cultural rules dictate where we can look, when we can look, for how long we can look, and at whom we can look. Eye contact conveys a personal interest in the other person. Staring or gazing can make another feel very uncomfortable.

F. Vocal cues or paralanguage. Paralanguage is the gestural component of the spoken word. It consists of pitch, tone, and loudness of spoken messages, the rate of speaking, expressively-placed pauses, and emphasis assigned to certain words. How a message is verbalized can be as important as what is verbalized.

V. Therapeutic Communication Techniques
   A. Using silence—allowing the client to take control of the discussion, if they so desire
   B. Accepting—conveying positive regard
   A. Giving recognition—acknowledging; indicating awareness.
   B. Offering self—making oneself available
   E. Giving broad openings—allowing the client to select the topic
   F. Offering general leads—encouraging the client to continue
   G. Placing the event in time or sequence—clarifying the relationship of events in time
   H. Making observations—verbalizing what is observed or perceived
   I. Encouraging description of perceptions—asking the client to verbalize what is being perceived
   J. Encouraging comparison—asking the client to compare similarities and differences in ideas, experiences, or interpersonal relationships
   K. Restating—letting the client know whether an expressed statement has been understood or not
   L. Reflecting—referring questions or feelings back to the client so that they may be recognized and accepted
   M. Focusing—taking notice of a single idea or even a single word
   N. Exploring—delving further into a subject, idea, experience, or relationship
   O. Seeking clarification and validation—striving to explain that which is vague and searching for mutual understanding
   P. Presenting reality—clarifying misperceptions that the client may be expression
   Q. Voicing doubt—expressing uncertainty as to the reality of the client's perceptions
   R. Verbalizing the implied—putting into words what the client has only implied
   S. Attempting to translate words into feelings—putting into words the feelings that client has expressed only indirectly
   T. Formulating a plan of action—striving to prevent anger or anxiety from escalating to an unmanageable level the next time the stressor occurs

VI. Nontherapeutic Communication Techniques
   A. Giving reassurance—may discourage the client from further expression or feelings if he or she believes they will only be belittled
   B. Rejecting—refusing to consider the client's ideas or behavior
   C. Giving approval or disapproval—implies that the nurse has the right to pass judgment on the "goodness" or "badness" of the client's behavior.
   D. Agreeing/disagreeing—implies that the nurse has the right to pass judgment on whether the client's ideas or opinions are "right" or "wrong"
   E. Giving advice—implies that the nurse knows what is best for the client and that the client is incapable of any self-direction.
   F. Probing—pushing for answers to issues the client does not wish to discuss causes the client to feel used and valued only for what is shared with the nurse
   G. Defending—to defend what the client has criticized implies that he or she has no right to express ideas, opinions, or feelings
   H. Requesting an explanation—asking "Why?" implies that the client must defend his or her behavior or feelings
   I. Indicating the existence of an external source of power—encourages the client to project blame for his or her thoughts or behaviors upon others.
   J. Belittling feelings expressed—causes the client to feel insignificant or unimportant
   K. Making stereotyped comments, cliches, and trite expressions— is meaningless in a nurse-client relationship
   L. Using denial—blocks discussion with the client and avoids helping the client identify and explore areas of difficulty
   M. Interpreting—results in the therapist telling the client the meaning of his experience
   N. Introducing an unrelated topic—causes the nurse to take over the direction of the discussion

VIII. Active Listening

     a.   To listen actively is to be attentive to what the client is saying, both verbally and nonverbally. Several nonverbal behaviors have been designed as facilitative skills for attentive listening. They can be identified by the acronym SOLER.

        1.   S–Sit squarely facing the client.

        2.   O–Observe an open posture.

        3.   L–Lean forward toward the client.

        4.   E–Establish eye contact.

        5.   R–Relax.

VIII. Process Recordings

    A.   Process recordings are written reports of verbal interactions with clients.

    B.   They are written by the nurse or student as a tool for improving communication techniques.

IX.   Feedback

    A.   Feedback is useful when it is conveyed in the following manner:

        1.   Feedback is descriptive rather than evaluative and focuses on the behavior rather than on the client.

        2.   Feedback should be specific rather than general.

        3.   Feedback should be directed toward behavior that the client has the capacity to modify.

        4.   Feedback should impart information rather than offering advice.

        5.   Feedback should be well timed.

X.   Summary

XI.   Review Questions

LEARNING ACTIVITIES

INTERPERSONAL COMMUNICATION TECHNIQUES

After reading the communication on the left, indicate what technique the nurse has used and whether the technique is therapeutic or nontherapeutic. Selections may be made from the list below. The first one has been completed as an example.

Giving recognition	Giving broad openings	Voicing doubt	Restating	Reflecting
Focusing	Verbalizing the implied	Exploring	Giving advice	Rejecting
Giving reassurance	Indicating an external source of power	Requesting an explanation	Belittling feelings	Defending

1. Pt: "The FBI wants to kill me."
   Ns: "I find that hard to believe."   _____Voicing doubt_____   T   N

2. Ns Asst: "Mr. J. always calls me sweetie pie. I get so angry when he does that."
   Ns: "Perhaps you should consider how he is feeling." _____   T   N

3. Pt: "My daddy always tucked me into bed at night."
   Ns: "I'd like to talk more about your relationship with your father." _____   T   N

4. Ns to Pt: "Good morning, Sue. I see you are wearing the hair bow you made in OT." _____   T   N

5. Pt: "I didn't really mean it when I said I wanted to die."
   Ns: "What makes you say those kinds of things?" _____   T   N

6. Pt: "Do you think I should get a divorce?"
   Ns: "What do you think would be best for you?" _____   T   N

7. Pt: "Whenever I ask for a different therapy, my doctor just ignores me!"
   Ns: "I'm sure he knows what's best for you." _____   T   N

8. Pt: "We always had such fun on holidays when I was growing up."
   Ns: "Tell me more about what it was like when you were a little girl." _____   T   N

9. Pt: (Mute refusing to talk)
   Ns: "It must have been a horrible experience for you being the only survivor of the automobile accident." _____   T   N

10. Pt: "I don't think my life will ever be the same again."
    Ns: "Cheer up. Everything's going to be okay." _____   T   N

11. Pt: "I feel like such a failure in the eyes of my family."
    Ns: "You feel as though you have let your family down." _____   T   N

12. Pt: "Do you think I should leave home and get an

apartment of my own?"
Ns: "I think you would be much better off away
from your parents." _____ T   N

13. Pt: "Good morning, nurse."
Ns: "Good morning, Patricia. What would you like
to talk about today?" _____ T   N

14. Pt: "I'd like to talk about my relationship with my
boyfriend, Jack."
Ns: "Oh, let's not talk about that. You talk about
that too much." _____ T   N

15. Pt: "I want to call my husband."
Ns: "Why do you want to talk to him after the way
he treated you?" _____ T   N

CHAPTER 6. TEST QUESTIONS

Situation: Roy is a client on the psychiatric unit. He has a diagnosis of antisocial personality disorder. Jack is assigned as Roy's nurse.

1. Occasionally, Roy loses his temper and expresses his anger inappropriately. Which of the following statements would be appropriate feedback for Roy's angry outbursts?
   a. "You were very rude to interrupt the group the way you did."
   b. "You accomplish nothing when you lose your temper like that."
   c. "Showing your anger in that manner is very childish and insensitive."
   • d. "You became angry in group, raised your voice, stomped out, and slammed the door."

2. Roy says to Jack, "I don't belong in this place with all these loonies. My doctor must be crazy!" Which of the following responses by Jack is most appropriate?
   • a. "You are here for a psychological evaluation."
   b. "I'm sure your doctor has your best interests in mind."
   c. "Why do you think you don't belong here?"
   d. "Just bide your time. You'll be out of here soon."

3. Nancy, a pregnant adolescent, asks the nurse on the psychiatric unit, "Do you think I should give my baby up for adoption?" Which of the following statements by the nurse is most appropriate?
   a. "It would probably be best for you and the baby."
   b. "Why would you want to give your baby up for adoption?"
   • c. "What do *you* think would be the best thing for you to do?"
   d. "I'm afraid you would feel very guilty afterward if you gave your baby away."

4. The purpose of providing feedback is to:
   a. Give the patient good advice
   b. Tell the patient how to behave
   c. Evaluate the patient's behavior
   • d. Give the patient information

5. When interviewing a psychiatric client, which of the following nonverbal behaviors should the nurse be careful to avoid?
   a. Maintaining eye contact
   • b. Leaning back with arms crossed
   c. Sitting directly facing the client
   d. Smiling

CHAPTER 7. THE NURSING PROCESS IN PSYCHIATRIC/MENTAL HEALTH NURSING

CHAPTER FOCUS

The focus of this chapter is to introduce the reader to each of the six steps of the nursing process and identify its use in psychiatric nursing. Documentation of the nursing process is discussed, and the concept of case management is described.

LEARNING OBJECTIVES

After reading this chapter, the student will be able to:

1. Define *nursing process*.
2. Identify the six steps of the nursing process and describe nursing actions associated with each.
3. Describe the benefits of using nursing diagnosis.
4. Discuss the list of nursing diagnoses approved by the North American Nursing Diagnosis Association (NANDA) for clinical use and testing.
5. Define and discuss the utilization of case management and critical pathways of care in the clinical setting.
6. Apply the six steps of the nursing process in the care of a client within the psychiatric setting.
7. Document client care that validates use of the nursing process.

KEY TERMS

nursing process
nursing diagnosis
case management
managed care
case manager
critical pathways of care
interdisciplinary
problem-oriented recording
Focus Charting®
PIE charting

CHAPTER OUTLINE/LECTURE NOTES

I. The Nursing Process
    A. A systematic framework for the delivery of nursing care.
    B. It uses a problem-solving approach.
    C. It is goal directed–the delivery of quality client care.
    D. It is dynamic, not static.
    E. Standards of care. The standards of care for psychiatric nursing are written around the six steps of the nursing process:
        1. Assessment— information is gathered from which to establish a client database
        2. Diagnosis—data from the assessment are analyzed. Diagnoses and potential problem statements are formulated and prioritized.
        3. Outcome identification—expected outcomes of care are identified. They must be measurable and estimate a time for attainment.

4. Planning—interventions for achieving the outcome criteria are selected.
5. Implementation—interventions selected during the planning stage are executed. Specific interventions include:
    a. Counseling to assist clients to improve coping skills and prevent mental illness and disability.
    b. Milieu therapy to provide and maintain a therapeutic environment for the client.
    c. Self-care activities to foster independence and mental and physical well-being.
    d. Psychobiological interventions to restore the client's health and prevent further disability.
    e. Health teaching to assist clients in achieving satisfying, productive, and healthy patterns of living.
    f. Case management to coordinate comprehensive health services and ensure continuity of care.
    g. Health promotion and health maintenance to promote and maintain mental health and prevent mental illness. Advanced practice interventions include:
        (1) Psychotherapy, including individual, group, family, child, and other treatments, to foster mental health and prevent disability
        (2) Prescription of pharmacological agents, in accordance with individual state practice acts, to treat symptoms of psychiatric illness and improve functional health status
        (3) Consultation with other health-care providers to enhance their abilities to provide emotional care for their clients.
6. Evaluation—success of the interventions in meeting the outcome criteria is measured.
II. Why Nursing Diagnosis?
    A. Identification and classification of nursing phenomena began in 1973 with the First National Conference on Nursing Diagnosis.
    B. Both general and specialty standards are written around the six steps of the nursing process, of which nursing diagnosis is an inherent part.
    C. It is defined in most state nursing practice acts as a legal responsibility of nursing.
    D. It promotes research in nursing.
III. Nursing Case Management
    A. Defined: a health-care delivery process whose goals are to provide quality health care, decrease fragmentation, enhance the client's quality of life, and contain costs (ANA, 1988).
    B. Managed care: a concept designed to control the balance between cost and quality of care. Individuals receive care based on need, which is determined by coordinators of the providership.
    C. Case manager: the individual responsible for negotiating with multiple health-care providers to obtain a variety of services for the client.
    D. Critical pathways of care (CPCs)
        1. CPCs are the tools for provision of care in a case management system. It is an abbreviated plan of care on which outcome-based guidelines for goal achievement within a designated length of time have been established.
        2. CPCs are used by the entire interdisciplinary team, which determines what categories of care are to be performed, by what date, and by whom.
        3. Nurses may be identified as case managers and will be ultimately responsible for ensuring that goals on the CPC are achieved within the designated time dimension.
        4. CPCs may be standardized, because they are intended to be used with uncomplicated cases. A CPC can be viewed as protocol for clients with problems for which a designated outcome can be predicted.
IV. Applying Nursing Process in the Psychiatric Setting
    A. Role of the nurse in psychiatry
        1. To assist the client to successfully adapt to stressors within the environment.
        2. Goals are directed toward change in thoughts, feelings, and behaviors that are age-appropriate and congruent with local and cultural norms.
        3. Nurses is a valuable member of the interdisciplinary team, providing a service that is unique and based on sound knowledge of psychopathology, scope of practice, and legal implications of the role.
V. Documentation to the Nursing Process
    A. Documentation of the steps of the nursing process is often considered as evidence in determining certain cases of negligence by nurses.

B. It is also required by some health-care organization accrediting agencies.
C. Examples of documentation that reflect use of the nursing process:
   1. Problem-oriented recording (POR)
      a. Has a list of problems as its basis.
      b. Uses subjective, objective, assessment, plan, intervention, and evaluation (SOAPIE) format.
   2. Focus Charting®
      a. Main perspective is to choose a "focus" for documentation. A focus may be:
         (1) A nursing diagnosis
         (2) A current client concern or behavior
         (3) A significant change in the client's status or behavior
         (4) A significant event in the client's therapy
      b. The focus cannot be a medical diagnosis..
      c. It uses a data, action, and response (DAR) format.
   3. The "A PIE" method
      a. A problem-oriented system.
      b. It uses flow sheets as accompanying documentation.
      c. It uses an assessment, problem, intervention, and evaluation (A PIE) format.
VI. Summary
VII. Review Questions

LEARNING ACTIVITIES

Read the following case study and follow the directions given below for application of the nursing process.

Case Study: Sam is admitted through the emergency department to the psychiatric unit of a major medical center. He was taken to the hospital by local police called by department store security when Sam frightened shoppers by yelling loudly to "imaginary" people and threatening to harm anyone who came close to him.

On the psychiatric unit, Sam keeps to himself and walks away when anyone approaches him. He talks and laughs to himself, and tilts his head to the side, as if listening. When the nurse attempts to talk to him, he shouts, "Get away from me. I know you are one of them!" He picks up a chair, as if to use it for protection.

Sam's appearance is unkempt. His clothes are dirty and wrinkled, his hair is oily and uncombed, and there is an obvious body odor about him. The physician admits Sam with a diagnosis of paranoid schizophrenia and orders chlorpromazine (Thorazine) and benztropine (Cogentin) on both a scheduled and as-needed basis.

1. Identify four segments of information from the assessment data that would be significant to nursing.

   a. _____
   b. _____
   c. _____
   d. _____

2. List the appropriate nursing diagnoses from analysis of the data described in question 1.

   a. _____
   b. _____
   c. _____
   d. _____

3. Provide outcome criteria for the four nursing diagnoses.

   a. _____
   b. _____
   c. _____
   d. _____

4. Select appropriate nursing interventions to achieve the outcome criteria.

CHAPTER 7. TEST QUESTIONS

1.   Laura is a nurse on an inpatient psychiatric unit. Much of her time is spent observing client activity, talking with clients, and striving to maintain a therapeutic environment in collaboration with other health-care providers. This specific example of the implementation step of the nursing process is called:
   a.   Health teaching
   b.   Case management
 • c.   Milieu therapy
   d.   Self-care activities

2.   Which of the following statements about nursing diagnosis is true?
   a.   Nursing diagnosis is a brand new concept.
   b.   All nurses are required by law to write nursing diagnoses.
   c.   All nursing diagnoses must be approved by NANDA.
 • d.   Nursing diagnoses are client responses to actual/potential health problems.

3.   Which of the following statements is *not* true about outcomes?
 • a.   Expected outcomes are specifically formulated by the nurse.
   b.   Expected outcomes are derived from the nursing diagnosis.
   c.   Expected outcomes must be measurable and estimate a time for attainment.
   d.   Expected outcomes must be realistic for the client's capabilities.

4.   Nursing diagnoses are prioritized according to:
   a.   The established goal of care
 • b.   Life-threatening potential
   c.   The nurse's priority of care
   d.   Specific focus on problem resolution

5.   The purpose of case management is to attempt to:
   a.   Improve the medical welfare system
   b.   Ensure that all individuals have medical coverage
 • c.   Maintain a balance between costs and quality of care
   d.   Increase hospital lengths of stay for chronically ill individuals

CHAPTER 8. THERAPEUTIC GROUPS

CHAPTER FOCUS

The focus of this chapter is on the dynamics and functions of therapeutic groups. The role of the nurse in this type of intervention is explored.

LEARNING OBJECTIVES

After reading this chapter, the student will be able to:

1. Define a *group.*
2. Discuss eight functions of a group.
3. Identify various types of groups.
4. Describe physical conditions that influence groups.
5. Discuss "curative factors" that occur in groups.
6. Describe the phases of group development.
7. Identify various leadership styles in groups.
8. Identify various roles that members assume within a group.
9. Discuss psychodrama as a specialized form of group therapy.
10. Describe the role of the nurse in group therapy.

KEY TERMS

altruism
autocratic
catharsis
democratic
group therapy
laissez-faire
psychodrama
universality

CHAPTER OUTLINE/LECTURE NOTES

I. The Group, Defined
   A. A collection of individuals whose association is founded upon shared commonalities of interest, values, norms, or purpose
II. Functions of a Group
   A. Socialization. The teaching of social norms.
   B. Support. Fellow members are available in time of need.
   C. Task Completion. Assistance is provided when completion is enhanced by group involvement.
   D. Camaraderie. Individuals receive joy and pleasure from interactions with significant others.
   E. Informational. Learning takes place when group members share their knowledge with the others in the group.
   F. Normative. Different groups enforce the established norms in various ways.
   G. Empowerment. Change can be effected by groups at times when individuals alone are ineffective.
   H. Governance. Large organizations often have leadership that is provided by groups rather than by a single individual.

III. Types of Groups
   A. Task groups. A group formed to accomplish a specific outcome.
   B. Teaching groups. Focus is to convey knowledge and information to a number of individuals.
   C. Supportive/therapeutic groups. The concern of these groups is to prevent possible future upsets by educating the participants in effective ways of dealing with emotional stress arising from situational or developmental crises.
      1. Therapeutic groups versus Group therapy
         a. Group therapy has a sound theoretical base, and its leaders generally have advanced degrees in psychology, social work, nursing, or medicine.
         b. Therapeutic groups are based to a lesser degree in theory. Focus is on group relations, interactions between group members, and the consideration of a selected issue.
         c. Leaders of both types of groups must be knowledgeable about group *process* (the way in which group members interact with each other), as well as group *content* (the topic or issue being discussed in the group).
   D. Self-help groups. Composed of individuals with a similar problem. Serve to reduce the possibilities of further emotional distress leading to pathology and necessary treatment. May or may not have a professional leader. Run by the members, and leadership often rotates from member to member.
IV. Physical Conditions that Influence Group Dynamics
   A. Seating. It is best when there is no barrier between the members. For example, a circle of chairs is better than chairs set around a table.
   B. Size. Size of the group makes a difference in the interaction among members. Seven or eight members provide a favorable climate for optimal group interaction and relationship development.
   C. Membership. Two types of groups exist: open-ended groups (those in which members leave and others join at any time during the existence of the group) and closed-ended groups (those in which all members join at the time the group is organized and terminate at the end of the designated length of time).
V. Curative Factors
   A. The instillation of hope. By observing the progress of others in the group with similar problems, a group member garners hope that his or her problems can also be resolved.
   B. Universality. Individuals come to realize that they are not alone in the problems, thoughts, and feelings they are experiencing.
   C. The imparting of information. Group members share their knowledge with each other. Leaders of teaching groups also provide information to group members.
   D. Altruism. Individuals provide assistance and support to each other, thereby helping to create a positive self-image and promote self-growth.
   E. The corrective recapitulation of the primary family group. Group members are able to re-experience early family conflicts that remain unresolved.
   F. The development of socializing techniques. Through interaction with and feedback from other members within the group, individuals are able to correct maladaptive social behaviors and learn and develop new social skills.
   G. Imitative behavior. Group members who have mastered a particular psychosocial skill or developmental task serve as valuable role models for others.
   H. Interpersonal learning. The group offers many and varied opportunities for interacting with other people.
   I. Group cohesiveness. Members develop a sense of belonging that separates the individual ("I am") from the group ("we are").
   J. Catharsis. Within the group, members are able to express both positive and negative feelings.
   K. Existential factors. The group is able to assist individual members to take direction of their own lives and to accept responsibility for the quality of their existence.
VI. Phases of Group Development
   A. Initial or orientation phase
      1. Leader and members work together to establish rules and goals for the group.
      2. The leader promotes trust and ensures that the rules do not interfere with the fulfillment of the goals.
      3. Members are superficial and overly polite. Trust has not yet been established.

B. Middle or working phase
  1. Productive work toward completion of the task is undertaken.
  2. Leader's role diminishes and becomes more one of facilitator.
  3. Trust has been established between the members and cohesiveness exists. Conflict is managed by the group members themselves.
C. Final or termination phase
  1. A sense of loss, precipitating the grief process, may be experienced by group members.
  2. The leader encourages the group members to discuss these feelings of loss and to reminisce about the accomplishments of the group.
  3. Feelings of abandonment may be experienced by some members. Grief for previous losses may be triggered.
VII. Leadership Styles
  A. Autocratic. The focus is on the leader, on whom the members are dependent for problem solving, decision making, and permission to perform. Production is high, but morale is low.
  B. Democratic. The focus is on the members, who are encouraged to participate fully in problem solving of issues that relate to the group, including taking action to effect change. Production is somewhat lower than it is with autocratic leadership, but morale is much higher.
  C. Laissez-faire. There is no focus in this type of leadership. Goals are undefined, and members do as they please. Productivity and morale is much higher.
VIII. Member Roles
  A. Members play one of three types of roles within a group:
    1. Task roles. Roles that serve to complete the task of the group.
    2. Maintenance roles. Roles that serve to maintain or enhance group processes.
    3. Individual (personal) roles. Roles that serve to fulfill personal or individual needs.
IX. Psychodrama
  A. It is defined as a type of group therapy that employs a dramatic approach in which clients become "actors" in life-situation scenarios.
  B. An identified client (called the protagonist) is selected to portray a life situation. Other members of the group play the roles of people with whom the protagonist has unresolved issues. Group members who do not participate in the drama act as the audience, and the group leader is called the director.
  C. The purpose is to provide the client with a safe place in which to confront unresolved conflicts, and hopefully progress toward resolution.
  D. Nurses who work as psychodramatists require specialist training beyond the master's degree.
X. The Role of the Nurse in Group Therapy
  A. Nurses who work in psychiatry may lead various type of therapeutic groups, such as client education groups, assertiveness training, support groups for clients with similar problems, parent groups, transition to discharge groups, and others.
  B. Guidelines set forth by the American Nurses' Association specify that nurses who serve as group psychotherapists should have a minimum of a master's degree in psychiatric nursing.
XI. Summary
XII. Review Questions

LEARNING ACTIVITIES

Allow students to use clinical time to attend various types of groups. Following attendance, students should report back to the clinical group in terms of
1. Type of group attended (task, teaching, supportive/therapeutic, self-help)
2. Type of leadership identified for the group (give rationale for determination)
3. Member roles identified (task roles, maintenance roles, personal roles)
4. Description of group dynamics

Suggestions for possible group attendance include:

1. Task groups:
    a. Various hospital committees
    b. Interdisciplinary treatment team meetings
    c. Nursing faculty curriculum committee meeting
    d. Discharge planning meetings

2. Teaching groups:
    a. Prepared childbirth classes
    b. Diabetes education classes
    c. Daily living skills groups
    d. Medication classes
    e. Transition to discharge groups

3. Supportive/therapeutic groups:
    a. Assertiveness training groups
    b. Survivors groups (victims of sexual abuse)
    c. Self-awareness groups
    d. Bereavement groups
    e. Groups for individuals coping with cancer

4. Self-help groups:
    a. Alcoholics Anonymous
    b. Al-Anon
    c. Parents Without Partners
    d. Weight Watchers
    e. Overeaters Anonymous
    f. Gamblers Anonymous
    g. Narcotics Anonymous

CHAPTER 8. TEST QUESTIONS

1. Jane, a psychiatric nurse, leads a supportive/therapeutic group on the psychiatric unit. It is an open group, and clients come and go within the group as they are admitted to and discharged from the unit. Members discuss unresolved issues and ways to cope with stress in their lives. One evening when the group was breaking up, Jane heard one client say to another, "I never thought that other people had the same problems that I have." This statement represents which of Yalom's curative factors?
   - a. Catharsis
   - b. Group cohesiveness
   - • c. Universality
   - d. Imitative behavior

2. Meredith has been in the group for 2 weeks now. She dominates the conversation and does not permit others to participate. Meredith is assuming which of the following roles within the group?
   - a. Aggressor
   - b. Dominator
   - c. Recognition seeker
   - • d. Monopolizer

3. One evening, several of the group members spoke up and expressed their dissatisfaction with Meredith's behavior in the group. They encouraged others in the group to express their feelings as well. Together, they decided that from then on all members who wished to do so would get a turn to talk in group and time would be monitored so that everyone would get their turn. Jane remained silent during this group interaction. Which type of leadership style does Jane demonstrate?
   - a. Autocratic
   - b. Democratic
   - • c. Laissez-faire

4. Although Meredith talks a lot in group, Jane notices that much of her expressions are kept on the superficial level. Jane decides that Meredith might benefit from psychodrama. She makes a referral for Meredith to the psychodramatist. Which of the following statements is *not* true about psychodrama?
   - a. It provides a safe setting in which to discuss painful issues.
   - b. Peers will act out roles that represent individuals with whom Meredith has unresolved conflicts.
   - • c. Meredith can choose who will play the role of *her*, while she observes the interaction from the audience.
   - d. After the drama has been completed, a discussion will be held with members of the audience.

5. Michael, an registered nurse with 3 years' experience on a psychiatric inpatient unit, has taken a position in a day treatment program where he will be leading some groups. Which of the following groups is Michael qualified to lead?
   - • a. A parenting group
   - b. A psychotherapy group
   - c. A psychodrama group
   - d. A family therapy group

CHAPTER 9. INTERVENTION WITH FAMILIES

CHAPTER FOCUS

The focus of this chapter is to introduce the student to the concept of psychotherapy with the family as a unit. Stages of family development and the characteristics of adaptive and maladaptive family functioning are discussed. Theoretical components of selected therapeutic approaches are described.

LEARNING OBJECTIVES

After reading this chapter, the student will be able to:

1. Define the term *family*.
2. Identify stages of family development.
3. Describe major variations to the American middle-class family life cycle.
4. Discuss characteristics of adaptive family functioning.
5. Describe behaviors that interfere with adaptive family functioning.
6. Discuss the essential components of family systems, structural, and strategic therapies.
7. Construct a family genogram.
8. Apply the steps of the nursing process in therapeutic intervention with families.

KEY TERMS

enmeshment	pseudomutuality
boundaries	pseudohostility
double-bind communications	marital schism
family system	marital skew
subsystems	paradoxical intervention
triangles	reframing
scapegoating	genogram
family structure	disengagement

CHAPTER OUTLINE/LECTURE NOTES

I.   Introduction
    A.   Family defined: The family are who they say they are.
    B.   Types of families
        1.   Biological family of procreation.
        2.   Nuclear family (that incorporates one or more members of the extended family()
        3.   The sole-parent family
        4.   The stepfamily
        5.   The communal family
        6.   The homosexual couple or family
    C.   Families may be more appropriately determined based on attributes of affection, strong emotional ties, a sense of belonging, and durability of membership.
    D.   Nurse generalists provide support and referrals to families of ill clients. They should be familiar with the tasks of adaptive family functioning.
    E.   Nurse specialists may perform family therapy.
    F.   Family therapy defined: the attempt to modify the relationships in a family to achieve harmony.

II. Stages of Family Development
   A. Stage 1. The single young adult
      1. Goal: Accepting separation from parents and responsibility for self.
      2. Tasks:
         a. Forming an identity separate from the parents
         b. Establishing intimate peer relationships
         c. Advancing toward financial independence
      3. Problems arise when either the young adult or the parents have difficulty separating from the previous interdependent relationship.
   B. Stage 2. The newly married couple
      1. Goal: Commitment to the new system.
      2. Tasks:
         a. Establishing a new identity as a couple
         b. Realigning relationships with members of the extended family
         c. Making decisions about having children
      3. Problems arise when either partner has difficulty separating from family of origin or when the couple cut themselves off completely from extended family.
   C. Stage 3. The family with young children
      1. Goal: Accepting a new generation of members into the system.
      2. Tasks:
         a. Adjusting the marital relationship to accommodate parental responsibilities while preserving the integrity of the couple relationship
         b. Sharing equally in the tasks of childrearing
         c. Integrating the roles of extended family members into the family
      3. Problems arise when the parents' lack of knowledge about normal childhood development interferes with satisfactory childrearing.
   D. Stage 4. The family with adolescents
      1. Goal: Increasing the flexibility of family boundaries to include children's independence and grandparents' increasing dependence.
      2. Tasks:
         a. Shifting of parent-child relationships to permit adolescents to move in and out of the system
         b. Refocusing on midlife marital and career issues
         c. Beginning a shift toward concerns for the older generation
      3. Problems arise when parents are unable to relinquish control and allow the adolescent increasing autonomy or when the parents cannot agree and support each other in this effort.
   E. Stage 5. The family launching grown children
      1. Goal: Accepting a multitude of exits from and entries into the family system.
      2. Tasks:
         a. Renegotiation of marital system as a dyad
         b. Development of adult-to-adult relationships between grown children and parents
         c. Dealing with disabilities and death of parents (grandparents)
      3. Problems arise when parents are unable to accept the departure of their children from the home and their status as adults, or the death of their own parents, or when the marital bond has deteriorated.
   F. Stage 6. The family in later life
      1. Goal: Accepting the shifting of generational roles.
      2. Tasks:
         a. Maintaining own and/or couple's functioning and interests in face of physiological decline
         b. Exploration of new familial and social role options
         c. Support for a more central role for the middle generation
         d. Dealing with loss of spouse, siblings, and other peers, and preparation for own death; life review and integration
      3. Problems arise when older adults have failed to fulfill the tasks of earlier stages and are dissatisfied with the way their lives have gone.
III. Major Variations

A. Divorce
   1. In the 1980s, nearly half of all American marriages ended in divorce.
   2. There is some indication that this trend is declining.
   3. Stages in the family life cycle of divorce:
      a. Deciding to divorce
      b. Planning the break-up of the system
      c. Separation
      d. Divorce
   4. Tasks:
      a. Accepting one's own part in the failure of the marriage
      b. Working cooperatively on problems related to custody and visitation of children and finances
      c. Realigning relationships with extended family
      d. Mourning the loss of the marriage relationship and the intact family
B. Remarriage
   1. Between two-thirds and three-fourths of those who divorce will eventually remarry.
   2. The rate of redivorce for remarried couples is even higher than the divorce rate following first marriages.
   3. Stages in the remarried family life cycle:
      a. Entering the new relationship
      b. Planning the new marriage and family
      c. Remarriage and reestablishment of family
   4. Tasks:
      a. Making a firm commitment to confronting the complexities of combining two families
      b. Maintaining open communication
      c. Facing fears
      d. Realigning relationships with extended family to include new spouse and children
      e. Encouraging healthy relationships with biological (noncustodial) parents and grandparents
   5. Problems arise when there is a blurring of boundaries between custodial and noncustodial families.
C. Cultural Variations
   1. Caution must be taken in generalizing about variations in family life-cycle development according to culture.
   2. Marriage
      a. Attitudes toward marriage are strongly influenced by Roman Catholicism in many Italian-American and Latino-American families.
      b. In Asian-American families, although marriages are no longer arranged, strong family influence on mate selection still exists.
      c. Jewish-Americans perceive intermarriage as a breach of family togetherness.
      d. In these ethnic subcultures, the father is considered the authority figure and head of the household, and the mother assumes the role of homemaker and caretaker.
   3. Children
      a. Roman Catholicism promotes marital relations for procreation, and large numbers of children are encouraged.
      b. In the traditional Jewish community, having children is seen as a scriptural and social obligation.
      c. In traditional Asian-American cultures, sons are more highly valued than are daughters, and the most important child is the oldest son.
   4. Extended Family
      a. Older family members are valued for their wisdom in Asian, Latino, Italian, and Iranian subcultures.
      b. Several generations within these subcultures may live together and share tasks of childrearing.
   5. Divorce
      a. In the Jewish community, divorce is often seen as a violation of family togetherness.
      b. Because of the opposition to divorce by Roman Catholicism, a low rate of divorce has existed among Italian-Americans, Latino-Americans, and Irish-Americans.

IV. Family Functioning
   A. Six elements on which families are assessed to be either functional or dysfunctional
      1. Communication
         a. Family members are encouraged to express honest feelings and opinions, and all members participate in decisions that affect the family system.
         b. Behaviors that interfere with functional communication include the following:
            (1) Making assumptions—assuming to know what another person is thinking or feeling without checking to make certain
            (2) Belittling feelings—ignoring or minimizing another's feelings when they are expressed
            (3) Failing to listen—one does not hear what the other individual is saying
            (1) Communicating indirectly—seeking to communicate to another through a third person
            (2) Presenting double-bind messages— sending conflicting messages to another (verbal communication may not be congruent with nonverbal communication)
      2. Self-concept reinforcement
         a. Functional families strive to reinforce and strengthen each member's self-concept, with the positive results being that family members feel loved and valued.
         b. Behaviors that interfere with self-concept reinforcement include:
            (1) Expressing denigrating remarks—"put-downs" that send messages that the individual is worthless or unloved
            (2) Withholding supportive messages—individuals who were not supported and reinforced by significant others are often unable to provide this type of support to others
            (3) Taking over—doing things for another and thereby failing to permit that person to develop a sense of responsibility and self-worth
      3. Family members' expectations
         a. In functional families, expectations are realistic, flexible, and individualized.
         b. Behaviors that interfere with adaptive functioning in terms of members' expectations include the following:
            (1) Ignoring individuality—expecting others to do things or behave in ways that do not fit with the latter's individuality or current life situation
            (2) Demanding proof of love—placing conditions on an individual's behavior as proof of love
      4. Handling differences
         a. Functional families understand that it is acceptable to disagree and deal with differences in an open, nonattacking manner.
         b. Behaviors that interfere with successful family negotiations are as follows:
            (1) Attacking—when differences of opinion become a personal attack by one individual on another
            (2) Avoiding—differences are not discussed by an individual who fears that the other person will withdraw love or approval or become angry in response to the disagreement
            (3) Surrendering—an individual avoids expressing a difference of opinion for fear of angering another person or of losing approval and support
      5. Family interactional patterns
         a. Family interactional patterns are functional when they are workable, are constructive, and promote the needs of all family members.
         b. They are dysfunctional when they become contradictory, self-defeating, and destructive. Examples include:
            (1) Patterns that cause emotional discomfort—behaviors such as never admitting making a mistake, rigidity in life situations, and making statements that devalue the worth of others
            (2) Patterns that perpetuate or intensify problems rather than solve them—occurs when unresolved problems are ignored, and then ignoring similar problems becomes the pattern of interaction
            (3) Patterns that are in conflict with each other—family rules that appear to be functional on the surface, but in practice may destroy healthy interactional patterns
      6. Family climate

  a. A positive family climate is founded on trust and is reflected in openness, appropriate humor and laughter, expressions of caring, mutual respect, a valuing of the quality of each individual, and a general feeling of well-being.

  b. A dysfunctional family climate is evidenced by tension, pain, physical disabilities, frustration, guilt, persistent anger, and feelings of hopelessness.

V. Therapeutic Modalities with Families

 A. The family as a system

  1. The family can be viewed as a system composed of various subsystems, such as the marital subsystem, parent-child subsystems, and sibling subsystems.

  2. A major contributor to this theory is Murray Bowen. He has identified the following major concepts:

   a. Differentiation of self—the ability to define oneself as a separate being, independent of others

   b. Triangles—a three-person emotional configuration that is considered the basic building block of the family system

   c. Nuclear family emotional process—the patterns of emotional functioning in a single generation

   d. Family projection process—the process of blaming a third person, usually a child, when anxiety occurs because of lack of differentiation on the part of one of the marital partners (called "scapegoating")

   e. Multigenerational transmission process—the manner in which interactional patterns are transferred from one generation to another

   f. Genograms— tool that provides an overall picture of the life of the family over several generations

   g. Sibling position profiles—the position one holds in a family influences the development of predictable personality characteristics

   h. Emotional cutoff—the degree to which individuals cut themselves off from the family of origin (often related to unresolved emotional attachment)

   i. Societal regression—comparison of society's response to stress to the same type of response seen in individuals and families in response to emotional crisis

  3. Goal and Techniques of Therapy

   a. Goal: to increase the level of differentiation of self, while remaining in touch with the family system

   b. Techniques:

    (1) Defining and clarifying the relationship between the spouses

    (2) Keeping the self (therapist) detriangled

    (3) Teaching family members about the functioning of emotional systems

    (4) Demonstrating differentiation by taking "I-position" stands during the course of therapy

 B. The structural model

  1. The family is viewed as a social system within which the individual lives and to which the individual must adapt.

  2. Major concepts:

   a. Systems—the structure of the family system is founded on a set of invisible principles that influence the interaction among family members.

   b. Transactional patterns—the "laws" that have been established over time that organize the ways in which family members relate to one another.

   c. Subsystems—smaller elements that make up the larger family system. Individual subsystems can be united by gender, relationship, generations, interest, or function

   d. Boundaries—the level of participation and interaction among subsystems. Boundaries may be rigid or diffuse. Rigid boundaries promote disengagement, or extreme separateness, among family members. Diffuse boundaries promote enmeshment, or exaggerated connectedness, among family members.

  3. Goals and techniques of therapy

   a. Goal: to facilitate change in the family structure

   b. Techniques:

    (1) Joining the family—the therapist becomes a part of the family system during therapy

    (2)   Evaluating the family structure—assessment is made of the family transactional patterns, system flexibility and potential for change, boundaries, family developmental stage, and role of the identified patient within the system

    (3)   Restructuring the family—the therapist manipulates the system and facilitates the circumstances and experiences that can lead to structural change (change of the family laws)

C. The strategic model
1. The strategic model uses the interactional or communications approach.
2. Communication theory is viewed as the foundation for this model.
3. Functional families are open systems with clear, precise messages that are congruent with the situation.
4. Dysfunctional families are viewed as closed or partially closed, communication is vague, and messages are often inconsistent and incongruent with the situation.
5. Major concepts:
    a. Double-bind communication—a pattern of communication that occurs when a statement is made and succeeded by a contradictory statement or nonverbal behavior that is inconsistent with the verbal communication
    b. Pseudomutuality—a facade of mutual regard that allows family members to deny underlying fears of hostility and separation.
    c. Pseudohostility—a facade of chronic conflict that allows family members to deny underlying fears of tenderness and intimacy
    d. Marital schism—a state of severe chronic disequilibrium and discord, with recurrent threats of separation
    e. Marital skew—a relationship in which one partner dominates the relationship and the other partner
6. Goal and techniques of therapy
    a. Goal: to create change in destructive behavior and communication patterns among family members. The identified problem is the focus of therapy.
    b. Techniques:
        (1) Paradoxical intervention—requesting that the family continue to engage in the behavior they are trying to change
        (2) Reframing—changing the conceptual and/or emotional setting or viewpoint in relation to which a situation is experienced and placing it in another frame that changes its entire meaning (sometimes referred to as positive reframing)

VI. The Nursing Process
A. A case study. The Marino family
  1. Assessment
    a. The Calgary Family Assessment Model
      (1) Structural assessment
        (a) Internal structure
        (b) External structure
        (c) Context
      (2) Developmental assessment
      (3) Functional assessment
        (a) Instrumental functioning
        (b) Expressive functioning
  2. Diagnosis
    a. Altered family processes
    b. Ineffective family coping
  3. Outcome Identification
  4. Planning/Implementation
  5. Evaluation
VII. Summary
VIII. Review Questions

LEARNING ACTIVITIES

Match the following tasks to the appropriate family developmental stage listed below.

_____ 1.   There is refocus on marital and career issues; a shift toward concerns for the older generation; and a relinquishing of some parental control, while still remaining responsive to children's needs.

_____ 2.   Dealing with loss of spouse, siblings, and other peers, and preparation for own death. Life review and integration occur.

_____ 3.   A differentiation of self in relation to family of origin occurs. Development of intimate peer relationships and the establishment of self in work.

_____ 4.   Adjustment of the marital system to include children. Realignment of relationships with extended family to include parenting and grandparenting roles.

_____ 5.   Renegotiation of the marital system as a dyad. Development of adult relationships with adult children. Dealing with aging parents.

_____ 6.   Formation of the marital system. Realignment of relationships with extended families and friends to include spouses.

        a.   Stage 1. The single young adult
        b.   Stage 2. The newly married couple
        c.   Stage 3. The family with young children
        d.   Stage 4. The family with adolescents
        e.   Stage 5. The family launching grown children
        f.   Stage 6. The family in later life

Construct a genogram of three generations of your family. Use the example in the textbook as a guideline.

CHAPTER 9. TEST QUESTIONS

Sam and Carla have been married for 18 years. They have two children: a boy, Franklin, age 17, and a girl, Natalie, age 15. Natalie recently took an overdose of alprazolam that she found in her parents' medicine cabinet. She was in the hospital for a week and diagnosed with depression. This family seeks counseling at the community mental health center.

1. Natalie says to the nurse, "I just want to go out and do things like all the rest of the kids. Mom says it's okay, but Dad says I'm too young." In the structural model of family therapy, which of the following has occurred?
    a. Multigenerational transmission
    b. Disengagement
    •   c. Mother-daughter subsystem
    d. Emotional cutoff

2. Sam and Natalie start to argue and Sam states, "Your brother never gave us this kind of trouble. Why can't you be more like him?" This is an example of:
    •   a. Triangulation
    b. Pseudohostility
    c. Double-bind communication
    d. Pseudomutuality

3. As the nurse continues to take notes of the initial family visit, she writes, "marital schism." What does this mean?
    a. Sam and Carla have a compatible marriage relationship.
    b. Sam has a dominant relationship over Carla.
    c. Sam and Carla have an enmeshed relationship.
    •   d. Sam and Carla have an incompatible marriage relationship.

4. Sam says to Carla, "What you need to do is spend more time with your family!" Carla responds, "Okay, I'll turn in my resignation at the office tomorrow." To this Sam replies, "Just as I thought! You've always been a quitter!" This is an example of:
    a. Emotional cutoff
    •   b. Double-bind communication
    c. Indirect messages
    d. Avoidance

5. Carla says to the nurse, "Every time we start to discuss rules for the children, we get into shouting matches. We can't ever settle on anything. We just shout at each other!" The nurse instructs Sam and Carla to shout at each other for the next 2 weeks on Tuesdays and Thursdays from 6:30 to 7 P.M. This intervention is called:
    a. Reframing
    b. Restructuring the family
    c. Expressive psychotherapy
    •   d. Paradoxical intervention

CHAPTER 10. MILIEU THERAPY—THE THERAPY COMMUNITY

CHAPTER FOCUS

The focus of this chapter is to introduce the student to the concept of milieu therapy. The role of the nurse in this therapeutic setting is emphasized.

LEARNING OBJECTIVES

After reading this chapter, the student will be able to:

1. Define *milieu therapy*.
2. Explain the goal of therapeutic community/milieu therapy.
3. Identify seven basic assumptions of a therapeutic community.
4. Discuss conditions that characterize a therapeutic community.
5. Identify the various therapies that may be included within the program of therapeutic community, and the health-care workers that make up the interdisciplinary treatment team.
6. Describe the role of the nurse on the interdisciplinary treatment team.

KEY TERMS

milieu
milieu therapy
therapeutic community

CHAPTER OUTLINE/LECTURE NOTES

I. Introduction
    A. Standard Vb of ANA Standards of Psychiatric-Mental Health Nursing Practice states that, "The psychiatric-mental health nurse provides, structures, and maintains a therapeutic environment in collaboration with the client and other health-care providers."
II. Defined
    A. Milieu therapy, or therapeutic community, is defined as a scientific structuring of the environment to effect behavioral changes and to improve the psychological health and functioning of the individual.
    B. Within the therapeutic community setting the client is expected to learn adaptive coping, interaction and relationship skills that can be generalized to other aspects of his or her life.
III. Basic Assumptions
    A. The health in each individual is to be realized and encouraged to grow.
    B. Every interaction is an opportunity for therapeutic intervention.
    C. The client owns his or her own environment.
    D. Each client owns his or her own behavior.
    E. Peer pressure is a useful and powerful tool.
    F. Inappropriate behaviors are dealt with as they occur.
    G. Restrictions and punishment are to be avoided.
IV. Conditions that Promote a Therapeutic Community
    A. Basic physiological needs are fulfilled.
    B. The physical facilities are conducive to achievement of the goals of therapy.
    C. A democratic form of self-government exists.
    D. Unit responsibilities are assigned according to client capabilities.

E.   A structured program of social and work-related activities is scheduled as part of the treatment program.

F.   Community and family are included in the program of therapy in an effort to facilitate discharge from the hospital.

V.   The Program of Therapeutic Community
   A.   Directed by an interdisciplinary team.
   B.   A treatment plan is formulated by the team.
   C.   All disciplines sign the treatment plan and meet weekly to update the plan as needed.
   D.   Disciplines may include psychiatry, psychology, nursing, social work, occupational therapy, recreational therapy, art therapy, music therapy, dietetics, and chaplain's service.

VI.   Role of the Nurse
   A.   Through use of the nursing process, nurses manage the therapeutic environment on a 24-hour basis.
   B.   Nurses have the responsibility for ensuring that clients' physiological and psychological needs are met.
   C.   Nurses also are responsible for:
      1.   Medication administration
      2.   Development of a one-to-one relationship
      3.   Setting limits on unacceptable behavior
      4.   Client education

VII.   Summary

VIII.   Review Questions

LEARNING ACTIVITIES

Identify the appropriate member of the interdisciplinary for the activity listed. Choices may be made from the following list.

Psychiatrist   Psychiatric staff nurse   Art therapist
Clinical psychologist   Occupational therapist   Dietitian
Psychiatric social worker   Recreational therapist   Chaplain
Psychiatric clinical nurse specialist   Music therapist   Mental health technician
                                                         Psychodramatist

1.   Accompanies clients to see a movie.   _____

2.   Helps clients identify unconscious feelings through their drawings.   _____

3.   Conducts psychological testing to assist the psychiatrist to determine a correct diagnosis.   _____

4.   Serves the spiritual needs of psychiatric clients.   _____

5.   Monitors nutritional needs for client with special requirements.   _____

6.   Teaches relaxation techniques through the use of music.   _____

7.   Conducts assertiveness training.   _____

8.   Prescribes electroconvulsive therapy for a depressed client.   _____

9.   Administers medication.   _____

10.   Locates appropriate placement for the client following hospital discharge.   _____

11.   Assists clients to increase self-esteem by providing small craft items for completion and display.   _____

12.   Assists a group of clients to perform in a safe environment, a situation that otherwise would be too painful in real life.   _____

13.   Works 1:1 with clients and assists the psychiatric nurse in running the day-to-day activities of the milieu unit.   _____

There are seven basic assumptions upon which a therapeutic community is based. Identify the assumption (from the column on the right) that is the foundation for each of the situations listed on the left.

_____ 1. John came into the TV room and changed the channel in the middle of a program that several others were watching. The group reprimanded him loudly, and returned the TV to the channel they had been watching. They told him they would not tolerate that kind of behavior.

a. The health in each individual is to be realized and encouraged to grow.

_____ 2. Even though she seemed unable to change, Nancy had a great deal of insight into her own behavior. She knew it was maladaptive and she knew it had psychological implications. The nurse focused on Nancy's insight and knowledge to help her find more adaptive ways of coping.

b. Every interaction is an opportunity for therapeutic intervention.

_____ 3. George always started an argument in group therapy. Each time, the group calmed him down with their discussion. However, when he became violent, he was placed in isolation for the safety of himself and others.

c. The client owns his or her own environment.

_____ 4. Fred becomes angry whenever anyone in the group disagrees with him. Members of the group examine Fred's defensiveness and help him to see how he is coming across to others. They help him to practice more appropriate ways of responding.

d. Each client owns his or her behavior.

_____ 5. Lloyd had always been unable to interact on a personal level with other people. In the milieu environment, he learned new communication skills and had the opportunity to practice relationship development that helped him when he left the hospital.

e. Peer pressure is a useful and powerful tool.

_____ 6. Kevin told the nurse of being arrested for driving the getaway car in an armed robbery. He stated, "I don't know why they grabbed me. Jack did the stealing! He made me drive the car." The nurse responded, "Kevin, no one made you drive the car. You made that choice yourself. Now you must own up to that decision."

f. Inappropriate behavior is dealt with as it occurs.

_____ 7. Carol was elected unit president at the community meeting. She assigns chores for the week and calls for a vote concerning late privileges for clients on Saturday night.

g. Restrictions and punishment are to be avoided.

CHAPTER 10. TEST QUESTIONS

1. Which of the following statements is true about milieu therapy?
    a. Punishments are used to eliminate negative behaviors.
    b. Interpersonal therapy is the foundation for the program of treatment.
    c. Staff perform all activities of care for the clients.
  • d. The environment is structured so that stresses are used as opportunities for learning.

2. To reinforce the democratic form of self-government on a milieu unit
    a. Clients are allowed to set forth the type of punishment for a peer who violates the rules.
    b. Clients may choose whether or not to attend daily community meetings.
  • c. Clients participate in decision making that affects management of the unit.
    d. Professional staff do not attend community meetings.

3. Jack is a client on the psychiatric unit. Jack expressed at community meeting which movie he wanted to see that night. His choice was denied because of majority rule. At movie time that evening, Jack put the tape he wanted to view into the VCR. He was reprimanded by his peers, who removed the tape and put in the one voted on by the majority. This is an example of which basic assumption of milieu therapy?
    a. Every interaction is an opportunity for therapeutic intervention.
  • b. Peer pressure is a useful and powerful tool.
    c. Restrictions and punishment are to be avoided.
    d. The client owns his or her own environment.

4. Jack's physician decides to have Jack undergo psychological testing. Which of the following members of the interdisciplinary team would Jack's physician consult for this purpose?
    a. The occupational therapist.
    b. The psychiatric social worker.
  • c. The clinical psychologist.
    d. The clinical nurse specialist.

5. Which of the following best describes the role of the nurse in the therapeutic milieu of a psychiatric unit?
  • a. The member of the treatment team who is responsible for management of the therapeutic milieu
    b. A member of the treatment team who develops the medical diagnosis for all clients on the unit
    c. The team member who provides for the spiritual and comfort needs of the client and his or he family
    d. The team member who conducts individual, group, and family therapy after an in-depth psychosocial history

CHAPTER 11. CRISIS INTERVENTION

CHAPTER FOCUS

The focus of this chapter is to introduce the student to the concept of crisis, and the therapy of crisis intervention. The role of the nurse in crisis intervention is emphasized.

LEARNING OBJECTIVES

After reading this chapter, the student will be able to:

1. Define *crisis.*
2. Describe four phases in the development of a crisis.
3. Identify types of crises that occur in people's lives.
4. Discuss the goal of crisis intervention.
5. Describe the steps in crisis intervention.
6. Identify the role of the nurse in crisis intervention.

KEY TERMS

crisis
crisis intervention

CHAPTER OUTLINE/LECTURE NOTES

I. Definition
    A. Crisis has been defined as a psychological disequilibrium in a person who confronts a hazardous circumstance that constitutes an important problem for that person and that cannot, for the time being, be escaped or solved with the person's customary problem-solving resources.
    B. Assumptions upon which the concept of crisis is based:
        1. Crisis occurs in all individuals at one time or another and is not necessarily equated with psychopathology.
        2. Crises are precipitated by specific identifiable events.
        3. Crises are personal by nature.
        4. Crises are acute, not chronic, and will be resolved in one way or another within a brief period.
        5. A crisis situation contains the potential for psychological growth or deterioration.
II. Phases in the Development of a Crisis
    A. The individual is exposed to a precipitating stressor.
    B. When previous problem-solving techniques do not relieve the stressor, anxiety increases further.
    C. All possible resources, both internal and external, are called upon to resolve the problem and relieve the discomfort.
    D. If resolution does not occur in previous phases, the tension mounts beyond a further threshold, or its burden increases over time to a breaking point. Major disorganization of the individual with drastic results often occurs.
III. Whether or not individuals experience a crisis in response to a stressful situation depends upon:
    A. The individual's perception of the event
    B. The availability of situational supports
    C. The availability of adequate coping mechanisms

IV. Types of Crises
    A. Dispositional crisis–an acute response to an external situational stressor
    B. Crisis of anticipated life transition–normal life-cycle transitions that may be anticipated, but over which the individual may feel a lack of control
    C. Crisis resulting from traumatic stress–a crisis that is precipitated by an unexpected, external stressor over which the individual has little or no control, and from which he or she feels emotionally overwhelmed and defeated
    D. Maturational/developmental crisis–crisis that occurs in response to situations that trigger emotions related to unresolved conflicts in one's life
    E. Crisis reflecting psychopathology—emotional crisis in which preexisting psychopathology has been instrumental in precipitating the crisis or in which psychopathology significantly impairs or complicates adaptive resolution
    F. Psychiatric emergencies—crisis situations in which general functioning has been severely impaired and the individual rendered incompetent or unable to assume personal responsibility
V. Crisis Intervention
    A. The minimum therapeutic goal of crisis intervention is psychological resolution of the individual's immediate crisis and restoration to at least the level of functioning that existed before the crisis period.
    B. A maximum goal is improvement in functioning above the precrisis level.
    C. It usually lasts from 4 to 6 weeks.
VI. Phases of Crisis Intervention: The Role of the Nurse
    A. Nurses may be called upon to function as crisis helpers in virtually any setting committed to the practice of nursing.
        1. Phase 1: Assessment. Information is gathered regarding the precipitating stressor and the resulting crisis that prompted the individual to seek professional help.
        2. Phase 2: Planning of therapeutic intervention. From the assessment data, the nurse selects appropriate nursing diagnoses that reflect the immediacy of the crisis situation. Desired outcome criteria are established. Appropriate nursing actions are selected taking into consideration the type of crisis, as well as the individual's strengths and available resources for support.
        3. Phase 3: Intervention. The actions identified in the planning phase are implemented. A reality-oriented approach is used. A rapid working relationship is established by showing unconditional acceptance, by active listening, and by attending to immediate needs. A problem-solving model becomes the basis for change.
        4. Phase 4: Evaluation of crisis resolution and anticipatory planning. A reassessment is conducted to determine if the stated objectives were achieved. A plan of action is developed for the individual to deal with the stressor should it recur.
VII. Summary
VIII. Review Questions

LEARNING ACTIVITIES

Match the situation on the left with the type of crisis listed on the right.

____ 1. Harriet, 24-years-old was informed that her husband was killed in an industrial accident at the plant where he works. An hour later, she was found walking down a busy highway saying, "I'm looking for my lucky rabbit's foot. Everything will be okay if I can just find my lucky rabbit's foot."

a. Dispositional crisis

____ 2. Ted was transferred on his job to a distant city. His wife Jane had never lived away from her family before. She became despondent, living only for daily phone calls to her relatives back in their home town.

b. Crisis of anticipated life transition

____ 3. Carrie knew when she married Matt that he had a drinking problem, but she believed he would change. Last night, after becoming intoxicated, Matt beat Carrie into unconsciousness. When she regained consciousness, he was gone. She took a taxi to the emergency department of the local hospital.

c. Crisis resulting from traumatic stress

____ 4. Linda had a history of obsessive-compulsive disorder. She was phobic about germs and washed her hands many times every day. Last night, after a party, she had sex with a fellow college student she barely knew. Today, she is extremely anxious, and keeps repeating that she knows she has AIDS. Her roommate cannot get her to come out of the shower.

d. Maturational/developmental crisis

____ 5. At age 13, Sue was raped by her uncle. The abuse continued for several years. He threatened to kill her mother if she told. She is 23-years-old now and recently became engaged. She has never had an intimate relationship and experiences panic attacks at the thought of her wedding night.

e. Crisis reflecting psychopathology

____ 6. Frank was very proud of his home. He had saved for many years to build it and had virtually built it from the ground up by himself. Last night, while he and his wife were visiting in a nearby town, a tornado ripped through his neighborhood and totally destroyed his home. Frank is devastated and for over a week has sat and stared into space, barely eating and rarely speaking.

f. Psychiatric emergency

You are a nurse in the mental health clinic in the town to which Ted and Jane (situation 2 in the previous activity) have moved. Ted brings Jane to your clinic and explains that she has become nonfunctional since their move. Use the steps of the problem-solving process with the objective of assisting Jane to overcome her despondency.

1.   Confront the problem.

2.   Identify realistic changes.

3.   Explore coping strategies for aspects about her situation that cannot be changed.

4.   Identify various alternatives for coping with situation.

5.   Weigh benefits and consequences of each alternative.

6.   Select most appropriate alternative.

CHAPTER 11. TEST QUESTIONS

Situation: On Thursday, Camille, a college junior, is accompanied to the student health center by her roommate, Nancy. Nancy explains to the nurse that for 3 days Camille has been unable to attend her classes, has cried constantly, and has become panicky whenever Nancy leaves to go to classes and meals. The nurse performs an assessment and finds that Camille does not know the date and has difficulty with short-term memory. Nancy is not aware that Camille has received any bad news recently, but she offers that Camille is a good student and has been spending long hours at the computer center for nearly 2 weeks working on a major class project, usually returning to the dorm after Nancy is asleep. This is the strategy she has successfully used when working on projects in the past and was the strategy employed through Monday of this week.

1. What crucial information is missing that will *most* assist the nurse to plan interventions that will be helpful for Camille?
    - • a. The precipitating stressor
      b. Camille's usual ability to cope with stress
      c. How far away Camille's home and parents are
      d. The due date of Camille's project

2. Based upon the correct answer in question 1, which of the following types of crises is the nurse most likely to suspect in Camille's case?
      a. A psychiatric emergency
      b. A crisis of anticipated life transition
      c. A crisis reflecting psychopathology
    - • d. A crisis resulting from traumatic stress

3. Camille eventually reports that she was nearly raped on Monday night when she took a shortcut on her way from the computer center to her dorm. She is referred to a nurse who is trained as a rape crisis counselor, who schedules appointments three times a week for 3 weeks. At the first session, Camille announces that she has decided to quit school and return home. What is the most therapeutic response for the counselor to make?
      a. "I'm confident you know what's best for you."
    - • b. "This is not a good time for you to make such an important decision."
      c. "Your mother and father will be terribly disappointed."
      d. "What will you do if you go home?"

4. In her interventions with Camille, which of the following therapeutic approaches would *best* be implemented by the nurse?
      a. A psychoanalytical approach
      b. A psychodynamic approach
    - • c. A reality-oriented approach
      d. A family-oriented approach

5. During the final two sessions, Camille and the counselor review the work they have done together. Which of the following statements by Camille would *most* clearly suggest that the goals of crisis intervention have been met?
      a. "Thanks a lot. You've really been helpful. I'll miss working with you."
      b. "My instructor gave me a 3-week extension on my project."
      c. "I'm really glad I didn't go home. It would have been hard to come back."
    - • d. "I'm wearing the whistle my dad gave me when I go out walking. I've practiced using it, too."

CHAPTER 12. RELAXATION THERAPY

CHAPTER FOCUS

The focus of this chapter is to introduce the student to the benefits of relaxation therapy. Various methods of achieving relaxation are presented, and emphasis is on the role of the nurse in relaxation therapy.

LEARNING OBJECTIVES

After reading this chapter, the student will be able to:

1. Identify conditions for which relaxation is appropriate therapy.
2. Describe physiological and behavioral manifestations of relaxation.
3. Discuss various methods of achieving relaxation.
4. Describe the role of the nurse in relaxation therapy.

KEY TERMS

stress management
progressive relaxation
meditation
mental imagery
biofeedback

CHAPTER OUTLINE/LECTURE NOTES

I.   The Stress Epidemic
    A. Stress is rapidly permeating our society.
    B. Individuals experience the "fight-or-flight" response on a regular basis.
    C. The fight-or-flight emergency response is inappropriate to today's psychosocial stresses that persist over long periods.
    D. Stress is known to be a major contributor, either directly or indirectly, to coronary heart disease, cancer, lung ailments, accidental injuries, cirrhosis of the liver, and suicide—six of the leading causes of death in the United States.
    E. An individual's predisposing factors (genetic influences, past experiences, and existing conditions) influence the degree of severity to which an individual perceives and responds to stress.
II. Physiological, Cognitive, and Behavioral Manifestations of Relaxation
    A. Physiological manifestations of stress include increases in heart rate, respirations, blood pressure, blood sugar, and metabolism.
    B. Behavioral manifestations of stress include restlessness, irritability, insomnia, and anorexia.
    C. Cognitive manifestations of stress include confusion and difficulty with concentration, problem solving, and learning.
    D. Relaxation can counteract these symptoms.
III. Methods of Achieving Relaxation
    A. Deep-breathing exercises
        1. Relaxation is accomplished by allowing the lungs to breathe in as much oxygen as possible. Air is breathed in slowly through the nose, held for a few seconds, and then exhaled slowly through the mouth.

2. Breathing exercises have been found to be effective in reducing anxiety, depression, irritability, muscular tension, and fatigue.
3. An advantage of these exercises is that they may be accomplished anywhere at any time.
B. Progressive relaxation
  1. Each muscle group is tensed for 5 to 7 seconds, and then relaxed for 20 to 30 seconds, during which time the individual concentrates on the difference in sensations between the two conditions.
  2. Excellent results have been observed with this method in the treatment of muscular tension, anxiety, insomnia, depression, fatigue, irritable bowel, muscle spasms, neck and back pain, high blood pressure, mild phobias, and stuttering.
C. Modified (or passive) progressive relaxation
  1 Relaxation is achieved with this method by passively concentrating on the feeling of relaxation within the muscle groups.
D. Meditation
  1. Meditation has been practiced for over 2000 years.
  2. The goal of meditation is to gain "mastery over attention."
  3. Relaxation is achieved through fulfillment of a special state of consciousness brought about by extreme concentration solely on one thought or object.
  4. It has been used successfully in the treatment of cardiovascular disease, obsessive thinking, anxiety, depression, and hostility.
E. Mental imagery
  1. This method of relaxation employs the imagination in an effort to reduce the body's response to stress.
  2. The individual follows his or her imagination in selecting an environment considered to be relaxing.
  3. The individual then concentrates on this relaxing image in an effort to achieve relaxation.
  4. Soft, background music enhances the effect.
F. Biofeedback
  1. Biofeedback is the use of instrumentation to become aware of processes in the body that usually go unnoticed and to help bring them under voluntary control. Some of these processes include blood pressure, muscle tension, skin surface temperature, and heart rate.
  2. Biofeedback has been used successfully in the treatment of spastic colon, hypertension, tension and migraine headaches, muscle spasms/pain, anxiety, phobias, stuttering, and teeth grinding.
G. Physical exercise
  1. Physical exertion provides a natural outlet for the tension produced by the body in the state of arousal for fight or flight.
  2. Following exercise, physiological equilibrium is restored resulting in a feeling of relaxation and revitalization.
  3. Aerobic exercises have been shown to be successful in strengthening the cardiovascular system.
  4. Low-intensity physical exercise can help prevent obesity, relieve muscular tension, prevent muscle spasms, and increase flexibility.
  5. Physical exercise can also be effective in reducing general anxiety and depression.
IV. The Role of the Nurse in Relaxation Therapy
  A. Nurses can help individuals recognize the sources of stress in their lives and identify methods of adaptive coping.
  B. Nurses can serve as educators to increase clients' knowledge regarding methods for achieving relaxation.
  C. Relaxation therapy provides alternatives to old, maladaptive methods of coping with stress.
  D. Nurses can help individuals analyze the usefulness of various relaxation techniques in the management of stress in their daily lives.
V. Summary
VI. Review Questions

LEARNING ACTIVITIES

Take the following self-test. Discuss the results in class or small student group.

How Vulnerable Are You To Stress?

Score each item from 1 (almost always) to 5 (never), according to how much of the time each statement applies to you.

_____ 1. I eat at least one hot, balanced meal a day.
_____ 2. I get 7 to 8 hours sleep at least four nights a week.
_____ 3. I give and receive affection regularly.
_____ 4. I have at least one relative within 50 miles on whom I can rely.
_____ 5. I exercise to the point of perspiration at least twice a week.
_____ 6. I smoke less than half a pack of cigarettes a day.
_____ 7. I take fewer than five alcoholic drinks a week.
_____ 8. I am the appropriate weight for my height.
_____ 9. I have an income adequate to meet basic expenses.
_____ 10. I get strength from my religious beliefs.
_____ 11. I regularly attend club or social activities.
_____ 12. I have a network of friends and acquaintances.
_____ 13. I have one or more friends to confide in about personal matters.
_____ 14. I am in good health (including eyesight, hearing, teeth).
_____ 15. I am able to speak openly about my feelings when angry or worried.
_____ 16. I have regular conversations with the people I live with about domestic problems (e.g., chores, money, and daily living issues).
_____ 17. I do something for fun at least once a week.
_____ 18. I am able to organize my time effectively.
_____ 19. I drink fewer than 3 cups of coffee (or tea or colas) a day.
_____ 20. I take quiet time for myself during the day.

_____ TOTAL

To get your score, add up the figures and subtract 20. Any number over 30 indicates a vulnerability to stress. You are seriously vulnerable if your score is between 50 and 75, and extremely vulnerable if it is over 75.

Keep a record for 1 week of situations that produce stress in your life. Rate the severity of each situation on a scale from 1 to 5 (with 5 being the most severe). Describe how you responded to the stress and whether your response was adaptive or maladaptive. If it was maladaptive, how could you have responded more adaptively?

Date	Situation	Rating (1–5)	How I Responded	Adaptive/ Maladaptive	How to Respond Adaptively

CHAPTER 12. TEST QUESTIONS

1. Which of the following is known to be a physiological manifestation of relaxation?
    a.   Increased levels of norepinephrine
    b.   Pupil dilation
    •   c.   Reduced metabolic rate
    d.   Increased blood sugar level

2. Ellen is a registered nurse who works in an employee health facility for a large corporation. She teaches many kinds of preventive health-care strategies to the employees, among them relaxation therapy. Which of the following is Ellen likely to teach as a *beginning* technique and is useful in conjunction with many other forms of relaxation therapy?
    •   a.   Deep-breathing exercises
    b.   Mental imagery
    c.   Biofeedback
    d.   Meditation

3. Physical exercise is an effective relaxation technique because it
    a.   Stresses and strengthens the cardiovascular system
    b.   Decreases the metabolic rate
    c.   Decreases levels of norepinephrine into the brain
    •   d.   Provides a natural outlet for release of muscle tension

4. Which of the following relaxation techniques is thought to improve concentration and attention?
    a.   Biofeedback
    b.   Physical exercise
    •   c.   Meditation
    d.   Mental imagery

CHAPTER 13. ASSERTIVENESS TRAINING

CHAPTER FOCUS

The focus of this chapter is to introduce the student to the concepts of assertiveness training. Various techniques to promote assertive behavior are discussed, and the role of the nurse in assertiveness training is emphasized.

LEARNING OBJECTIVES

After reading this chapter, the student will be able to:

1. Define assertive behavior.
2. Discuss basic human rights.
3. Differentiate between nonassertive, assertive, aggressive. and passive-aggressive behaviors.
4. Describe techniques that promote assertive behavior.
5. Demonstrate thought-stopping techniques.
6. Discuss the role of the nurse in assertiveness training.

KEY TERMS

assertiveness
nonassertiveness
aggressiveness
passive-aggressive
thought stopping

CHAPTER OUTLINE/LECTURE NOTES

I. Assertive Communication
   A. Assertiveness is behavior that enables individuals to act in their own best interests, to stand up for themselves without undue anxiety, to express their honest feelings comfortably, or to exercise their own rights without denying the rights of others.
   B. Honesty is basic to assertive behavior and is expressed in a manner that promotes self-respect and respect for others.
II. Basic Human Rights
   A. Basic human rights include:
      1. The right to be treated with respect
      2. The right to express feelings, opinions, and beliefs
      3. The right to say "no" without feeling guilty
      4. The right to make mistakes and to accept responsibility for them
      5. The right to be listened to and taken seriously
      6. The right to change your mind
      7. The right to ask for what you want
      8. The right to put yourself first, sometimes
      9. The right to set your own priorities
      10. The right to refuse justification for your feelings or behavior
   B. If one is to accept these rights, he or she must also accept the responsibilities that accompany them.
III. Response Patterns
   A. Individuals develop, in certain ways, patterns of responding to others. These ways include:

1. By watching other people (role modeling)
2. By being positively reinforced or punished for a certain response
3. By inventing a response
4. By not thinking of a better way to respond
5. By not developing the proper skills for a better response
6. By consciously choosing a response style
   B. Four common response patterns are as follows:
   1. Nonassertive behavior. Sometimes called passive, these individuals seek to please others at the expense of denying their own basic human rights.
   2. Assertive behavior. These individuals stand up for their own rights while protecting the rights of others. Feelings are expressed openly and honestly. Self-respect and respect for others are maintained.
   3. Aggressive behavior. These individuals defend their own basic rights by violating the basic rights of others. Aggressive behavior hinders interpersonal relationships.
   4. Passive-aggressive behavior. These individuals defend their own rights by expressing resistance to social and occupational demands. Sometimes called *indirect aggression,* this behavior takes the form of passive, nonconfrontive action. These individuals use actions instead of words to convey their message, and the actions express covert aggression.

IV. Behavioral Components of Assertive Behavior
   A. Intermittent eye contact
   B. Body posture. Sitting and leaning slightly toward the other person in a conversation.
   C. Distance/physical contact. Appropriate physical distance is culturally determined. Invasion of personal space may be interpreted by some individuals as aggressive.
   D. Gestures may also be culturally related. Gestures can add meaning to the spoken word.
   E. Facial expression. Various facial expressions convey different messages.
   G. Fluency. Being able to discuss a subject with ease and with obvious knowledge conveys assertiveness and self-confidence.
   H. Timing. Assertive response are most effective when they are spontaneous and immediate.
   I. Listening. Assertive listening means giving the other individual full attention.
   J. Thoughts. One's attitudes about the appropriateness of assertive behavior influences one's responses.
   K. Content. Many times it is not what is being said that is as important as how it is said.

V. Techniques that Promote Assertive Behavior
   A. Standing up for one's basic human rights.
   B. Assuming responsibility for own statements.
   C. Responding as a "broken record." Persistently repeating in a calm voice what is wanted.
   D. Agreeing assertively. Assertively accepting negative aspects about oneself. Admitting when an error has been made.
   E. Inquiring assertively. Seeking additional information about critical statements.
   F. Shifting from content to process. Changing the focus of the communication from discussing the topic at hand to analyzing what is actually going on in the interaction.
   G. Clouding/fogging. Concurring with the critic's argument without becoming defensive and without agreeing to change.
   H. Defusing. Putting off further discussion with an angry individual until he or she is calmer.
   I. Delaying assertively. Putting off further discussion with an angry individual until he or she is calmer.
   J. Responding assertively with irony.

VI. Thought-Stopping Techniques
   A. Techniques that were developed to eliminate intrusive, unwanted thoughts.
   B. The individual practices interrupting negative thought processes with the word "stop" and shifting his or her thoughts to those that are considered pleasant and desirable.

VII. Role of the Nurse
   A. Nurses must understand and use assertive skills to effect change that will improve the status of nursing and the system of health-care provision in our country.
   B. Nurses who understand and use assertiveness skills themselves can in turn assist clients who wish to effect behavioral change in an effort to increase self-esteem and improve interpersonal relationships.

C. Nurses can teach clients assertive skills on a one-to-one basis or in a group situation.

D. Information should include examples of various behavioral responses (assertive, nonassertive, aggressive, and passive-aggressive), as well as techniques that can be used to promote assertive behavior.

E. Clients should be given the opportunity to practice their newly learned skills through role playing, to facilitate the behavior when the actual situation arises.

VIII. Summary

IX. Review Questions

LEARNING ACTIVITIES

Match the responses on the left to the assertive technique being used.

_____ 1. Wife: "You let that guy walk all over you. What a wimp!"
Husband: "Yes, I admit I didn't handle that situation very well."

a. Standing up for one's basic human rights.

_____ 2. Husband: "Would you please re-sew this seam. Its coming loose again."
Wife: "I can never do anything to please you!"
Husband: "Seems we need to discuss the real issue here."

b. Assuming responsibility for own statements.

_____ 3. Man: "If I were your husband, I'd keep my eye on you all the time."
Woman: "It's so nice to know you care."

c. Responding as a "broken record."

_____ 4. Male board member: "How dare you suggest we hire homosexuals! What kind of company do you think this is?"
Female board member: "I would like to discuss this further with you when you have had a chance to cool off."

d. Agreeing assertively

_____ 5. Woman No. 1: "How can you be in favor of abortion? Can't you see it's murder?"
Woman No. 2: "I have a right to my opinion just as you have."

e. Inquiring assertively.

_____ 6. Door-to-door salesman: "I'd like to demonstrate this steam cleaner by cleaning one of your rugs for you."
Housewife: "I'm not interested in seeing a demonstration of a steam cleaner."
Door-to-door salesman: "But surely you have a rug you'd like to have cleaned!"
Housewife: "I'm not interested in seeing a demonstration of a steam cleaner."

f. Shifting from content to process.

_____ 7. Husband: "Boy, I can't believe you screwed up that audition so badly."
Wife: "Just what do you think I did that was so wrong?"

g. Clouding/fogging.

_____ 8. Male staff nurse: "I think the changes I have proposed for the unit will improve staff relations, not to mention client care. I'm surprised they haven't been thought of before."
Female head nurse: "Thank you for your suggestions. I will study them and talk to you about them later."

h. Defusing.

_____ 9. Husband: "If you'd just slow down, you wouldn't make so many mistakes!"
Wife: "You are probably right. It probably would help if I slowed down some."

i. Delaying assertively.

_____ 10. Head nurse: "I need someone to stay on and work an extra shift."
Staff nurse: "I don't want to work an extra shift tonight."

j. Responding assertively with irony.

ROLE-PLAYING

Have students rate their behavior on the assertiveness evaluation tool presented in the text (Fig. 13–1). Instruct them to identify areas in which they could be more assertive. In small groups have them practice increasing their assertive skills by role playing situations that represent areas in which they rated themselves as nonassertive on the tool. This may also be accomplished in larger groups by asking the observers to critique the responses given during role playing.

CHAPTER 13. TEST QUESTIONS

1. Tracy, a new graduate from the local university, is beginning her first position on a medical-surgical unit where clients from the psychiatric unit often receive care. Which of the following best describes Tracy's use of assertive behavior?
    - a. Tracy attempts to please others and apologizes for her awkwardness in her new role.
    - b. Tracy frequently stands up for herself by defending her behavior to the nurse manager.
    - c. Tracy has some problems making decisions and has a tendency to procrastinate with her work.
    - • d. Tracy is open and direct with the nurse manager when asked to complete her assignments.

2. Tracy is working with a male client who is complaining about the attention he is receiving. She responds to him calmly and non-defensively, "You are very angry right now. I don't want to discuss this with you while you are so upset. I will be back in 1 hour to meet with you and we will talk about it then. "This is an example of which of the following assertive techniques?
    - • a. Defusing
    - b. Clouding/fogging
    - c. Responding as a broken record
    - d. Shifting from content to process

3. Tracy works with her clients to teach assertiveness and ways in which they can improve their communication. Which of the following nursing diagnoses is selected for clients needing assistance with assertiveness?
    - a. Impaired adjustment
    - b. Altered though process
    - • c. Defensive coping
    - d. Impaired verbal communication

4. The goal of assertive skills training is to:
    - a. Help clients explain themselves and their life-cycle events and assist them in resolving problems
    - b. Give reliable, expert information so that clients may correct faulty behaviors
    - c. Clarify misconceptions and misperceptions that have caused clients to distort reality
    - • d. Improve communication skills in an effort to improve interpersonal relationships

5. Tracy has worked 10 days straight when her nurse manager approaches her with a request to stay on the 3 to 11 shift and work a double shift. Which of the following represents a passive-aggressive response on Tracy's part?
    - a. "Get someone else to work 3 to 11! I've been working 10 days straight and I need a break!"
    - • b. "Okay. I'll do it." Then purposefully leaving tasks undone when she leaves the unit at 11 A.M.
    - c. "I have worked 10 days straight and I cannot work tonight. I will work for you tomorrow if you need me."
    - d. "Yes, I'll do it. Anything to keep peace with the staff is a good thing, I guess."

CHAPTER 14. PROMOTING SELF-ESTEEM

CHAPTER FOCUS

The focus of this chapter is on the developmental progression of self-esteem. Verbal and behavioral manifestations of self-esteem are described, and the concept of boundaries and its relationship to self-esteem is explored. Nursing care of clients with disturbances in self-esteem is described in the context of the nursing process.

LEARNING OBJECTIVES

After reading this chapter, the student will be able to:

1. Identify and define components of the self-concept.
2. Discuss influencing factors in the development of self-esteem and its progression through the life span.
3. Describe the verbal and nonverbal manifestations of low self-esteem.
4. Discuss the concept of boundaries and its relationship to self-esteem.
5. Apply the nursing process with clients who are experiencing disturbances in self-esteem.

KEY TERMS

self-concept	self-ideal
physical self	self-expectancy
body image	focal stimuli
personal self	contextual stimuli
personal identity	residual stimuli
self-esteem	boundaries
moral-ethical self	rigid boundaries
self-consistency	flexible boundaries
	enmeshed boundaries

CHAPTER OUTLINE/LECTURE NOTES

I. Introduction
   A. Healthy self-esteem has been described as essential for psychological survival.
   B. An awareness of self is an important differentiating factor between humans and other animals.
II. Components of Self-Concept
   A. Self-concept has been defined as the composite of beliefs and feelings that one holds about oneself at a given time, formed from perceptions particularly of others' reactions and from directing one's behavior.
   B. The self-concept consists of the following three components:
      1. The physical self or body image—a personal appraisal by an individual of his or her physical being and includes physical attributes, functioning, sexuality, wellness-illness state, and appearance
         a. Personal body image may not necessarily coincide with actual physical appearance.
         b. Disturbances in body image may occur when individuals undergo alterations in structure or function. These include conditions such as colostomy, paralysis, and impotence and may be perceived as losses.
      2. Personal identity consists of three parts:
         a. The moral-ethical self functions as observer, standard setter, dreamer, comparer, and most of all, evaluator of who the individual says he or she is.
         b. Self-consistency is striving to maintain a stable self-image, whether it is positive or negative.

        c.   Self-ideal/self-expectancy relates to an individual's perception of what he or she wants to be, to do, or to become.

     3.   Self-esteem—the degree of regard or respect that individuals have for themselves and is a measure of worth that they place on their abilities and judgments

III.   The Development of Self-Esteem

    A.   The following antecedent conditions of positive self-esteem have been identified by Coopersmith:

       1.   Power—a feeling of control over own life situation

       2.   Significance—a feeling of being loved, respected, and cared for by significant others

       3.   Virtue—knowledge that actions reflect a set of personal, moral, and ethical values

       4.   Competence—The ability to perform successfully or achieve self-expectations and the expectations of others

    B.   Warren lists the following as important for parents and others who work with children to emphasize and encourage healthy self-esteem:

       1.   A sense of competence—the feeling that they are skilled at something

       2.   Unconditional love— the knowledge that they are loved regardless of success or failure

       3.   A sense of survival—the ability to learn and grow from having experienced failure

       4.   Realistic goals—having expectations that are attainable by the child

       5.   A sense of responsibility—expectations to complete tasks that they perceive are valued by others

       6.   Reality orientation—achieving a healthy balance between what they can possess and achieve and what is beyond their capability or control

    C.   Driever cites the following factors as influential in the development of self-esteem:

       1.   The perceptions of responses by others, particularly significant others

       2.   Genetic factors

       3.   Environmental factors

IV.   Developmental Progression of the Self-Esteem Through the Life Span

    A.   Erikson's theory of personality development provides a useful framework for illustration of self-esteem development.

       1.   Trust versus mistrust. Achievement of trust results in positive self-esteem, whereas dissatisfaction with the self and suspiciousness of others promotes negative self-esteem.

       2.   Autonomy versus shame and doubt. Achievement of autonomy results in a feeling of self-confidence in one's ability to perform, whereas negative self-esteem is promoted by failure to achieve this task and a lack of pride in the ability to perform and a sense of being controlled by others.

       3.   Initiative versus guilt. Positive self-esteem is gained through initiative when creativity is encouraged and performance is recognized and positively reinforced. Guidance and discipline that relies heavily on shaming the child creates guilt and results in a decrease in self-esteem.

       4.   Industry versus inferiority. Positive self-esteem is gained at this stage by performing and receiving recognition from others. Negative self-esteem is the result of nonachievement or when accomplishments are met with negative feedback.

       5.   Identity versus role confusion. Positive self-esteem occurs when individuals are allowed to experience independence by making decisions that influence their lives. Failure to develop a new self-definition results in a sense of self-consciousness, doubt, and confusion about one's role in life.

       6.   Intimacy versus isolation. Positive self-esteem is promoted through the capacity for giving of oneself to another. When one has been deprived of unconditional love in the younger years, he or she has difficulty with this task, and social isolation occurs.

       7.   Generativity versus stagnation. Generativity promotes positive self-esteem through gratification from personal and professional achievements and from meaningful contributions to others. When previous tasks to unfulfilled, the individual lacks self-worth and becomes withdrawn and isolated.

       8.   Ego integrity versus despair. Ego integrity results in a sense of self-worth and self-acceptance as one reviews life goals, accepting that some were achieved and some were not. When earlier developmental tasks of self-confidence, self-identity, and concern for others remain unfulfilled, a sense of despair and negative self-esteem prevail.

V.   The Manifestation of Low Self-Esteem

    A.   Behaviors that reflect low self-esteem manifest themselves according to three types of stimuli:

1. Focal stimuli—the immediate concern that is causing the threat to self-esteem and the stimulus that is engendering the current behavior
2. Contextual stimuli—all of the other stimuli present in the person's environment that contribute to the behavior being caused by the focal stimulus
3. Residual stimuli—factors that may influence one's maladaptive behavior in response to focal and contextual stimuli
   B. Symptoms of low self-esteem are many, and are listed in Table 14–2 of the text.

VI. Boundaries
   A. Boundaries are the personal space, both physical and psychological, that individuals identify as their own.
   B. Sometimes they are referred to as "limits."
   C. Individuals who are aware of their boundaries have a healthy self-esteem because they must know and accept their inner selves.
   D. Types of physical boundaries include physical closeness, touching, sexual behavior, eye contact, privacy, and pollution. Touching someone who does not want to be touched is an example of an invasion of a physical boundary.
   E. Types of psychological boundaries include beliefs, feelings, choices, needs, time alone, interests, confidences, individual differences, and spirituality. Being criticized for doing something differently than others is an example of an invasion of a psychological boundary.
   F. Boundary pliancy
      1. Boundaries can be rigid, flexible, or enmeshed.
         a. Rigid boundaries—occur when people having a very narrow perspective on life. They perceive that things must be one way and refuse to change for any reason.
         b. Flexible boundaries—occur when people are able to let go of their boundaries when appropriate. Healthy boundaries are flexible.
         c. Enmeshed boundaries—occur when two people's boundaries are so blended together that neither can be sure where one stops and the other begins. An individual with an enmeshed boundary is unable to differentiate his or her wants and needs from the other person's.
   G. Establishing boundaries
      1. Boundaries are established in childhood.
      2. Unhealthy boundaries are the products of unhealthy, troubled, or dysfunctional families.
         a. Negative role modeling
         b. Abuse or neglect

VII. The Nursing Process
   A. Assessment
      1. The Self-Esteem Inventory
   B. Diagnosis/outcome identification
      1. Self-esteem disturbance
      2. Chronic low self-esteem
      3. Situational low self-esteem
      4. Outcome criteria
   C. Planning/implementation
   D. Evaluation

VIII. Summary
IX. Review Questions

LEARNING ACTIVITY

Have students fill out this form. Emphasize the importance of complete honesty. The content is intended for discussion in small groups (no more than 4 to 6 students), and preferably with the instructor as group leader. This may be used as alternative clinical time, and groups may want to meet more than once. Students should be encouraged (but not required) to share.

SELF-CONCEPT
How I Was . . . How I Am . . . How I Want To Be

My earliest memory of being praised is

_____

My earliest memory of being criticized is

_____

My favorite relationship in my childhood was with

_____

I remember that when I was with this person, I felt

_____

As a teenager, I felt good about myself when

_____

As a teenager, I felt disappointed with myself when

_____

As a teenager, I liked being with _____ because _____

_____

What I like most about myself now is

_____

What I like least about myself now is

_____

When I am alone, I feel

_____

I get angry when

_____

I am happiest when

_____

If my relationship with _____ were to end, _____

_____

The one thing I most want to accomplish is

_____

If I could change one thing about myself, it would be

_____

CHAPTER 14. TEST QUESTIONS

Situation: Allen is a 37-year-old man who has never married and has remained at home with his aging mother. He has not worked since he had a paper route as a teenager so that he can remain at home to care for his mother. She gives him a weekly allowance out of an estate left to her by her late husband, who died when Allen was age 15. A community health nurse visits the family once a month to administer Vitamin B$_{12}$ injections to the mother.

1. On one of these visits, Allen confides to the nurse that he is terrified of what will happen to him should his mother die. The nurse recognizes that Allen has low self-esteem related to failure at which of Erikson's developmental tasks?
    a. Trust versus mistrust
    b. Initiative versus guilt
    • c. Identity versus role confusion
    d. Ego integrity versus despair

2. The community health nurse notices that Allen demonstrates certain behaviors consistent with low self-esteem. Which of the following behaviors is Allen *not* likely to exhibit?
    a. Hostility
    • b. Meticulous grooming
    c. Rumination about his situation
    d. Complaints of various aches and pains

3. What kind of boundaries does Allen appear to have relative to his mother?
    a. Loose
    b. Rigid
    c. Flexible
    • d. Enmeshed

4. Although Allen's mother is the community health nurse's primary client, she identifies Allen's need for intervention regarding his low self-esteem. The nursing diagnosis she selects from which to identify goals and interventions is:
    a. Self-esteem disturbance
    • b. Chronic low self-esteem
    c. Situational low self-esteem
    d. Social isolation

5. The community health nurse talks with Allen about his situation over the next several months, and he finally agrees to see a psychotherapist. After several more months, the nurse notices some changes in Allen's behavior. Which of the following behaviors *most clearly* indicates improvement in Allen's self-esteem?
    a. He decides to save his money to buy a dog.
    b. He asks his mother for permission to buy a dog.
    • c. He tells his mother he plans to buy a dog.
    d. He buys a dog and hides it in the garage.

CHAPTER 15. ANGER/AGGRESSION MANAGEMENT

CHAPTER FOCUS

The focus of this chapter is on the concepts of anger and aggression. Predisposing factors to the maladaptive expression of anger are discussed, and the nursing process as a vehicle for delivery of care to assist clients in the management of anger and aggression is described.

LEARNING OBJECTIVES

After reading this chapter, the student will be able to:

1. Define and differentiate between *anger* and *aggression*.
2. Identify when the expression of anger becomes a problem.
3. Discuss predisposing factors to the maladaptive expression of anger.
4. Apply the nursing process to clients and psychological responses to anger.
   a. Assessment: Describe physical and psychological responses to anger.
   b. Diagnosis/Outcome Identification: Formulate nursing diagnoses and outcome criteria for clients expressing anger and aggression.
   c. Planning/Intervention: Describe nursing interventions for clients demonstrating maladaptive expressions of anger.
   d. Evaluation: Evaluate achievement of the projected outcomes in the intervention with clients demonstrating maladaptive expression of anger.

KEY TERMS

anger
aggression
modeling
operant conditioning
preassaultive tension state

CHAPTER OUTLINE/LECTURE NOTES

I. Introduction
   A. Anger need not be a negative expression.
   B. Anger is a normal human emotion that, when handled appropriately and expressed assertively, can provide an individual with a positive force to solve problems and make decisions concerning life situations.
   C. Anger becomes a problem when it is not expressed and when it is expressed aggressively.
II. Anger and Aggression, Defined
   A. Anger.
      1. Anger is the emotional response to one's perception of a situation. Anger is:
         a. Not a primary emotion
         b. Typically experienced as an automatic inner response to hurt, frustration, or fear
         c. A physiological arousal mechanism, instilling feelings of power and generating preparedness
         d. Significantly different from aggression
         e. Learned
         f. Capable of being under personal control

2. Anger has both positive and negative functions (see Table 156–1 in text).
 B. Aggression.
    1. Aggression is one way that individuals express anger.
    1. Aggression is a behavior that is intended to threaten or injure the victim's security or self-esteem.
    2. Aggression can cause damage with words, fists, or weapons, but it is virtually always designed to inflict punishment or pain.
III. Predisposing Factors to Anger and Aggression
 A. Modeling
    1. Role modeling is one of the strongest forms of learning.
    2. Role models can be positive or negative.
    3. Earliest role models are the primary caregivers.
    4. As the child matures, role models can be celebrities or any other influential individual in the child's life.
 B. Operant conditioning.
    1. Operant conditioning occurs when a specific behavior is positively or negatively reinforced.
       a. A positive reinforcement is a response to the specific behavior that is pleasurable or produces the desired results.
       b. A negative reinforcement is à response to the specific behavior that prevents an undesirable result from occurring.
    2. Anger and aggression can be learned through operant conditioning.
 C. Neurophysiological disorders.
    1. Several disorders of or conditions within the brain have been implicated in episodic aggression and violent behavior. They include:
       a. Temporal lobe epilepsy
       b. Brain tumors
       c. Brain trauma
       d. Encephalitis
 D. Biochemical factors.
    1. Aggressive behavior may have some correlation to alterations in brain chemicals. These include:
       a. Hormonal dysfunction associated with hyperthyroidism.
       b. Alterations in the neurotransmitters epinephrine, norepinephrine, dopamine, acetylcholine, and serotonin. These chemicals may play a role in either the facilitation or inhibition of aggression.
 E. Socioeconomic factors
    1. High rates of violence exist within the subculture of poverty in the United States.
    2. Poverty is thought to encourage aggression because of the associated deprivation, disruption of families, and unemployment.
 F. Environmental factors
    1. Several environmental factors have been associated with an increase in aggressive behavior. They include:
       a. Physical crowing of people
       b. Discomfort associated with a moderate increase in environmental temperature
       c. Use of alcohol and some other drugs, particularly cocaine, amphetamines, hallucinogens, and minor tranquilizers/sedatives
       d. Availability of firearms
IV. The Nursing Process
 A. Assessment
    1. Anger can be identified by a cluster of characteristics that include:

a. Intense distress	g. Increased energy
b. Frowning	h. Fatigue
c. Gritting teeth	i. Withdrawal
d. Pacing	j. Flushed face
e. Eyebrow displacement	k. Emotional overcontrol
f. Clenched fists	l. Change in voice tone

    2. Aggression can be identified by a cluster of characteristics that include:

a. Sarcasm
b. Verbal/physical threats
c. Change in voice tone
d. Degrading comments
e. Pacing
f. Throwing objects
g. Striking objects/people
h. Suspiciousness

i. Homicidal ideation
j. Self-mutilation
k. Invasion of personal space
l. Increased agitation
m. Disturbed thought process/perception
n. Misinterpretation of stimuli
o. Exaggerated anger
p. Suicidal ideation

    3. Assessing risk factors
       a. Prevention is the key issue in the management of aggressive or violent behavior.
       b. Three factors are important considerations in identifying degree of risk:
          (1) Past history of violence is considered the most widely recognized risk factor for violence in a treatment setting.
          (2) Client diagnosis. The most common diagnoses associated with violence include:
             (a) Substance abuse/intoxication
             (b) Schizophrenia
             (c) Posttraumatic stress disorder
             (d) Organic brain disorders
             (e) Epilepsy
             (f) Temporal lobe abnormalities
       c. Certain behaviors are predictive of impending violence and have been termed the "preassaultive tension state." They include:
          (1) Agitation and pacing
          (2) Pounding and slamming
          (3) Tense posture
          (4) Grim, defiant affect
          (5) Clenched teeth and fists
          (6) Arguing and demanding
          (7) Talking in rapid, raised voice
          (8) Challenging and threatening staff
B. Diagnosis/outcome identification
    1. Nursing diagnoses for inappropriate expression of anger or for aggressive behavior include:
       a. Ineffective individual coping
       b. Risk for violence, self-directed or directed at others
    2. Outcome behaviors are identified as criteria for evaluation.
C. Planning/implementation
D. Evaluation
V. Summary
VI. Review Questions

LEARNING ACTIVITY

Have students:

1. Write about a time that they can remember when anger was a positive response for them.
2. Write about a time that they can remember when anger turned out to be a maladaptive or destructive response. What would have been a more adaptive response?

These papers may be discussed in group situations; however, students should not be *required* to share their personal experiences with others.

CHAPTER 15. TEST QUESTIONS

1. Anna is the charge nurse on a psychiatric unit in a large, inner city hospital. She carefully reviews clients' histories when making assignments so that the most experienced staff are assigned to clients who may become violent. Which of the following risk factors does Anna recognize as the *most* reliable indicator for a client becoming violent?
    a. Diagnosis of schizophrenia
    •   b. Past history of violence
    c. Family history of violence
    d. Tense posture and agitation

2. John, who has a diagnosis of paranoid schizophrenia, is admitted to Anna's unit after attempting to injure his father with a butcher knife. The nurse who writes John's care plan gives him the priority nursing diagnosis of Risk for violence toward others. Which of the following is the priority goal for John during his hospitalization?
    a. The client will not verbalize anger or hit anyone.
    b. The client will verbalize anger rather than hit others.
    •   c. The client will not harm self or others.
    d. The client will be restrained if he becomes verbally or physically abusive.

3. Because of the frequency with which they deal with violent clients, staff on this unit has a violence intervention protocol. Which of the following interventions would be *contraindicated* as part of such a protocol?
    a. Administration of psychotropic medication
    •   b. Soothing the client by stroking an arm or shoulder
    c. Application of leather restraints
    d. Observation for symptoms of the preassaultive tension state

4. John begins to lose control of his anger and the nurse decides intervention must occur. John cannot be "talked down," and he refuses medication. The nurse should then:
    •   a. Call for assistance from the assault team
    b. Ask the ward clerk to put in a call for the physician
    c. Make John go to his room
    d. Tell John if he doesn't calm down, he will be placed in restraints

5. John is placed in restraints, after which the nurse administers the as-needed neuroleptic medication that the client had previously refused. Which of the following statements is *true* regarding this intervention?
    a. The physician must leave a standing order for this intervention to be appropriate.
    b. The nurse who intervenes in this manner is setting himself or herself up for a lawsuit, because the client always has a right to refuse medication.
    c. The physician must write an order to cover the nurse's actions after the intervention has taken place.
    •   d. Most states consider this intervention appropriate in emergency situations or if a client would likely harm self or others.

CHAPTER 16. THE SUICIDAL CLIENT

CHAPTER FOCUS

The focus of this chapter is on the care of the suicidal client. Epidemiological and etiologic aspects of suicide are also explored.

LEARNING OBJECTIVES

After reading this chapter, the student will be able to:

1. Discuss epidemiological statistics and risk factors related to suicide.
2. Describe predisposing factors implicated in the etiology of suicide.
3. Differentiate between facts and fables regarding suicide.
4. Apply the nursing process to individuals exhibiting suicidal behavior.

KEY TERMS

egoistic suicide
altruistic suicide
anomic suicide

CHAPTER OUTLINE/LECTURE NOTES

I.   Introduction
   A. Suicide is not a diagnosis or a disorder; it is a behavior.
   b. More than 90 percent of suicides are by individuals who are psychiatrically ill at the time of the suicide.
II. Epidemiological factors
   A. Approximately 30,000 persons in the United States end their lives each year by suicide.
   B. Suicide is the ninth leading cause of death among adults and the third leading cause of death among adolescents.
III. Risk factors
   A. Marital status
      1. The suicide rate for single persons is twice that of married persons.
   B. Gender
      1. Women attempt suicide more, but more men succeed.
      2. Men commonly choose more lethal methods than women.
   C. Age
      1. Risk of suicide increases with age, particularly so with men.
      2. Suicide is the third leading cause of death (following motor vehicle accidents and homicides) among the 15- to 24-year-old age group.
   D. Religion
      1. Protestants have significantly higher rates of suicide than Catholics or Jews.
   E. Socioeconomic status
      1. Individuals in the very highest and lowest social classes have higher suicide rates than those in the middle classes.
   F. Ethnicity
      1. Whites are at higher risk for suicide, followed by Native-Americans, African-Americans, Hispanic-Americans, and Asian Americans.

G. Other risk factors
  1. Psychiatric illness
     a. Mood disorders are the most common psychiatric illnesses that precede suicide. Other psychiatric disorders that account for suicidal behavior include substance-related disorders, schizophrenia, organic brain disorders, personality disorders, and panic disorders.
  2. Severe insomnia is associated with increased risk of suicide.
  3. Homosexual individuals, especially if depressed, aging, or alcoholic, have a high risk of suicide.
  4. Affliction with a chronic painful or disabling illness increases the risk of suicide.
  5. Family history of suicide, particularly a same-sex parent, increases the risk of suicide.
  6. Having attempted suicide previously increases the risk of a subsequent attempt. Fifty to 80 percent of those who ultimately commit suicide have a history of a previous attempt.
  7. Loss of a loved one through death or separation is a risk factor.
  8. Lack of employment or increased financial burden increases the risk of suicide.
IV. Predisposing Factors: Theories of Suicide
  A. Psychological theories
     1. Anger turned inward. Freud believed that suicide was a result of an earlier repressed desire to kill someone else. Anger that was previously directed to another person is turned inward on the self.
     2. Hopelessness. Studies indicate a high correlation between feelings of hopelessness and suicide.
     3. Desperation and guilt. Desperate feelings occur when an individual feels the need for change but feels helpless to bring about that change. Guilt and self-recrimination are other aspects of desperation.
     4. History of aggression and violence. Rage and violent behavior have been identified as important psychological factors underlying suicidal behavior.
     5. Shame and humiliation. Some individuals view suicide as a "face-saving" mechanism, following a social defeat such as a sudden loss of status or income.
     6. Developmental stressors. Certain life stressors that occur during various developmental levels have been identified as precipitating factors to suicide.
  B. Sociological theory
     1. Durkheim believed that suicide was correlated to the cohesiveness of a society in which the individual lived. He described three social categories of suicide:
        a. Egoistic suicide—the response of the individual who felt separate and apart from the mainstream of society. Integration was lacking.
        b. Altruistic suicide—the opposite of egoistic suicide. The individual is excessively integrated into the group, and allegiance to the group is governed by cultural, religious, or political ties.
        c. Anomic suicide—the response to changes in the individual's life that disrupt feelings of relatedness to the group. The interruption in the customary norms of behavior instills feelings of "separateness," and fears of being without support from the formerly cohesive group.
  C. Biological theories
     1. Genetics. Twin studies have indicated a possible genetic predisposition toward suicidal behavior.
     2. Neurochemical factors. Some studies have revealed decreased levels of serotonin (measured by decreased levels of S-HIAA in cerebrospinal fluid) in depressed clients who attempted suicide.
V. Application of the Nursing Process with the Suicidal Client
  A. Assessment
     1. The aspects of information that are gathered during a suicidal assessment include:
        a. Demographics
           (1) Age
           (2) Gender
           (3) Ethnicity
           (4) Marital status
           (5) Socioeconomic status
           (6) Occupation
           (7) Lethality and availability of method
           (8) Religion
           (9) Family history of suicide

  b. Presenting symptoms/medical-psychiatric illness
  c. Suicidal ideas or acts
    (1) Seriousness of intent
    (2) Plan
    (3) Means
    (4) Verbal or behavioral clues
  d. Interpersonal support system
  e. Analysis of the suicidal crisis
    (1) The precipitating stressor
    (2) Relevant history
    (3) Life-stage issues
  f. Psychiatric/medical/family history
  g. Coping strategies
 B. Diagnosis/outcome identification
  1. Nursing diagnoses for the suicidal client may include the following:
   a. Risk for self-directed violence
   b. Hopelessness
 C. Planning/Implementation
  1. Establish a therapeutic relationship.
  2. Communicate the potential for suicide to team members.
  3. Stay with the person.
  4. Accept the person.
  5. Listen to the person.
  6. Secure a no-suicide contract.
  7. Give the person a message of hope.
  8. Give the person something to do.
 D. Evaluation
VI. Summary
VII. Review Questions

LEARNING ACTIVITY

FACTS AND FABLES ABOUT SUICIDE

Indicate with a T or F whether each of the following statements is true or false.

_____ 1. Suicide is an inherited trait.

_____ 2. Gunshot wounds are the leading cause of death among suicide victims.

_____ 3. Most people give clues and warnings about their suicidal intentions.

_____ 4. If a person has attempted suicide, he or she will not do it again.

_____ 5. Suicide is the act of a psychotic person.

_____ 6. Once a person is suicidal, he or she is suicidal forever.

_____ 7. Most suicides occur when the severe depression has started to improve.

_____ 8. Most suicidal people have ambivalent feelings about living and dying.

_____ 9. If a suicidal person is intent upon dying, he or she cannot be stopped.

_____ 10. People who talk about suicide do not commit suicide.

CHAPTER 16. TEST QUESTIONS

Situation: Edward is a 67-year-old white lawyer who has been diagnosed with major depression. He was widowed 3 years ago, and has had no interest in attending synagogue services since that time. He has taken fluoxetine (Prozac) for several years. He made a suicide attempt 45 years ago during his first year in law school. He has been transported to the emergency department by ambulance after telling his son he was thinking of swallowing his whole bottle of fluoxetine.

1. How many risk factors for suicide will the triage nurse document?
   - a. Three
   - b. Five
   - • c. Seven
   - d. Nine

2. Edward is admitted to the psychiatric unit. The nurse initiates suicidal precautions for Edward. She understands that which of the following statements regarding suicide is correct?
   - • a. The more specific the plan, the more likely the client will attempt suicide.
   - b. Clients who talk about suicide never actually commit it.
   - c. The client who fails to complete a suicide attempt will not try again.
   - d. The nurse should refrain from actually saying the word "suicide," because this may give the client ideas.

3. In creating the care plan for Edward, which of the following would be the *priority* nursing diagnosis?
   - a. Risk for self-mutilation related to low self-esteem
   - • b. Risk for self-directed violence related to depressed mood.
   - c. Dysfunctional grieving related to loss of wife
   - d. Powerlessness related to dysfunctional grieving process

4. What is the *most* immediate outcome criterion for Edward?
   - • a. The client will not physically harm himself.
   - b. The client will express hope for the future.
   - c. The client will reveal his suicide plan.
   - d. The client will establish a trusting relationship with the nurse.

5. Which of the following interventions is *not* consistent with the established outcome criteria for Edward?
   - a. Accept Edward with unconditional positive regard.
   - b. Encourage Edward to talk about his pain.
   - c. Provide Edward with tasks to occupy him.
   - • d. Provide Edward with ample privacy.

6. Edward says to the nurse, "There's nothing to live for anymore." What is the nurse's most therapeutic response?
   - a. "Now Edward, you know that isn't true."
   - b. "In your situation, I might feel the same way."
   - c. "Things will look better in the morning."
   - • d. "It sounds like you are feeling pretty hopeless."

CHAPTER 17. BEHAVIOR THERAPY

CHAPTER FOCUS

The focus of this chapter is on various concepts associated with learning and on techniques for modification of learned behaviors. The role of the nurse in behavior therapy is emphasized.

LEARNING OBJECTIVES

After reading this chapter, the student will be able to:

1. Discuss the principles of classical and operant conditioning as foundations for behavior therapy.
2. Identify various techniques used in the modification of client behavior.
3. Implement the principles of behavior therapy using the steps of the nursing process.

KEY TERMS

classical conditioning	shaping
unconditioned response	modeling
conditioned response	Premack principle
unconditioned stimulus	extinction
conditioned stimulus	flooding
stimulus generalization	token economy
operant conditioning	time-out
positive reinforcement	reciprocal inhibition
negative reinforcement	overt sensitization
aversive stimulus	covert sensitization
discriminative stimulus	systematic desensitization
contingency contracting	

CHAPTER OUTLINE/LECTURE NOTES

I   Introduction
    A. A behavior is considered to be maladaptive when it:
        1. is age-inappropriate
        2. interferes with adaptive functioning
        3. is misunderstood by others in terms of cultural inappropriateness
    B. The behavioral approach to therapy is that people have become what they are through learning processes, or through the interaction of the environment with their genetic endowment.
    C. The basic assumption is that problematic behaviors occur when there has been inadequate learning and, therefore, can be corrected through the provision of appropriate learning experiences.

II.   Classical Conditioning
    A. Concept was introduced by Russian physiologist Pavlov in his experiments with dogs
    B. Pavlov related that the dogs salivated when presented with food (unconditioned response).
    C. He soon learned that dogs salivated when food came into view (conditioned response).
    D. He introduced an unrelated stimulus (the sound of a bell) with presentation of food.
    E. He learned that the dogs soon began salivating (conditioned response) at the sound of the bell alone (conditioned stimulus).
    F. When a similar response is elicited from similar stimuli, it is called stimulus generalization.

III. Operant Conditioning
   A. Concept was introduced by American psychologist B.F. Skinner.
   B. Basic assumption: that the connection between a stimulus and a response is strengthened or weakened by the consequences of the response.
   C. A stimulus that follows a behavior (or response) is called a reinforcer.
   D. When the reinforcing stimulus increases the probability that the behavior will recur, it is called a positive reinforcer.
   E. When the reinforcing stimulus increases the probability that a behavior will recur by removal of an undesirable reinforcing stimulus, it is called a negative reinforcer.
   F. A stimulus that follows a behavioral response and decreases the probability that the behavior will recur is called an aversive stimulus or punisher.
IV. Techniques for Modifying Client Behavior
   A. Shaping. In shaping the behavior of another, reinforcements are given for increasingly closer approximations to the desired response.
   B. Modeling. Modeling refers to the learning of new behaviors by imitating the behavior of others.
   C. Premack principle. This principle states that a frequently occurring response can serve as a positive reinforcement for a response.
   D. Extinction. The gradual decrease in frequency or disappearance of a response when the positive reinforcement is withheld.
   E. Contingency contracting. A contract for behavioral change is developed. Positive and negative reinforcers for performing the desired behaviors, as well as aversive reinforcers for failure to perform, are stated explicitly in the contract.
   F. Token economy. A type of contingency contracting in which the reinforcers for desired behaviors are presented in the form of tokens. The tokens may then be exchanged for designated privileges.
   G. Time-out. An aversive stimulus or punishment during which the client is removed from the environment where the unacceptable behavior is being exhibited. The client is usually isolated so that reinforcement from the attention of others is absent.
   H. Reciprocal inhibition. Also called counterconditioning, this technique serves to decrease or eliminate a behavior by introducing a more adaptive behavior, but one that is incompatible with the unacceptable behavior.
   I. Overt sensitization. An aversion therapy that produces unpleasant consequences for undesirable behavior.
   J. Covert sensitization. This aversion technique relies on the individual's imagination to produce unpleasant symptoms as consequences for undesirable behavior.
   K. Systematic desensitization. A technique to assist an individual to overcome fear of a phobic stimulus. A systematic hierarchy of events associated with the phobic stimulus is used to gradually desensitize the individual.
   L. Flooding. Sometimes called implosive therapy, a technique used to desensitize an individual to a phobic stimulus. It differs from systematic desensitization in that, instead of working through a hierarchy of anxiety-producing stimuli, the individual is "flooded" with a continuous presentation of the phobic stimulus until it no longer elicits anxiety.
V. Role of the Nurse in Behavior Therapy
   A. The nursing process is the vehicle for delivery of nursing care with clients requiring assistance with behavior modification.
   B. Assessment of behaviors that are unacceptable for age and cultural inappropriateness is conducted.
   C. Nursing diagnoses are formulated and outcome criteria are established.
   D. A plan for behavior modification is devised using techniques thought to be most appropriate for the client. The plan may be devised by the nurse alone, the physician alone, the nurse and physician together, or with input from the client and various members of the treatment team.
   E. All members of the treatment team must be made aware of the behavior modification plan. Consistency among all staff is required for implementation to be successful.
   F. Evaluation of care is based upon achievement of the outcome criteria.
VI. Summary
VII. Review Questions

LEARNING ACTIVITY

TECHNIQUES FOR MODIFYING CLIENT BEHAVIOR

Match the techniques listed on the left to the situations described on the right.

_____ 1. Shaping

a. John had tried many times without success to stop drinking. His physician has suggested trying disulfiram therapy, and John has agreed.

_____ 2. Modeling

b. Two-year-old Missy has had temper tantrums for 6 months. They have become progressively worse, because her Mother always gives in and lets Missy have what she wants to end the tantrum. The therapist suggested that Mom turn and walk away when a tantrum occurs.

_____ 3. Premack principle

c. The therapist is trying to teach 3-year-old Billy to use sign language. She rewards him when he watches her sign; then rewards him when he attempts to sign himself; and finally rewards him only when he signs correctly.

_____ 4. Extinction

d. Nancy has a phobia of flying. The therapist asks Nancy to imagine, as she is confronted with a continuous presentation of stimuli associated with flying, until she no longer feels anxious by the images elicited.

_____ 5. Contingency contracting

e. Eleven-year-old Timmy likes to bully the younger kids. He refuses to do anything his parents ask and talks back to the teachers when they give him direction. The therapist outlines for Timmy which behaviors are acceptable and which are not. She explains to Timmy that he will receive a "chip" each time he behaves appropriately, and he may use the chips to buy certain privileges.

_____ 6. Token Economy

f. Ten-year-old Sonja begged her Mother to let her take piano lessons. Her Mother agreed, but now Sonja wants to watch TV all the time instead of practicing her piano lesson. Her Mother tells Sonja she can only watch TV after she has practiced her piano lesson.

_____ 7. Time-out

g. Thirteen-year-old Lisa is a client on the adolescent psychiatric unit. Each time she is with a group of her peers she begins using offensive, vulgar language. Her peers provide positive reinforcement by laughing at her. The therapist tells Lisa that each time this occurs she will spend time alone in the isolation room.

_____ 8. Reciprocal inhibition

h. Janet, age 25, has been obese since childhood. The therapist is helping Janet in her effort to lose weight. The therapist teaches Janet to visualize in her mind foods that are offensive to her and that make her feel nauseated. Each time Janet is tempted to eat more than her reducing diet allows, she is to conjure up this image in her mind.

_____ 9. Overt sensitization

i. Angie has been in trouble with her parents and school authorities for inappropriate behavior. Angie strongly admires her Aunt Sylvia, her mother's sister, who is a successful newspaper reporter in a nearby city. Angie is sent to live with her aunt in hopes that she will imitate her cherished aunt's behavior and lifestyle.

_____ 10. Covert sensitization

j. Sixteen-year-old Andy loses his temper at the slightest provocation on the adolescent psychiatric unit. The therapist draws up a written contract with Andy. Rewards for managing his anger are explicitly stated, as are punishments for losing his temper.

_____ 11. Systematic desensitization

k. Sandy experiences test anxiety. She becomes overwhelmed with anxiety each time she is faced with an examination. The therapist teaches Sandy to perform relaxation exercises before, and sometimes even during an exam when she feels anxiety escalating.

_____ 12. Flooding

l. Barbara has an extreme fear of dogs. She panics when she sees one. The therapist attempts to help Barbara overcome her fear by exposing her to a step-by-step process in which she gradually is able to look at a dog, touch one, and be in the presence of one without experiencing panic anxiety.

CHAPTER 17. TEST QUESTIONS

1. Gloria, a single mother, has been attending parenting classes with her 9-year-old son Phil. She wants him to begin doing some chores, and asks him to clean his room. When she checks on him, she discovers he has picked up everything on the floor and tossed it on a chair. She says, "You've done a nice job of picking up things off the floor." This is consistent with which technique of behavior modification?
   - a. Shaping
   - b. Modeling
   - c. Contracting
   - d. Premack Principle

2. Gloria responds to an advertisement in the local newspaper soliciting subjects for a research program to investigate effective ways to stop smoking. She is told that she will be assigned to a group that will use a reciprocal inhibition technique. Which of the following exercises is based on reciprocal inhibition?
   - a. Before she can smoke, she must first take a half-hour walk.
   - b. When she has the urge to smoke, she is to imagine herself as short of breath.
   - c. She will be paid $1 for each cigarette she does not smoke, and must forfeit $2 for each cigarette that she does smoke.
   - d. When she has the urge to smoke, she must first hold her breath to a count of 30, then perform a rhythmic breathing exercise to a count of 100.

3. Claudia has been seeing a psychotherapist for treatment of a phobia for spiders. Her therapist has begun a program of systematic desensitization. Which of the following interventions would *not* be a part of this behavior modification technique?
   - a. Breathing exercises
   - b. One-hour audiotape describing being in a room full of spiders
   - c. A visit to an insect zoo with the psychotherapist
   - d. Self-paced computer program presenting progressively more anxiety-producing scenarios regarding spiders

4. The correct answer in question 3 describes which behavior modification technique?
   - a. Flooding
   - b. Shaping
   - c. Extinction
   - d. Reciprocal inhibition

5. Tony is a 20-year-old man with a history of suicide attempts of low-to-moderate lethality. He has been seeing Norman, a nurse psychotherapist, for 4 years. Late one Friday evening, Norman receives a telephone call from Tony, who informs Norman that he has ingested half a bottle of aspirin. Norman advises Tony to call 911 for emergency assistance and says that he (Norman) will be available to reschedule a psychotherapy appointment when Tony has recovered. What is the explanation for Norman's behavior?
   - a. Norman is using an aversive stimulus in response to Tony's suicide attempt.
   - b. Norman is using a negative reinforcement in response to Tony's suicide attempt.
   - c. Norman is minimizing reinforcement of Tony's suicidal behavior with the goal of extinction.
   - d. Norman lacks empathy for Tony's recurring suicidal behavior.

CHAPTER 18. COGNITIVE THERAPY

CHAPTER FOCUS

The focus of this chapter is to introduce the student to the concepts of cognitive therapy. Various techniques of therapy are discussed, and the role of the nurse in cognitive therapy is highlighted.

LEARNING OBJECTIVES

After reading this chapter, the student will be able to:

1. Discuss historical perspectives associated with cognitive therapy.
2. Identify various indications for cognitive therapy.
3. Describe goals, principles, and basic concepts of cognitive therapy.
4. Discuss a variety of cognitive therapy techniques.
5. Apply techniques of cognitive therapy within the context of the nursing process.

KEY TERMS

automatic thoughts
arbitrary inference
overgeneralization
dichotomous thinking
selective abstraction
magnification
minimization
catastrophic thinking
personalization
schemas
Socratic questioning
distraction
decastastrophizing

CHAPTER OUTLINE/LECTURE NOTES

I.   Introduction
     A. The foundation upon which cognitive therapy is established can be identified by the statement, "Men are disturbed not by things, but by the views which they take of them."
II. Historical Background
     A. Cognitive therapy has its roots in the early 1960s research on depression conducted by Aaron Beck.
     B. Beck's concepts have been expanded to include active, direct dialogues with clients and behavioral techniques such as reinforcement and modeling.
     C. Lazarus' concept of personal appraisal of an event by an individual has also contributed to the cognitive therapy approach.
     D. Cognitive therapy is aimed at modifying distorted cognitions about a situation.
III. Indications for Cognitive Therapy
     A. Cognitive therapy was originally developed for use with depression.
     B. Today, it is also used with panic disorder, generalized anxiety disorder, social phobias, obsessive-compulsive disorder, posttraumatic stress disorder, eating disorders, substance abuse, personality

disorders, schizophrenia, couples' problems, bipolar disorder, hypochondriasis, and somatoform disorder.

IV. Goals and Principles of Therapy

    A. The goal of cognitive therapy is for the client to learn to identify and alter the dysfunctional beliefs that predispose him or her to distort experiences.

    B. Cognitive therapy is highly structured and short term, lasting from 12 to 16 weeks.

    C. The following principles underlie cognitive therapy for all clients:

        1. Cognitive therapy is based on an ever-evolving formulation of the client and his or her problems in cognitive terms.

        2. Cognitive therapy requires a sound therapeutic alliance.

        3. Cognitive therapy emphasizes collaboration and active participation.

        4. Cognitive therapy is goal oriented and problem focused.

        5. Cognitive therapy initially emphasizes the present.

        6. Cognitive therapy is educative, aims to teach the client to be his or her own therapist, and emphasizes relapse prevention.

        7. Cognitive therapy aims to be time limited.

        8. Cognitive therapy sessions are structured.

        9. Cognitive therapy teaches clients to identify, evaluate, and respond to their dysfunctional thoughts and beliefs.

        10. Cognitive therapy uses a variety of techniques to change thinking, mood, and behavior.

    D. Basic concepts. The general thrust of cognitive therapy is that emotional responses are largely dependent on cognitive appraisals of the significance of environmental cues. Basic concepts include:

        1. Automatic thoughts. Thoughts that occur rapidly in response to a situation, and without rational analysis. Sometimes called cognitive errors. Examples include:

            a. Arbitrary inference. In this type of error, the individual automatically comes to a conclusion about an incident without the facts to support it, or even sometimes despite contradictory evidence to support it.

            b. Overgeneralization (absolutistic thinking). Sweeping conclusions are made based on one incident—a type of "all-or-nothing" thinking.

            c. Dichotomous thinking. Situations are viewed in all-or-nothing, black-or-white, good-or-bad terms.

            d. Selective abstraction (sometimes referred to as mental filter). A conclusion is drawn based only on only a selected portion of the evidence.

            e. Magnification. Exaggerating the negative significance of an event.

            f. Minimization. Undervaluing the positive significance of an event.

            g. Catastrophic thinking. Always thinking that the worst will occur without considering the possibility of more likely, positive outcomes.

            h. Personalization. Taking complete responsibility for situations without considering that other circumstances may have contributed to the outcome.

        2. Schemas (core beliefs). Cognitive structures that consist of the individual's fundamental beliefs and assumptions, which develop early in life from personal experiences and identification with significant others. These concepts are reinforced by further learning experiences and, in turn, influence the formation of other beliefs, values, and attitudes. Schemas may be adaptive or maladaptive, general or specific, and positive or negative.

V. Techniques of Therapy

    A. Didactic (educational) aspects

        1. Client must be prepared to become own therapist.

        2. Therapist provides information about cognitive therapy and provides assignments to reinforce learning.

        3. A full explanation about correlation between distorted thinking and the client's mental illness is provided.

    B. Cognitive techniques

        1. Recognizing automatic thoughts

   a. Socratic questioning (also called guided discovery). The client is asked to describe feelings associated with specific situations. Questions are stated in such a way that may stimulate a recognition of possible dysfunctional thinking and produce a dissonance about the validity of the thoughts.

   b. Imagery. Through guided imagery, the client is asked to "relive" the stressful situation through his or her imagination.

   c. Role playing. With role playing, the therapist assumes the role of an individual within a situation that produces a maladaptive response in the client. The situation is played out in an effort to elicit recognition of automatic thinking on the part of the client.

   d. Thought recording. In thought recording, the client is asked to keep a written record of situations that occur and the automatic thoughts that are elicited by the situation.

  2. Modifying automatic thoughts. Techniques include:

   a. Generating alternatives. Helping the client see a broader range of possibilities than had originally been considered.

   b. Examining the evidence. The client and therapist set for the automatic thought as the hypothesis and study the evidence both for and against the hypothesis.

   c. Decatastrophizing. The therapist assists the client to examine the validity of a negative automatic thought.

   d. Reattribution. This technique is aimed at helping clients decrease the tendency of attributing adverse life events to themselves.

   e. Daily record of dysfunctional thoughts (DRDT). A common tool used in cognitive therapy to modify automatic thoughts. An extended thought-recording instrument in which the client is asked to record more rational cognitions than the automatic thoughts that occurred. Changes in emotional responses are also recorded.

VI. Behavioral interventions

 A. It is believed that cognitions affect behavior and behavior influences cognitions.

 B. The following procedures are directed toward helping the client learn more adaptive behavioral strategies that will, in turn, have a more positive effect on cognitions.

  1. Active scheduling. The client is asked to keep a daily log of activities on an hourly basis and rate each activity for mastery and pleasure. The schedule is then used to determine important areas needing concentration during therapy.

  2. Graded task assignments. When a client perceives a task to be overwhelming, it is broken down into smaller subtasks, with a goal and time interval attached to each. This helps to make the client feel less powerless.

  3. Behavioral rehearsal. Often used in conjunction with cognitive rehearsal, this technique uses role-play to "rehearse" a modification of maladaptive behaviors that may be contributing to dysfunctional cognitions.

  4. Distraction. Use of activities to distract the client and divert him or her from the intrusive thoughts or depressive ruminations that are contributing to the client's maladaptive responses.

  5. Others. Relaxation exercises, assertiveness training, role modeling, social skills training, and thought-stopping techniques may also be used to modify dysfunctional cognitions.

VII. Role of the Nurse: Application of the Nursing Process

 A. Cognitive therapy techniques are within the scope of nursing practice.

 B. These concepts are often not a part of basic nursing education.

 C. It is important for nurses to understand the basic concepts of cognitive therapy, as the scope of nursing practice continues to expand.

 D. A case study presented the role of the nurse in cognitive therapy in the context of the nursing process.

VIII. Summary

IX. Review Questions

LEARNING ACTIVITIES

Match the cognitive distortions described in the left-hand column to the appropriate basic concept listed on the right.

_____ 1. "No matter what I do, I will fail."

a. Overgeneralization (absolutistic thinking)

_____ 2. Nancy has kept in touch with Emma since their college days, but the letters are becoming less frequent, and Nancy hasn't heard from Emma for almost a year now. Nancy thinks, "She obviously doesn't think of me as a friend anymore."

b. Unloveability category

_____ 3. Janet has been invited to apply for membership in an exclusive women's club in her town. She is very flattered when they invite her to a luncheon at the country club. During lunch, she accidentally spills some water on the tablecloth. She is mortified and thinks, "That's it. I will never be accepted now!"

c. Magnification

_____ 4. Janet (from the situation in No. 3) thinks, "Not only will this club not want me, but no other club in town will want me now!"

d. Personalization

_____ 5. Carol is a nursing student. She has always made A's in her prenursing classes. When she makes a B on her first nursing examination, she thinks, "I will never be a good nurse!"

e. Minimization

_____ 6. "I'm stupid. No one would love me."

f. Helplessness schema

_____ 7. Jane has joined a duplicate bridge club. Last week she was assigned to play with Sara as her partner. When she arrives at the bridge club this week, Sara has already signed up to be partners with Linda. Jane thinks, "She didn't like playing with me. She thinks I'm a lousy bridge player!"

g. Arbitrary inference

_____ 8. The residents of a suburban neighborhood have been told that a possible escaped convict may be in their neighborhood and not talk to or let any strangers in their homes. Sam is a college student walking door-to-door attempting to sell magazine subscriptions. No one will talk to him. He thinks, "I'm a lousy salesman. I'll never earn any money!"

h. Selective abstraction

_____ 9. Alice has had two dates with Hank. She is very attracted to him. He must go out of town on business, but he told her he would take her out before he left. The day arrived for his departure, and she had not heard from him. She was very disappointed. He was out of town for a week and called her twice during that time. Nevertheless, Alice still felt betrayed by his not having taken her out before he left town.

i. Dichotomous thinking

_____ 10. Harry just retired after 30 years in a very successful career as an architect. He worked for a large firm, led many projects, made a lot of money, and is financially comfortable in his retirement. "But I was never considered to be a partner in the firm."

j. Catastrophic thinking

THOUGHT RECORDING

All individuals experience cognitive distortions from time to time. Have students keep a record of thought patterns that they recognize as negative. Use the format of the DRDT as presented below. An example of this record appears in Table 18–3 of the text.

Situation	Automatic Thought	Emotional Response	Rational Response	Outcome: Emotional Response

CHAPTER 18. TEST QUESTIONS

Situation: Nancy is an 18-year-old college senior. She has dreamed of attending a large Ivy League college when she graduates. She has received rejection letters from all to which she has applied, owing to inadequate GPA and SAT scores. She is devastated and becomes depressed. She is referred to Carol, a nurse psychotherapist.

1. Nancy says to Carol, "I guess I'll just have to forget about going to college. I'm just not good enough." This is an example of:
    a. Arbitrary inference
    • b. Overgeneralization
    c. Dichotomous thinking
    d. Personalization

2. Carol responds to Nancy's statement, "I thought you had received a scholarship to the local university." To this, Nancy replies, "Oh, that doesn't count." This is an example of:
    a. Magnification
    b. Minimization
    • c. Selective abstraction
    d. Catastrophic thinking

3. Carol wants to help Nancy by using problem solving. Which of the following represents intervention with this technique?
    • a. "Let's look at what your alternatives are."
    b. "I know you are feeling unhappy now, but things will get better."
    c. "Tell me what you are thinking now."
    d. "When you start to think about the rejections, I want you to switch to thinking about something else."

4. Carol asks Nancy to keep a DRDT. The purpose of this tool in cognitive therapy is to:
    a. Identify automatic thoughts
    • b. Modify automatic thoughts
    c. Identify rational alternatives
    d. All of the above

5. The nursing diagnosis that Carol would most likely choose to work with Nancy during this period would be:
    a. Chronic low self-esteem
    b. Risk for self-directed violence
    c. Powerlessness
    • d. Situational low self-esteem

CHAPTER 19. PSYCHOPHARMACOLOGY

CHAPTER FOCUS

The focus of this chapter is to introduce the student to the major drugs used in the psychiatric setting. Those presented include anxiolytics, antidepressants, antimanic agents, antipsychotics, antiparkinsonian agents, sedative-hypnotics, and central nervous system stimulants. The role of the nurse in administration of these medications and in client education is emphasized.

LEARNING OBJECTIVES

After reading this chapter, the student will be able to:

1. Discuss historical perspectives related to psychopharmacology.
2. Describe indications, actions, contraindications, precautions, side effects, and nursing implications for the following classifications of drugs:
    a. Antianxiety agents
    b. Antidepressants
    c. Antimanics
    d. Antipsychotics
    e. Antiparkinsonian agents
    f. Sedative-hypnotics
    g. Central nervous system stimulants
3. Apply the steps of the nursing process to the administration of psychotropic medications.

KEY TERMS

hypertensive crisis
priapism
retrograde ejaculation
gynecomastia
amenorrhea
agranulocytosis
extrapyramidal symptoms
akinesia
akathisia
dystonia
oculogyric crisis
tardive dyskinesia
neuroleptic malignant syndrome

CHAPTER OUTLINE/LECTURE NOTES

I. Historical Perspectives
    A. Neuroleptics were introduced into the United States in the 1950s.
    B. They are intended to be used as an adjunct to individual or group psychotherapy.
II. Applying the Nursing Process in Psychopharmacological Therapy
    A. Antianxiety agents
        1. Background assessment data

    a. Indications: anxiety disorders, anxiety symptoms, acute alcohol withdrawal, skeletal muscle spasms, convulsive disorders, status epilepticus, and preoperative sedation.
    b. Examples
    c. Action: depression of the central nervous system (CNS).
    d. Contraindications/precautions: contraindicated in known hypersensitivity and in combination with other CNS depressants. Caution with elderly and debilitated clients, clients with renal or hepatic dysfunction, clients with a history of drug abuse or addiction, and those who are depressed or suicidal.
    e. Interactions
  2. Diagnoses
    a. Risk for injury
    b. Risk for activity intolerance
    c. Risk for acute confusion
  3. Planning/Implementation
    a. Side effects and nursing implications
      (1) Drowsiness, confusion, lethargy
      (2) Tolerance; physical and psychological dependence
      (3) Potentiation of other CNS depressants
      (4) Aggravation of depression
      (5) Orthostatic hypotension
      (6) Paradoxical excitement
      (7) Dry mouth
      (8) Nausea and vomiting
      (9) Blood dyscrasias
      (10) Delayed onset (with buspirone only)
    b. Client/family education
  4. Outcome criteria/evaluation
B. Antidepressants
  1. Background assessment data
    a. Indications: dysthymic disorder, major depression; depression associated with organic disease, alcoholism, schizophrenia, or mental retardation; depressive phase of bipolar disorder; and depression accompanied by anxiety.
    b. Examples
    c. Action: block the reuptake of norepinephrine and serotonin by the neurons, thereby increasing their concentrations.
    d. Contraindications/precautions: contraindicated in known hypersensitivity, acute phase of recovery from myocardial infarction, and in angle-closure glaucoma. Caution should be taken in prescribing for elderly or debilitated clients or in clients with hepatic, cardiac, or renal insufficiency. Caution also should be exercised with psychotic clients, clients with benign prostatic hypertrophy, and those with history of seizures.
    e. Interactions
  2. Diagnoses
    a. Risk for self-directed violence
    b. Risk for injury
    c. Social isolation
    d. Constipation
  3. Planning/Implementation
    a. Side effects and nursing implications
      (1) May occur with all chemical classes
        (a) Dry mouth
        (b) Sedation
        (c) Nausea
      (2) Most commonly occur with tricyclics
        (a) Blurred vision

            (b) Constipation
            (c) Urinary retention
            (d) Orthostatic hypotension
            (e) Reduction of seizure threshold
            (f) Tachycardia; arrhythmias
            (g) Photosensitivity
            (h) Weight gain
        (3) Most commonly occur with selective serotonin reuptake inhibitors (SSRIs):
            (a) Insomnia; agitation
            (b) Headache
            (c) Weight loss
            (d) Sexual dysfunction
        (4) Most commonly occurs with monoamine oxidase inhibitors (MAOIs):
            (a) Hypertensive crisis
        (5) Miscellaneous side effects:
            (a) Priapism (with trazodone [Desyrel])
     b. Client/family interaction
   4. Outcome criteria/evaluation
C. Antimanic agents
   1. Background assessment data
     a. Indications: prevention and treatment of manic episodes associated with bipolar disorder;
     b. Examples: lithium carbonate; clonazepam; carbamazepine; valproic acid; verapamil.
     c. Action: Lithium enhances the reuptake of norepinephrine and serotonin in the brain, lowering levels in the body and resulting in decreased hyperactivity. The role of clonazepam, carbamazepine, valproic acid, and verapamil in the treatment of bipolar mania is not fully understood.
     d. Interactions
     e. Contraindications/precautions
   2. Diagnoses
     a. Risk for injury
     b. Risk for violence
     c. Rick for activity intolerance
   3. Planning/implementation
     a. Side effects and nursing implications
     b. Lithium toxicity
     c. Client/family education
   4. Outcome criteria/evaluation
D. Antipsychotics
   1. Background assessment data
     a. Indications: treatment of acute and chronic psychoses. Selected agents are also used as antiemetics, in the treatment of intractable hiccoughs, and for the control of tics and vocal utterances in Tourette's disorder.
     b. Examples
     c. Action: unknown. Thought to block postsynaptic dopamine receptors in the basal ganglia, hypothalamus, limbic system, brainstem, and medulla.
     d. Contraindications/precautions: contraindicated in clients with known hypersensitivity, CNS depression, and blood dyscrasias; in clients with Parkinson's disease; or in those with liver, renal, or cardiac insufficiency. Exercise caution with elderly, debilitated, or diabetic clients, or those with respiratory insufficiency, prostatic hypertrophy, or intestinal obstruction.
     e. Interactions
   2. Diagnoses
     a. Risk for violence
     b. Risk for injury
     c. Risk for activity intolerance

      d.   Noncompliance
   3.   Planning/Implementation
      a.   Side effects and nursing implications
         (1)   Anticholinergic effects
         (2)   Nausea; gastrointestinal (GI) upset
         (3)   Skin rash
         (4)   Sedation
         (5)   Orthostatic hypotension
         (6)   Photosensitivity
         (7)   Hormonal effects
         (8)   Reduction of seizure threshold
         (9)   Agranulocytosis
         (10) Salivation (with Clozapine)
         (11) Extrapyramidal symptoms (EPS)
         (12) Tardive dyskinesia
         (13) Neuroleptic malignant syndrome (NMS)
      b.   Client/family education
   4.   Outcome criteria/evaluation
E. Antiparkinsonian agents
   1.   Background Assessment Data
      a.   Indications: treatment of parkinsonism of various causes, including degenerative, toxic, infective, neoplastic, or drug-induced.
      b.   Examples
      c.   Action: works to restore the natural balance of acetylcholine and dopamine in the CNS.
      d.   Contraindications/Precautions: contraindicated in known hypersensitivity; angle-closure glaucoma; pyloric, duodenal, or bladder neck obstructions; prostatic hypertrophy; or myasthenia gravis. Caution is advised in clients with hepatic, renal, or cardiac insufficiency; in elderly and debilitated clients; in those with tendency toward urinary retention; or in those exposed to high environmental temperatures.
   2.   Planning/Implementation
      a.   Side effects
         (1)   Anticholinergic effects
         (2)   Nausea; GI upset
         (3)   Sedation, drowsiness, dizziness
         (4)   Exacerbation of psychoses
         (5)   Orthostatic hypotension
F. Sedative-hypnotics
   1.   Background assessment data
      a.   Indications: short-term management of various anxiety states and to treat insomnia.
      b.   Examples
      c.   Action: depression of the CNS.
      d.   Contraindications/precautions: contraindicated in known hypersensitivity. Caution advised with in clients with hepatic dysfunction or severe renal impairment. Caution is also advised with suicidal clients and with clients who have been previously addicted to drugs.
      e.   Interactions
   2.   Diagnoses
      a.   Risk for injury
      b.   Sleep pattern disturbance
      c.   Risk for activity intolerance
      d.   Risk for acute confusion
   3.   Planning/implementation (refer to section on antianxiety medications)
      a.   Side effects and nursing implications
      b.   Client/family education
   4.   Outcome criteria/evaluation

G. CNS stimulants
  1. Background assessment data
     a. Indications: in the management of narcolepsy, attention-deficit disorder with hyperactivity in children, and as adjunctive therapy to caloric restriction in the treatment of exogenous obesity.
     b. Examples
     c. Action: stimulate the CNS by increasing levels of norepinephrine, dopamine, and serotonin.
     d. Contraindications/precautions: contraindicated in individuals with hypersensitivity to sympathomimetic amines; in individuals with advanced arteriosclerosis, symptomatic cardiovascular disease, hypertension, hyperthyroidism, glaucoma, agitated or hyperexcitability states, in clients with a history of drug abuse during or within 14 days of receiving therapy with MAOIs, in children under 3 years of age, and in pregnant women. Exercise caution with lactating women, with psychotic children, in clients with Tourette's disorder, in clients with anorexia or insomnia, in elderly, debilitated, or asthenic clients, and in those with a history of suicidal or homicidal tendencies.
     e. Interactions
  2. Diagnoses
     a. Risk for injury
     b. Risk for self-directed violence
     c. Alteration in nutrition, less than body requirements
     d. Alteration in nutrition, more than body requirements
     e. Sleep pattern disturbance
  3. Planning/implementation
     a. Side effects and nursing implications
        (1) Overstimulation, restlessness, insomnia
        (2) Palpitations, tachycardia
        (3) Anorexia, weight loss
        (4) Tolerance, physical and psychological dependence
     b. Client/family education
  4. Outcome criteria/evaluation
III. Summary
IV. Review Questions

LEARNING ACTIVITY

PSYCHOTROPIC MEDICATION QUIZ

Please fill in the blanks and answer the questions in the space provided.

1. What is the mechanism of action by which antidepressant medications achieve the desired effect (regardless of the different physiological processes by which this action is accomplished)?

2. For what must the nurse be on the alert with the client who is receiving antidepressant medication?

3. As the nurse, when would you expect the client to begin showing signs of symptomatic relief after the initiation of antidepressant therapy?

4. Name an example of a tricyclic antidepressant

    _____

    Name an example of a MAOI.

    _____

    Name an example of an SSRI.

    _____

5. Describe some common side effects and nursing implications for tricyclic antidepressants.

6. _____ is the most potentially life-threatening adverse effect of MAOIs. Symptoms for which the nurse and client must be on the alert include: _____ _____. What must be done to prevent these symptoms from occurring? (Your answer must include some examples.)

7. Lithium carbonate is the drug of choice for _____. Many times when these individuals are started on lithium therapy, the physician also orders an antipsychotic medication. Why might he or she do so?

8. There is a narrow margin between the therapeutic and toxic serum levels of lithium carbonate. What is the therapeutic range, and list the initial signs and symptoms of lithium toxicity.

9. Describe some nursing implications for the client on lithium therapy.

10. What is the mechanism of action for antianxiety medications?

11. What is the most commonly-used group of antianxiety drugs? Give two examples.

12. What are the most common side effects of antianxiety drugs?

13. What must the client on long-term antianxiety therapy be instructed to prevent a potentially life-threatening situation?

14. What is thought to be the mechanism of action that produces the desired effect with antipsychotic medications?

15. Phenothiazines are the most commonly used antipsychotic group. Give two examples of phenothiazines.

16. Describe potential adverse hormonal effects associated with antipsychotic therapy.

17. Agranulocytosis is a potentially very serious side effect of antipsychotic therapy. The nurse and client should be on the alert for symptoms of _____, _____, and _____.

18. Neuroleptic malignant syndrome is a rare, but potentially fatal, side effect of antipsychotic drugs. List symptoms for which the nurse must be on the alert when assessing for NMS.

19. Describe the symptoms of extrapyramidal side effects associated with antipsychotic therapy.

20. What is the classification of medication that is commonly prescribed for drug-induced extrapyramidal reactions? Give two examples of these medications.

21. Describe a life-threatening situation that could occur in the client who abruptly withdraws from long-term use of CNS stimulants.

CHAPTER 19. TEST QUESTIONS

1. Carol has made an appointment to see her primary care provider because of increased anxiety. She sees a nurse practitioner who does a physical examination and takes a detailed history. The psychiatrist diagnoses Carol with anxiety disorder. Which of the following medications is prescribed for anxiety?
   - a. Chlorpromazine (Thorazine)
   - b. Imipramine (Elavil)
   - • c. Diazepam (Valium)
   - d. Methylphenidate (Ritalin)

2. Which of the following data would suggest that caution is necessary in prescribing the medication of choice to Carol?
   - • a. The client has a history of alcohol dependence.
   - b. The client has a history of diabetes mellitus.
   - c. The client has a history of schizophrenia.
   - d. The client has a history of hypertension.

3. Peter has been diagnosed with major depression. His psychiatrist prescribes imipramine (Tofranil). What information is specifically related to *this* class of antidepressants and should be included in client/family education?
   - a. The medication may cause dry mouth.
   - b. The medication may cause constipation.
   - c. The medication should not be discontinued abruptly.
   - • d. The medication may cause photosensitivity.

4. When Peter did not achieve relief from his depression, his psychiatrist decided to try Parante, an MAOI. When teaching Peter about the effects of tyramine, which of the following foods and/or medications will the nurse caution Peter not to consume?
   - • a. Pepperoni pizza and red wine
   - b. Bagels with cream cheese and tea
   - c. Apple pie and coffee
   - d. Potato chips and diet Coke

5. Alex, a 24-year-old graduate student, is taken to the emergency department by one of his classmates because of increased suspiciousness and auditory hallucinations. He keeps asking others what they are whispering about him. The nurse who takes his history discovers that he has a history of depression and has been taking desipramine (Norpramine) for 3 years. He is in good physical health but has allergies to penicillin, prochlorperazine maleate (Compazine), and beestings. Although a definitive diagnosis is not made, it is clear that Alex is experiencing a psychotic episode. Using the assessment data gathered upon admission, which of the following antipsychotic medications would be contraindicated for Alex?
   - a. haloperidol (Haldol)
   - b. clozapine (Clozaril)
   - c. risperidone (Risperdal)
   - • d. thioridazine (Mellaril)

6. Which of the following is the rationale for the correct answer in the previous question?
   - • a. Cross-sensitivity is common among the phenothiazines.
   - b. The drug is new and not adequately tested.
   - c. The drug is old and more effective ones have been developed.
   - d. It is one of the phenothiazines that is least effective for the treatment of psychosis.

7. The physician prescribes a medication for Alex described as "prn for EPS." When should the nurse give this medication?
    - a. When Alex's white cell count falls below 3000 mm^3
    - • b. When Alex exhibits tremors and shuffling gait
    - c. When Alex complains of dry mouth
    - d. When Alex experiences a seizure

8. Which of the following medications would the physician have prescribed for the EPS described in the previous question?
    - a. Diazepam (Valium)
    - b. Amitriptyline (Elavil)
    - • c. Benztropine (Cogentin)
    - d. Methylphenidate (Ritalin)

9. Nancy takes a maintenance dosage of lithium carbonate for a history of bipolar disorder. She has come to the community health clinic stating that she "has had the flu for over a week." She describes her symptoms as coughing, runny nose, chest congestion, fever, and GI upset. Her temperature is 100.9F. She is complaining of blurred vision and "ringing in my ears." What might the nurse suspect in Nancy's case?
    - a. She has consumed some foods high in tyramine.
    - b. She has stopped taking her lithium carbonate.
    - c. She has probably developed a tolerance to the lithium.
    - • d. She may have become toxic on the lithium carbonate.

10. Joey, age 8, takes methylphenidate for attention-deficit-hyperactivity disorder. His mother complains to the nurse that Joey has a very poor appetite, and she struggles to help him gain weight. Which of the following would be appropriate for the nurse to advise Joey's mother?
    - • a. Administer Joey's medication immediately after meals.
    - b. Administer Joey's medication at bedtime.
    - c. Skip a dose of the medication when Joey doesn't eat anything.
    - d. Assure Joey's mother that Joey will eat when he is hungry.

CHAPTER 20. ELECTROCONVULSIVE THERAPY

CHAPTER FOCUS

The focus of this chapter is to introduce the student to the use of electroconvulsive therapy in psychiatry. The role of the nurse in the administration of electroconvulsive therapy is described.

LEARNING OBJECTIVES

After reading this chapter, the student will be able to:

1. Define *electroconvulsive therapy.*
2. Discuss historical perspectives related to electroconvulsive therapy.
3. Discuss indications, contraindications, mechanism of action, and side effects of electroconvulsive therapy.
4. Identify risks associated with electroconvulsive therapy.
5. Describe the role of the nurse in the administration of electroconvulsive therapy.

KEY TERMS

electroconvulsive therapy
insulin coma therapy
pharmacoconvulsive therapy

CHAPTER OUTLINE/LECTURE NOTES

I.   Electroconvulsive Therapy (ECT) Defined
    A.   ECT is the induction of a grand mal (generalized) seizure through the application of electrical current to the brain.
    B.   Applied through electrodes placed bilaterally in the frontotemporal region, or unilaterally on the same side as the dominant hand.
    C.   Dose of stimulation is based on the client's seizure threshold, which is highly variable among individuals. The duration of the seizure should be at least 25 seconds.
    D.   Most clients require an average of 6 to 12 treatments, but some may require up to 20 treatments.
    E.   Usually administered every other day, three times per week.
II.   Historical Perspectives
    A.   The first treatment was performed in 1938 in Rome.
    B.   Other types of somatic therapies had been tried prior to that time: insulin coma therapy and pharmacoconvulsive therapy.
    C.   With insulin coma therapy, an injection of insulin produced a hypoglycemic coma, which was believed to alleviate the symptoms of schizophrenia. A number of fatalities occurred with insulin therapy, and its use has been discontinued in the treatment of mental illness.
    D.   Pharmacoconvulsive therapy involved induction of convulsions with intramuscular injections of camphor in oil. The originator of this therapy believed this treatment also alleviated schizophrenic symptoms. He switched to the use of pentylenetetrazol when camphor was found to be unreliable. Some successes were reported in terms of reduction of psychotic symptoms, and this method was used until the advent of ECT.
    E.   ECT was widely accepted from around 1940 to 1955. This period was followed by a 20-year span during which ECT was considered objectionable by both the psychiatric profession and the lay public alike. A second peak of acceptance began around 1975 and has been increasing to the present.

F. An estimated 50,000 to 100,000 people per year receive ECT treatments in the United States.

III. Indications
A. ECT has been shown to be effective in the treatment of severe depression. It is usually not considered the treatment of choice for depression, but may be administered following a trial of therapy with antidepressant medication.
B. ECT is also indicated in the treatment of acute manic episodes of bipolar affective disorder. It has been shown to be effective in treating manic clients who are refractory to antimanic drug therapy.
C. ECT can induce a remission in some clients who present with acute schizophrenia. It seems to be of little value in the treatment of chronic schizophrenia.

IV. Contraindications
A. The only absolute contraindication for ECT is increased intracranial pressure (from brain tumor, recent cerebrovascular accident [CVA], or other cerebrovascular lesion).
B. Individuals at high risk with ECT include those with myocardial infarction or CVA within the preceding 3 months, aortic or cerebral aneurysm, severe underlying hypertension, or congestive heart failure.

V. Mechanism of Action
A. The exact mechanism of action by which ECT effects a therapeutic response is unknown. Some credibility has been given to the biochemical theory that ECT results in significant increases in the circulating levels of serotonin, norepinephrine, and dopamine.

VI. Side Effects
A. Most common side effects: temporary memory loss and confusion.

VII. Risks Associated with Electroconvulsive Therapy
A. Mortality
1. Mortality rate from ECT falls somewhere in the range of 0.01% to 0.04%. Although death is rare, when it does occur, it is usually related to cardiovascular complications.
B. Permanent memory loss
1. Studies have shown that a small subgroup of clients receiving ECT may suffer permanent memory impairment.
C. Brain Damage
1. Critics of ECT remain adamant in their belief that the procedure always results in some degree of immediate brain damage. There are, however, no current data to substantiate that ECT produces any permanent changes in brain structure or functioning.

VIII. Role of the Nurse in Electroconvulsive Therapy
A. The nursing process is the method of delivery of care for the client receiving ECT.
B. The client must receive a thorough physical examination prior to initiation of therapy. This examination should include assessment of cardiovascular and pulmonary status, as well as laboratory blood and urine studies. A skeletal history and x-ray assessment should also be considered.
C. The nurse must ensure that informed consent has been granted. The nurse must also assess mood, level of anxiety, thought and communication patterns, and vital signs. Appropriate nursing diagnoses are formulated based on assessment data.
D. Nurses prepare the client for the treatment by having him or her void and remove dentures, eyeglasses or contact lenses, jewelry, and hairpins. Atropine sulfate or glycopyrrolate is administered according to physician's orders approximately 30 minutes prior to the treatment.
E. In the treatment room, the anesthesiologist administers a muscle relaxant (usually succinylcholine) and a short-acting anesthetic (such as thiopental sodium or methohexital sodium). The client receives oxygen during and after the treatment.
F. An airway/bite block is used to facilitate the client's airway patency. Electrodes are placed on the temples to deliver the electrical stimulation.
G. The nurse assists the psychiatrist and the anesthesiologist as required, as well as providing support to the client, both physically and emotionally.
H. Following the treatment, the nurse remains with the client until he or she is fully awake. Vital signs are taken every 15 minutes for the first hour. The client is oriented to time and place and given an explanation of what has occurred.
I. Evaluation of changes in client behavior is made to determine improvement and provide assistance in deciding the number of treatments that will be administered.

IX. Summary
X. Review Questions

LEARNING ACTIVITY

ELECTROCONVULSIVE THERAPY

Match the terms on the left with the descriptions listed on the right.

_____ 1. Atropine sulfate

_____ 2. Succinylcholine

_____ 3. Thiopental sodium

_____ 4. Increased intracranial pressure

_____ 5. Temporary memory loss and confusion

_____ 6. Major depression

_____ 7. Oxygen

_____ 8. Informed consent

_____ 9. Norepinephrine and serotonin

_____ 10. Recent myocardial infarction

a. Major indication for ECT

b. The only absolute contraindication for ECT

c. Given prior to ECT to decrease secretions and increase heart rate

d. Administered prior to, during, and after ECT

e. Most common cause of mortality associated with ECT

f. Administered as a short-acting anesthetic

g. Thought to be increased by ECT

h. Most common side effects of ECT

i. Required before treatment can be initiated

j. Muscle relaxant given to prevent bone fractures

CHAPTER 20. TEST QUESTIONS

Situation: Sarah, age 70, is a client on the psychiatric unit with a diagnosis of major depression. She has been seeing her psychiatrist on an outpatient basis for several months and has been taking an antidepressant medication, with no improvements in symptoms. Her physician has suggested hospitalization with a series of ECT treatments.

1. The nurse is doing some pretreatment teaching with Sarah and her family. Sarah's daughter asks, "Isn't this treatment dangerous?" Which is the most appropriate response by the nurse?
   a. "No, this treatment is absolutely safe."
   b. "There are some risks involved, but in your mother's case, the benefits outweigh the risks."
   - c. "There are some risks involved, but your mother will have a thorough examination in advance to ensure that she is a good candidate for the treatment."
   d. "There are some side effects to the treatment, but they are not life threatening."

2. The nurse explains to Sarah and her family what will happen in association with a treatment. Which of the following statements is true regarding ECT?
   - a. Electrical stimulation to the brain produces a grand mal seizure.
   b. Maximal muscle movement is required to ensure efficacy of the treatment.
   c. The client will sleep for about 12 hours following a treatment.
   d. The client will have full recall of what has occurred during the treatment.

3. The nurse explains to Sarah and her family what she can expect immediately following the ECT. Which of the following statements is true regarding ECT?
   a. Sarah will most likely wake up right away and no longer be depressed.
   - b. Sarah will likely be confused and somewhat disoriented.
   c. Sarah will be sleepy and very likely sleep for a number of hours following the treatment.
   d. Sarah may experience some soreness in her muscles and joints following the treatment.

4. The nurse tells Sarah that she will receive an injection of medication called atropine sulfate about 30 minutes before she gets her treatment. She explains to Sarah that this is for:
   a. Alleviating her anxiety.
   b. Relaxing her muscles.
   - c. Decreasing secretions.
   d. Putting her to sleep.

5. The nurse constructs a plan of care for Sarah's hospital stay and includes the following nursing diagnoses. Which must receive priority attention?
   a. Anxiety related to receiving ECT
   b. Knowledge deficit related to ECT
   c. Confusion related to side effects of ECT
   - d. Risk for injury related to risks and side effects of ECT

CHAPTER 21. COMPLEMENTARY THERAPIES

CHAPTER FOCUS

The focus of this chapter is to introduce the student to various alternatives to allopathic medicine. The historical background and techniques of each are presented.

LEARNING OBJECTIVES

After reading this chapter, the student will be able to:

1.   Describe the philosophies behind various complementary therapies, including herbal medicine, acupressure and acupuncture, diet and nutrition, chiropractic medicine, therapeutic touch and massage, yoga, and pet therapy.
2.   Discuss the historical background of various complementary therapies.
3.   Describe the techniques used in various complementary therapies.

KEY TERMS

allopathic medicine
alternative medicine
complementary medicine
acupressure
acupuncture
acupoints
chiropractic
subluxation
chi
meridians
yoga

CHAPTER OUTLINE/LECTURE NOTES

I.   Introduction
    A.   The connection between mind and body is well recognized.
    B.   Traditional medicine practiced in the United States today is based on scientific methodology and is known as allopathic medicine.
    C.   Practices that differ from the usual traditional practices are known as alternative medicine.
    D.   The Office of Alternative Medicine was established by the National Institutes of Health in 1991 to study nontraditional therapies and to evaluate their usefulness and their effectiveness.
    E.   Increasing numbers of third-party payers are bowing to public pressure and including alternative therapies in their coverage.
    F.   Some clinicians view these therapies not as alternatives, but as complementary therapies, in partnership with traditional medicine.
    G.   Complementary medicine is viewed as holistic health care, which deals not only with the physical perspective, but also the emotional and spiritual components of the individual.
    H.   Most complementary therapies are not founded in scientific principle, but they have been shown to be effective in the treatment of certain disorders and, therefore, merit further examination as a viable component of holistic health care.

II. Types of Complementary Therapies
   A. Herbal medicine
      1. Virtually every culture in the world has relied on herbs and plants to treat illness.
      2. Twenty-five percent of all prescription drugs in the United States today are derived from plants.
      3. The Food and Drug Administration (FDA) classifies herbal remedies as dietary supplements or food additives. Therefore, their labels cannot indicate medicinal uses, and they are not subjected to FDA approval.
      4. The Commission E of the German Federal Health Agency has been researching and regulating the safety and efficacy of herbs and plant medicines in Germany. Recently, all 380 German Commission E monographs of herbal medicines have been translated into English.
      5. Just because a substance is called "natural" does not mean that it is necessarily completely safe. All herbal medicines must be approached with caution.
      6. The following cautions are offered:
         a. Be careful of sources.
         b. Choose the most reliable forms.
         c. More is not better.
         d. Monitor your reactions.
         e. Take no risks by self-medicating with herbal remedies.
      7. Examples of herbal medicines, their uses, action, and safety profile are included.
   B. Acupressure and acupuncture
      1. Acupressure and acupuncture are healing techniques based on the ancient philosophies of traditional Chinese medicine dating back to 3000 B.C.
      2. The main concept is that healing energy (chi) flows through the body along specific pathways called meridians. The meridians connect a series of acupoints to which the clinician applies pressure.
      3. Pressure to these acupoints is thought to dissolve any obstructions in the flow of healing energy (chi), and to restore the body to a healthier functioning.
      4. In acupuncture, hair-thin, sterile, disposable, stainless-steel needles are inserted into acupoints to dissolve the obstructions along the meridians.
      5. The Western medical philosophy regarding acupressure and acupuncture is that they stimulate the body's own painkilling chemicals, the morphinelike substances known as endorphins.
      6. The treatment has been found to be effective in the treatment of asthma, headaches, dysmenorrhea, cervical pain, insomnia, anxiety, depression, substance abuse, stroke rehabilitation, nausea of pregnancy, postoperative and chemotherapy-induced nausea and vomiting, tennis elbow, fibromyalgia, low back pain, and carpal tunnel syndrome.
   C. Diet and nutrition
      1. Many diseases today are linked to poor nutritional habits.
      2. The U.S. Departments of Agriculture and Health and Human Services have collaborated on a set of guidelines to help individuals understand what types of foods to eat in order to promote health and prevent disease. They include:
         a. Eat a variety of foods. Most of the daily servings of food should be selected from the food groups that comprise the largest areas of the pyramid pictured below, and are closest to the base.
         b. Balance the food you eat with physical activity to maintain or improve your weight. Thirty minutes or more of moderate physical activity, such as walking, regularly 3 to 5 days a week can help to increase calorie expenditure and assist in maintaining a healthy weight.
         c. Choose a diet with plenty of grain products, vegetables, and fruits. Consumption of these foods is associated with a substantially lower risk for many chronic diseases, including certain types of cancer.
         d. Choose a diet low in fat, saturated fat, and cholesterol. Heart disease and some types of cancer (e.g., breast, colon) have been linked to high-fat diets. Choose foods with mono- and polyunsaturated fat sources, and keep daily cholesterol intake below 300 mg. Fats should comprise no more than 30 percent of the total daily calorie intake.

      e. Choose a diet moderate in sugars. Sugars should be used in moderation by most healthy people and sparingly by people with low calorie needs. Problems correlated with eating too much sugar include tooth decay and the risk for heart disease in women 35 and older.

      f. Choose a diet moderate in salt and sodium. Some studies indicate that a high intake of salt is associated with high blood pressure.

      g. If you drink alcoholic beverages, do so in moderation. High levels of alcohol intake raise the risk for high blood pressure, stroke, heart disease, certain cancers, accidents, violence, suicides, birth defects, cirrhosis of the liver, inflammation of the pancreas, damage to the brain, and overall mortality.

   3. Essential vitamins and minerals

      a. Examples

      b. Functions

      c. Recommended daily allowance requirements

      d. Food Sources

D. Chiropractic medicine

   1. It is probably the most widely used form of alternative healing in the United States. It was developed in the late 1800s.

   2. Theory behind this type of healing is that energy flows from the brain to all parts of the body through the spinal cord and spinal nerves. When vertebrae of the spinal column become displaced, they may press on a nerve and interfere with the normal nerve transmission.

   3. Displacements of vertebrae are called "subluxations." To restore normal function, the vertebrae are manipulated back into their normal positions.

   4. The manipulations are called "adjustments."

   5. Adjustments are made by hand or facilitated by the use of special treatment tables.

   6. Muscle relaxation may be achieved with massage, with the application of heat or cold, and through the use of ultrasound treatments.

   7. The most common type of ailment for which individuals seek chiropractic treatment is back pain. Others include headaches, sciatica, shoulder pain, tennis and golfer's elbow, leg and foot pain, hand and wrist pain, allergies, asthma, stomach disorders, and menstrual problems.

   8. Chiropractors are licensed to practice in all 50 states.

E. Therapeutic touch and massage

   1. The technique of therapeutic touch was developed in the 1970s by Dolores Krieger, a nurse associated with the New York University School of Nursing.

   2. This therapy is based on the philosophy that the human body projects a field of energy around it, which when blocked, produces pain or illness.

   3. Therapeutic touch is used to correct the blockages and relieve the discomfort.

   4. Because therapeutic touch is based on the premise that the energy field extends beyond the surface of the body, the practitioner need not actually touch the client's skin.

   5. Slow, rhythmic hand motions are swept over the entire body while the hands remain 2 to 4 inches from the skin. Heat should be felt where the energy is blocked.

   6. The therapist "massages" the energy field in that area, smoothing it out, and thus correcting the obstruction.

   7. Therapeutic touch is thought to reduce pain and anxiety and to promote relaxation and health maintenance. It has been useful in the treatment of chronic health conditions.

F. Massage

   1. Massage is the technique of manipulating the muscles and soft tissues of the body.

   2. It has been used by Chinese physicians for the treatment of disease more than 5000 years ago.

   3. The Eastern style of massage focuses on balancing the body's vital energy (chi) as it flows through pathways called meridians.

   4. The Western style of massage affects muscles, connective tissues, such as tendons and ligaments, and the cardiovascular system.

   5. A variety of gliding and kneading strokes, along with deep circular movements and vibrations, are used to relax the muscles, improve circulation, and increase mobility.

6. Massage is helpful in reducing anxiety and in relieving chronic back and neck pain, arthritis, sciatica, migraine headaches, muscle spasms, insomnia, pain of labor and delivery, stress-related disorders, and whiplash.
7. Massage is contraindicated in high blood pressure, acute infection, osteoporosis, phlebitis, skin conditions, varicose veins, or over the site of a recent injury, bruises, or burns.

G. Yoga
   1. Yoga is thought to have been developed in India some 5000 years ago.
   2. The ultimate goal of yoga is to unite the human soul with the universal spirit.
   3. Yoga is helpful in relieving stress and in improving overall physical and psychological wellness.
   4. Yoga breathing is a deep, diaphramatic breathing that increases oxygen to brain and body tissues, thereby easing stress and fatigue, and boosting energy.
   5. Another component of yoga is meditation, used to achieve a profound feeling of relaxation.
   6. Western yoga uses body postures, along with meditation and breathing exercises, to achieve a balanced, disciplined workout that releases muscle tension, tones the internal organs, and energizes the mind, body, and spirit, so that natural healing can occur.

H. Pet therapy
   1. Evidence has shown that animals can directly influence a person's mental and physical well-being.
   2. Pets have been shown to:
      a. Reduce the death rate from recurrence of heart attack
      b. Lower blood pressure, which can occur simply by petting a dog or cat
      c. Enhance mood and improve social interaction among nursing home clients
   3. Some researchers believe that animals actually may retard the aging process among those who live alone.

III. Summary
IV. Review Questions

LEARNING ACTIVITY

Fill in the food pyramid with the appropriate food groups for each level and the number of servings suggested for each group.

CHAPTER 21. TEST QUESTIONS

1. Carol went to the community mental health clinic because she was feeling depressed. She told the therapist that she had broken up with her boyfriend 6 weeks ago and that she has been feeling depressed since that time. She wants to feel better, but she does not want to take medication. She told the therapist she would be willing to take an herbal medication if there was something that might help her feel better. The therapist may suggest which of the following for Carol?
   - a. Chamomile
   - b. Echinacea
   - • c. St. John's Wort
   - d. Feverfew

2. Carol decided to see a chiropractor for a recurring pain in her lower back. The chiropractor took X-rays and told Carol he saw some displacement of vertebrae in her spine. In chiropractic medicine, these displacements are called:
   - a. Maladjustments
   - b. Manipulations
   - c. Meridians
   - • d. Subluxations

3. The therapist suggested that Carol see a physician for a complete physical examination. Part of the examination included a health risk assessment. Carol's medical history revealed that her father had died of colon cancer and her mother has had surgery for breast cancer, both of which may have a link to high-at diet. The nurse does health teaching about diet with Carol. In terms of her risk factors, which of the following food groups should Carol modify her intake of?
   - a. Fruit and grain
   - • b. Meat and cheese
   - c. Meat and starches
   - d. Milk and cereal

4. Which of the following herbal remedies is thought to improve memory and blood circulation?
   - • a. Ginkgo
   - b. Ginseng
   - c. Kava Kava
   - d. St. John's Wort

5. The technique of yoga uses which of the following?
   - a. Deep breathing
   - b. Meditation
   - c. Balanced body postures
   - • d. All of the above
   - e. C only

CHAPTER 22.   DISORDERS USUALLY FIRST DIAGNOSED IN INFANCY, CHILDHOOD, OR ADOLESCENCE

CHAPTER FOCUS

The focus of this chapter is on psychiatric disorders usually first evident in infancy, childhood, or adolescence. Symptomatology and predisposing factors are described. Role of the nurse in care of these clients is emphasized.

LEARNING OBJECTIVES

After reading this chapter, the student will be able to:

1.   Identify psychiatric disorders usually first diagnosed in infancy, childhood, or adolescence.
2.   Discuss predisposing factors implicated in the etiology of mental retardation, autistic disorder, attention-deficit hyperactivity disorder, conduct disorder, oppositional defiant disorder, Tourette's disorder, and separation anxiety disorder.
3.   Identify symptomatology and use the information in the assessment of clients with the aforementioned disorders.
4.   Identify nursing diagnoses common to clients with these disorders, and select appropriate nursing interventions for each.
5.   Discuss relevant criteria for evaluating nursing care of clients with selected infant, childhood, and adolescent psychiatric disorders.
6.   Describe treatment modalities relevant to selected disorders of infancy, childhood, and adolescence.

KEY TERMS

aggression
autistic disorder
temperament
impulsivity
negativism
clinging
palilalia
echolalia

CHAPTER OUTLINE/LECTURE NOTES

I.   Introduction
    A. It is often difficult to determine if a child's behavior is indicative of emotional problems.
    B. The *DSM-IV* suggests that an emotional problem exists if the behavioral manifestations:
        1.   Are not age-appropriate
        2.   Deviate from cultural norms
        3.   Create deficits or impairments in adaptive functioning
II.   Mental Retardation (MR)
    A. It is defined by deficits in general intellectual functioning (as measured by IQ examinations) and adaptive functioning (the ability to adapt to the requirements of daily living and the expectations of age and cultural group).
    B. Predisposing Factors
        1.   Hereditary

         a.   Implicated in approximately 5% of the cases.

             (1)   Inborn errors of metabolism, such as Tay-Sachs disease, phenylketonuria, and hyperglycinemia

             (2)   Chromosomal disorders, such as Down's syndrome and Klinefelter's syndrome

             (3)   Single-gene abnormalities, such as tuberous sclerosis and neurofibromatosis

    2. Early alterations in embryonic development

         a.   Account for 30% of MR cases

         b.   Damages may occur in response to:

             (1)   Toxicity associated with maternal ingestion of alcohol or other drugs

             (2)   Maternal illnesses and infections during pregnancy

             (3)   Complications of pregnancy, such as toxemia and uncontrolled diabetes

    3. Pregnancy and perinatal factors

         a.   Account for approximately 10% of cases of MR

         b.   Can be caused by:

             (1)   Fetal malnutrition, viral or other infections during pregnancy

             (2)   Trauma or complications of the birth process that result in deprivation of oxygen to the infant

             (3)   Premature birth

    4. General medical conditions acquired in infancy or childhood

         a.   Account for approximately 5% of cases of MR

         b.   Can be caused by:

             (1)   Infections, such as meningitis and encephalitis

             (2)   Poisonings, such as from insecticides, meditations, lead

             (3)   Physical traumas, such as head injuries, asphyxiation, and hyperpyrexia

    5. Environmental influences and other mental disorders

         a.   Account for approximately 20% of cases of MR

         b.   May be attributed to:

             (1)   Deprivation of nurturance and social, linguistic, and other stimulation

             (2)   Severe mental disorders, such as autistic disorder

C. Application of the nursing process

    1. Degree of severity of mental retardation is identified by level of IQ.

    2. Four levels have been delineated: mild, moderate, severe, and profound.

    3. Nurses must assess strengths as well as limitations in order to encourage the client to be as independent as possible.

    4. It is important to include family members in the planning and implementation of care.

    5. Family members should receive information regarding the scope of the condition, realistic expectations and client potentials, methods for modifying behavior as required, community resources from which they may seek assistance and support.

    6. Evaluation of care given to the mentally retarded client should reflect positive behavioral change.

III. Autistic Disorder

  A. It is characterized by a withdrawal of the child into the self and into a fantasy world of his or her own creation.

  B. The disorder is relatively rare and occurs 4 to 5 times more often in boys than in girls. Onset occurs prior to age 3 and in most cases runs a chronic course with symptoms persisting into adulthood.

  C. Predisposing factors

    1. Social environment. Causative factors are thought to include parental rejection, child responses to deviant parental personality characteristics, family breakup, family stress, insufficient stimulation, and faulty communication patterns. Little credibility given to social factors at present.

    2. Biological factors.

         a.   Genetics. Sibling and twin studies have revealed strong evidence that genetic factors play a significant role.

         b.   Neurological factors. Early developmental problems have been implicated:

             (1)   Postnatal neurological infections, congenital rubella, phenylketonuria, and fragile X syndrome.

       (2)   Various structural and functional abnormalities, including ventricular enlargement, left temporal abnormalities, increased glucose metabolism, and elevated blood serotonin level may also be involved.

  D. Application of the nursing process
     1. Background assessment data (symptomatology)
       a. Impairment in social interaction
       b. Impairment in communication and imaginative activity
       c. Restricted activities and interests
     2. Nursing intervention is aimed at protection of the child from self-directed violence and improvement in social functioning, verbal communication, and personal identity.

IV.   Attention-Deficit Hyperactivity Disorder (ADHD)
  A. Essential features include developmentally inappropriate degrees of inattention, impulsiveness, and hyperactivity.
  B. The disorder is further categorized into three subtypes:
     1. ADHD, combined type
     2. ADHD, predominantly inattentive type
     3. ADHD, predominantly hyperactive-impulsive type
  C. Predisposing factors
     1. Biologic influences
       a. Genetics. Frequency among family members has been noted.
       b. Biochemical theory. Implicates a deficit of dopamine and norepinephrine in the brain
       c. Prenatal, perinatal, and postnatal factors:
         (1) Prenatal factors include maternal smoking during pregnancy
         (2) Perinatal factors include prematurity, signs of fetal distress, prolonged labor, and perinatal asphyxia
         (3) Postnatal factors include cerebral palsy, epilepsy, and central nervous system (CNS) trauma or infections
     2. Environmental influences
       a. Environmental lead
       b. Diet factors, including food dyes and additives, and sugar
     3. Psychosocial influences
       a. Disorganized or chaotic environments
       b. Disruption in bonding during the first 3 years of life
       c. Family history of alcoholism, hysterical or sociopathic behaviors
       d. Parental history of hyperactivity
       e. Developmental learning disorders
  D. Application of the nursing process
     1. Background assessment data (symptomatology)
       a. Highly distractible with extremely limited attention span
       b. Difficulty forming satisfactory interpersonal relationships
       c. Low frustration tolerance and outbursts of temper
       d. Excessive levels of activity, restlessness, and fidgeting
     2. Nursing intervention is aimed at protection from injury due to excessive hyperactivity, improvement in social interaction, self-esteem, and compliance with task expectations.
     3. Psychopharmacological intervention
       a. Drugs of choice: CNS stimulants.
       b. Examples: dextroamphetamine, methylphenidate, and pemoline.
       c. Effects on children with ADHD: increased attention span, control of hyperactive behavior, and improvement in learning ability.
       d. Side effects: insomnia, anorexia, weight loss, tachycardia, and temporary decrease in rate of growth and development. Tolerance can occur. The drug should not be withdrawn abruptly.
       e. A drug "holiday" should be attempted periodically under direction of the physician to determine effectiveness of the medication and need for continuation.

V.   Conduct Disorder

A. A persistent pattern of conduct in which the basic rights of others and major age-appropriate societal norms or rules are violated. Two subtypes based on age at onset:
   1. Childhood-onset type: defined by the onset of at least one criterion characteristic of conduct disorder prior to age 10
   2. Adolescent-onset type: defined by the absence of any criteria characteristic of conduct disorder prior to age 10
B. Predisposing factors
   1. Biological influences
      a. Genetics. Twin and nontwin sibling studies indicate a higher incidence among those who have family members with the disorder.
      b. Temperament. Children who are born with "difficult" temperaments were found to have a significantly higher degree of aggressive behavior later in life.
      c. Biochemical. Elevated levels of plasma testosterone have been correlated with aggressive behavior.
   2. Psychosocial Influences
      a. Impaired Social-Cognition. Rejection by peers may predispose to aggressive behavior.
      b. Family Influences.
         (1) The following family dynamics may contribute to the development of conduct disorder:
             (a) Parental rejection
             (b) Inconsistent management with harsh discipline
             (c) Early institutional living
             (d) Frequent shifting of parental figures
             (e) Large family size
             (f) Absent father
             (g) Parents with antisocial personality disorder or alcohol dependence
             (h) Association with a delinquent subgroup
             (i) Marital conflict and divorce
             (j) Inadequate communication patterns
             (k) Parental permissiveness
C. Application of the nursing process
   1. Background assessment data (symptomatology)
      a. Physical aggression in the violation of the rights of others
      b. Use of drugs and alcohol
      c. Sexual permissiveness
      d. Use of projection as a defense mechanism
      e. Low self-esteem manifested by "tough-guy" image
      f. Inability to control anger
      g. Low academic achievement
   2. Nursing intervention is aimed at protection of others from client's physical aggression, improvement in social interaction and self-esteem, and acceptance of responsibility for own behavior.
VI. Oppositional Defiant Disorder (ODD)
   A. It is characterized by a pattern of negativism, defiant, disobedient, and hostile behavior toward authority figures that occurs more frequently than is typically observed in individuals of comparable age and developmental level, and interferes with social, academic, or occupational functioning.
   B. Predisposing factors
      1. Biological Influences. Role not established.
      2. Family influences. If power and control are issues for parents, or if they exercise authority for their own needs, a power struggle can be established between the parents and the child that sets the stage for the development of ODD.
   C. Application of the nursing process
      1. Background assessment data (symptomatology)
         a. Symptoms include passive-aggression, exhibited by obstinacy, procrastination, disobedience, carelessness, negativism, dawdling, provocation, resistance to change, violation of minor rules, blocking out communications from others, and resistance to authority.

b. Other symptoms may include enuresis, encopresis, elective mutism, running away, school avoidance, school underachievement, eating and sleeping problems, temper tantrums, fighting, and argumentativeness.

c. Interpersonal relationships are impaired and school performance is often unsatisfactory.

2. Nursing intervention is aimed at compliance with therapy, acceptance of responsibility for own behavior, increase in self-esteem, and improvement in social interaction.

VII. Tourette's disorder

A. The essential feature is the presence of multiple motor tics and one or more vocal tics.

B. Onset of the disorder is before age 18 and is more common in boys than in girls.

C. Predisposing factors

1. Biological factors

a. Genetics. Twin studies suggest an inheritable component. The familial predisposition to tic disorders appears to be governed by a single gene with autosomal dominant transmission.

b. Biochemical factors. Abnormalities in levels of dopamine, serotonin, dynorphin, gamma-aminobutyric acid, acetylcholine, and norepinephrine have been associated with Tourette's disorder.

c. Structural Factors. Brain studies in Tourette's disorder have found enlargement in the caudate nucleus and decreased cerebral blood flow in the left lenticular nucleus.

2. Environmental factors

a. Increased prenatal complications and lower birth weight.

b. Greater emotional stress during pregnancy and more nausea and vomiting during the first trimester of pregnancy have been noted in the mothers of these children.

D. Application of the nursing process

1. Background assessment data (Symptomatology)

a. Simple motor tics include eye blinking, neck jerking, shoulder shrugging, facial grimacing, and coughing.

b. Complex motor tics include touching, squatting, hopping, skipping, deep knee bends, retracing steps, and twirling when walking.

c. Vocal tics include words or sounds such as clicks, grunts, yelps, barks, sniffs, snorts, coughs, and rarely, the uttering of obscenities.

d. Vocal tics may also include repeating one's own sounds or words (called palilalia), or repeating the words of others (called echolalia).

2. Nursing intervention is aimed at protection of the client and others, improvement in social interaction, and improvement in self-esteem.

3. Pharmacological intervention with Tourette's disorder is most effective when it is combined with other forms of therapy, such as education and supportive intervention, individual counseling or psychotherapy, and family therapy. The most common medications used are:

a. Haloperidol (Haldol). Because of the severe side effects, this medication should be reserved for children with severe symptoms or with symptoms that impede their ability to function in school, socially, or with the family setting.

b. Pimozide (Orap). Similar in response rate and side effect profile to haloperidol. Used only with severe cases. Not recommended for children under age 12.

c. Clonidine (Catapres). Sometimes used as drug of first choice because of few side effects. Results of studies on the efficacy of clonidine in the treatment of Tourette's disorder have been mixed.

VIII. Separation anxiety disorder

A. Essential feature of this disorder is excessive anxiety concerning separation from the home or from those to whom the person is attached.

B. Predisposing factors

1. Biological influences

a. Genetics. Studies show that a greater number of children with relatives who manifest anxiety problems develop anxiety disorders themselves than do children with no such family patterns.

b. Temperament. It is believed that certain individuals inherit a "disposition" toward developing anxiety disorders.

2. Environmental influences

a. Stressful life events. It is thought that children who are already predisposed to developing anxiety disorders may be affected significantly by stressful life events.

3. Family influences

          a.   Possible overattachment to the mother

          b.   Separation conflicts between parent and child

          c.   Families that are very close-knit

          d.   Overprotection by parents

          e.   Transfer of fears and anxieties from parents to child through role modeling

C.   Application of the nursing process

    1.   Background assessment data (symptomatology)

          a.   Onset of separation anxiety disorder may occur as early as preschool age, rarely as late as adolescence.

          b.   Child has difficulty separating from mother.

          c.   Separation results in tantrums, crying, screaming, complaints of physical problems, and "clinging" behaviors.

          d.   School reluctance or refusal.

          e.   Fear of sleeping away from home.

          f.   Fear of harm to self or attachment figure.

          g.   Nightmares may occur.

          h.   Phobias and depressed mood are not uncommon.

    2.   Nursing intervention is aimed at maintaining anxiety at moderate level or below; improvement in social interaction; and development of adaptive coping strategies that prevent maladaptive symptoms of anxiety in response to separation from attachment figure.

IX.   Summary

X.   Critical Thinking Exercise

XI.   Review Questions

ANSWERS TO CRITICAL THINKING EXERCISE

1. Assessment data: behavior unmanageable, yells, interrupts, is physically aggressive, cannot sit still, jumps from topic to topic, no insight into his own behavior, refusing to cooperate.

2. Risk for violence toward others.

3. Noncompliance and defensive coping.

CASE STUDIES FOR USE WITH STUDENT LEARNING

Case Study No. 1: Autistic Disorder*

Seth, age 3, is the third child (and only boy) of Tom and Sue. He has been referred to a psychiatrist by their family physician at the request of the parents. Sue reports that she had a very difficult delivery of Seth, and he had needed oxygen at birth. Tom and Sue report that, from the very beginning, Seth has been "different" from their other children, who have always enjoyed social interaction. Seth has tended to be aloof with a lack of response to social contact. When left with a babysitter, he often screams much of the time. His speech is limited and often confusing. For example, he often echoes words and phrases he hears or has heard in the past. He may state, "Do you want to eat?" to indicate that he is hungry. His words are monotonistic and carry little, if any, inflection. He is fascinated by two things: objects that turn and music. He loves to listen to music and often dances in circles when listening. He has a favorite spinning top that he likes to carry around with him at all times. He is an expert at putting together jigsaw puzzles. He also likes to distribute kitchen utensils (particularly those with spinning parts) to various places around the house, and retrieval by Mom for their original use may precipitate temper tantrums lasting an hour or more, with screaming, kicking, and biting of himself or others. Restoration of the status quo, playing his favorite music, or a long car ride is often the only way to interrupt these tantrums. The psychiatrist admits Seth to the child psychiatric unit with a diagnosis of autistic disorder. Design a nursing plan of care for Seth.

---

    *Adapted from Spitzer, R. L., et al. (1994). *DSM-IV Case Book*. Washington, D.C.: American Psychiatric Press.

Case Study No. 2: Attention-Deficit Hyperactivity Disorder*

Frankie is a 9-year-old boy who, according to his teacher, is constantly "into everything." He keeps the class in an uproar, and has been suspended from school three times this year, most recently for swinging from a light fixture. He wanders around the classroom talking to all the children, so that not only does Frankie not accomplish *his* work, the other students cannot complete *theirs* either. Frankie's mother reports that Frankie's behavior has been difficult since he was a toddler, when he became unbearably restless and demanding. He slept very little and "got into everything." When he was 4-years-old, he was rejected by a preschool because of his difficult behavior. He has few friends because he is unable to participate in fair play. He is unable to watch TV or participate in games that require quiet concentration. His activities at home essentially include riding his bike or playing outdoors with his dog. His room stays messy and he is destructive of his possessions. The psychiatrist admits Frankie to the child psychiatric unit with a diagnosis of ADHD. He orders initiation of therapy with methylphenidate (Ritalin). Design a nursing plan of care for Frankie.

---

    *Adapted from Spitzer, R.L. et al. (1994). *DSM-IV Case Book*. Washington, D.C.:American Psychiatric Press.

LEARNING ACTIVITY

DISORDERS OF INFANCY, CHILDHOOD, OR ADOLESCENCE

Match the disorders listed on the left to the behaviors associated with each on the right.

____	1. Mild mental retardation	a.	Has no capacity for independent functioning, IQ below 20
____	2. Autistic disorder	b.	Violates the rights of others and societal norms and rules. Displays physical aggression and inability to control anger
____	3. Moderate mental retardation	c.	Displays negativistic and defiant behavior, including obstinacy, procrastination, disobedience, resistance to change and authority
____	4. Conduct Disorder	d.	May be trained in elementary hygiene skills. Requires complete supervision. Has IQ of 20 to 34
____	5. Severe mental retardation	e.	Characterized by withdrawal of the child into the self and into a fantasy world of his or her own creation
____	6. Separation anxiety disorder	f.	Shows developmentally inappropriate degrees of inattention, impulsiveness, and hyperactivity
____	7. ADHD	g.	Screams and throws temper tantrums at anticipated separation from mother. Fears harm to self or mother
____	8. Tourette's disorder	h.	Is capable of developing social skills and independent living, with assistance. Has IQ of 50 to 70
____	9. Oppositional defiant disorder	i.	Has multiple motor tics and one or more vocal tics.
____	10. Profound mental retardation	j.	Is capable of academic skill to second grade level. IQ 35 to 49.

CHAPTER 22. TEST QUESTIONS

1. Glenda, diagnosed as mentally retarded, recently scored 47 on IQ testing. Her parents have called a local agency that serves the developmentally disabled and asked for advice regarding Glenda's potential. Which of the following statements from the nurse who counsels them is the *best* estimate of Glenda's eventual level of development?
   a. "Glenda may develop minimal verbal skills."
   • b. "Glenda may be able to work at an unskilled job."
   c. "Glenda may eventually function at about a sixth-grade level."
   d. "Glenda will require constant supervision and care."

2. The nurse counselor develops a long-term plan for Glenda, based on nursing diagnoses appropriate to her potential level of function. Which of the following nursing diagnoses is *most appropriate* for Glenda?
   • a. Self-care deficit related to lack of maturity
   b. Impaired social interaction related to speech difficulties
   c. Risk for injury related to aggressive behavior
   d. Altered growth and development related to inadequate environmental stimulation

3. Tommy, age 9, has been diagnosed with autistic disorder. The cause of this disorder is thought to be:
   a. Refrigerator parents
   b. Fragile X syndrome
   c. Increased glucose metabolism
   • d. Unknown

4. A psychiatric nurse frequently visits Tommy and his family, who also have a second son, Ronnie, age 3. Which of the following behaviors would the nurse regard as age-appropriate and *not* indicative of autistic disorder?
   a. Intense fascination with fans
   • b. Parallel play
   c. Lack of eye contact
   d. Drinking large quantities of fluid

5. Tommy's mother tells the psychiatric nurse that Ronnie is in constant motion and is unable to sit long enough to listen to a story or even to watch TV. She asks the nurse if she thinks he could be "hyperactive." The nurse's *best* response is:
   a. "I wouldn't worry about it."
   b. "It's certainly possible."
   • c. "It's hard to tell with a 3-year-old."
   d. "Why would you think that?"

6. Which of the following factors would prompt the nurse to continue to evaluate Ronnie for ADHD?
   a. Ronnie's father smokes.
   • b. Ronnie was born 7 weeks prematurely.
   c. Ronnie develops hives when he eats food with red food coloring added.
   d. Ronnie has a cousin on his father's side who has ADHD.

7. Calming effects on hyperactive children have been found to occur with the administration of which of the following classifications of medications?
   • a. CNS stimulants
   b. CNS depressants
   c. Nonsterioidal anti-inflammatory drugs
   d. Antimanic drugs, such as lithium

8. A potential side effect from prolonged use of methylphenidate (Ritalin) is which of the following?
    a. Psychosis
    b. Decreased intelligence
    c. Dry mouth and sore throat
•   d. Decrease in rate of growth and development

9. The *primary* nursing intervention in working with a child with a conduct disorder is to:
    a. Plan activities that provide opportunities for success
    b. Give the child unconditional acceptance for good behaviors that occur
•   c. Recognize behaviors that precede the onset of aggression and intervene before violence occurs
    d. Provide immediate positive feedback for acceptable and unacceptable behaviors

10. Which of the following classes of medications is effective in the treatment of Tourette's disorder?
•   a. Neuroleptics
    b. Antimanics
    c. Tricyclic antidepressants
    d. Monoamine oxidase inhibitors

11. In providing care for the adolescent with an overanxious disorder, the *primary* goal of the nurse is:
    a. To set very strict limits on what behavior can be tolerated
    b. To make the adolescent aware of the outcome of his or her desire to excel
•   c. To establish an atmosphere of calm trust and unconditional acceptance
    d. To accept all "nervous habit" behavior and extinguish somatic symptoms

12. The essential feature that distinguishes ODD from other disorders is:
    a. Gender ratio
•   b. Passive-aggressiveness
    c. Violence toward others
    d. The role of genetic predisposition

CHAPTER 23. DELIRIUM, DEMENTIA, AND AMNESTIC DISORDERS

CHAPTER FOCUS

The focus of this chapter is on predisposing factors, symptomatology, and nursing interventions for the care of clients with delirium, dementia, and amnestic disorders. These disorders were identified in previous editions of the *Diagnostic and Statistical Manual of Mental Disorders (DSM)* as organic mental syndromes and disorders.

LEARNING OBJECTIVES

After reading this chapter, the student will be able to:

1. Define and differentiate among *delirium, dementia,* and *amnestic disorders.*
2. Discuss predisposing factors implicated in the etiology of delirium, dementia, and amnestic disorders.
3. Identify symptomatology and use the information to assess clients with delirium, dementia, and amnestic disorders.
4. Identify nursing diagnoses common to clients with delirium, dementia, and amnestic disorders, and select appropriate nursing interventions for each.
5. Identify topics for client and family teaching relevant to these disorders.
6. Discuss relevant criteria for evaluating nursing care of clients with delirium, dementia, and amnestic disorders.
7. Describe various treatment modalities relevant to care of clients with delirium, dementia, and amnestic disorders.

KEY TERMS

aphasia
praxia
delirium
dementia
ataxia
amnesia
pseudodementia
confabulation
primary dementia
secondary dementia
sundowning

CHAPTER OUTLINE/LECTURE NOTES

I. Introduction
   A. This chapter discusses disorders in which a clinically significant deficit in cognition or memory exists, representing a significant change from a previous level of functioning.
   B. The numbers of individuals with these disorders is growing because more people now survive into the high-risk period for dementia, which is middle age and beyond.
II. Delirium

A. It is characterized by a disturbance of consciousness and a change in cognition that develop rapidly over a short period.
B. Symptoms include:
   1. Difficulty sustaining and shifting attention
   2. Extreme distractibility
   3. Disorganized thinking
   4. Speech that is rambling, irrelevant, pressured, and incoherent
   5. Impaired reasoning ability and goal-directed behavior
   6. Disorientation to time and place
   7. Impairment of recent memory
   8. Misperceptions of the environment, including illusions and hallucinations
   9. Disturbance in level of consciousness, with interruption of the sleep-wake cycle
   10. Psychomotor activity that fluctuates between agitation and restlessness and a vegetative state
   11. Emotional instability
   12. Autonomic manifestations, such as tachycardia, sweating, flushed face, dilated pupils, and elevated blood pressure
C. Delirium usually begins abruptly, such as following a head injury or seizure. It can have a slower onset if the underlying etiology is systemic illness or metabolic imbalance.
D. Duration is usually brief (e.g., 1 week; rarely more than 1 month) and subsides completely upon recovery from the underlying determinant.
E. Predisposing factors:
   1. Delirium due to a general medical condition, such as systemic infections, metabolic disorders (e.g., hypoxia, hypercarbia, and hypoglycemia), fluid or electrolyte imbalances, hepatic or renal disease, thiamine deficiency, postoperative states, hypertensive encephalopathy, postictal states, and sequelae of head trauma.
   2. Substance-induced delirium. Symptoms are attributed to side effects of analgesics, anticonvulsants, antiparkinsonian agents, neuroleptics, sedative-hypnotics, anxiolytics, antidepressants, cardiovascular medications, anticoagulants, antineoplastics, respiratory drugs, hormones, and diuretics.
   3. Substance-intoxication delirium. Symptoms may occur following ingestion of high doses of cannabis, cocaine, hallucinogens, alcohol, anxiolytics, or narcotics.
   4. Substance-withdrawal delirium. Withdrawal delirium symptoms develop after reduction or termination of sustained, usually high-dose use of certain substances such as alcohol, sedatives, hypnotics, or anxiolytics.
   5. Delirium due to multiple etiologies. The delirium symptoms may be related to more than one general medical condition or to the combined effects of a general medical condition and substance use.

III. Dementia
A. It is defined as a syndrome of acquired, persistent intellectual impairment with compromised function in multiple spheres of mental activity, such as memory, language, visuospatial skills, emotion or personality, and cognition.
B. Dementias can be classified as either primary or secondary.
   1. Primary—the dementia itself is the major sign of some organic brain disease, such as Alzheimer's disease
   6. Secondary—the dementia is caused by, or related to, another disease or condition, such as HIV disease or a cerebral trauma
C. Symptoms include:
   1. Impairment in abstract thinking, judgment, and impulse control
   2. Disregard for the conventional rules of social conduct
   3. Neglect of personal appearance and hygiene
   4. Language may or may not be affected
   5. Personality change is common
D. Truly reversible dementia occurs in only 2% to 3% of cases and is determined by the underlying pathology and timely application of effective treatment.

E. As the disease progresses, symptoms may include:
1. Aphasia (absence of speech).
2. Apraxia (inability to carry out motor activities despite intact motor functioning).
3. Irritability and moodiness, with sudden outbursts over trivial issues.
4. Inability to care for personal needs independently.
5. Wandering away from the home may become a problem
6. Incontinence.
F. Dementia of the Alzheimer's type (DAT) accounts for about 70% of all cases of dementia. DAT progresses according to stages.
1. Stage 1: No apparent symptoms.
2. Stage 2: Forgetfulness. Experiences loss of short-term memory. Anxiety and depression common.
3. Stage 3: Early confusion. Has difficulty concentrating. Individual may become lost while driving.
4. Stage 4: Late confusion. Forgets important dates. Unable to perform tasks or understand current events. May use confabulation.
5. Stage 5: Early dementia. Unable to perform activities of daily living independently. May forget names of close relatives. Requires assistance to manage on an ongoing basis.
6. Stage 6: Middle dementia. May be unable to recall recent major life events, or even name of spouse. Disoriented to time and place. Incontinence, agitation; and sleeping may be a problem. Wandering is common. Institutional care is usually required at this time.
7. Stage 7: Late dementia. Unable to recognize family. Commonly bedfast and aphasic.
G. Predisposing factors
1. DAT
   a. Onset is slow and insidious and the course of the disorder is generally progressive and deteriorating.
   b. Definitive diagnosis requires biopsy or autopsy examination of brain tissue.
   c. Etiologies may include:
      (1) Acetylcholine alterations
      (2) Accumulation of aluminum
      (3) Alterations in the immune system
      (4) Head trauma
      (5) Genetic factors
2. Vascular dementia
   a. Dementia is due to significant cerebrovascular disease (significant number of small strokes).
   b. More abrupt onset than Alzheimer's disease, and course is more variable.
   c. Etiologies may include:
      (1) Arterial hypertension
      (2) Cerebral emboli
      (3) Cerebral thrombosis
3. Dementia due to HIV disease
   a. Dementia is due to brain infections by opportunistic organisms or by the HIV-1 virus directly.
   b. Symptoms may range from barely perceptible changes to acute delirium to profound dementia.
4. Dementia due to head trauma
   a. Posttrauma symptoms include headache, irritability, dizziness, diminished concentration, and hypersensitivity to certain stimuli. Intellectual functioning and memory may also be impaired.
5. Dementia due to Parkinson's disease
   a. It is caused by a loss of nerve cells located in the substantia nigra and a decrease in dopamine activity.
   b. Cerebral changes in dementia of Parkinson's disease sometimes resemble those of Alzheimer's disease.
6. Dementia due to Huntington's disease
   a. Damage from this disease occurs in the areas of the basal ganglia and the cerebral cortex.
   b. A profound state of dementia and ataxia occur within 5 to 10 years of onset.
7. Dementia due to Pick's disease

        a.   Pathology results from atrophy in the frontal and temporal lobes of the brain.

        b.   Clinical picture is very similar to that of Alzheimer's disease.

    8.   Dementia due to Creutzfeldt-Jacob disease

        a.   Onset of symptoms occurs between ages 40 and 60, and course is extremely rapid, with progressive deterioration and death within 1 year.

        b.   Etiology is thought to be a transmissible agent known as a "slow virus." Five to 15 percent of cases have a genetic component.

    9.   Dementia due to other general medical conditions

        a.   Other medical conditions that can cause dementia include:

           (1) Endocrine conditions

           (2) Pulmonary disease

           (3) Hepatic or renal failure

           (4) Cardiopulmonary insufficiency

           (5) Fluid and electrolyte imbalances

           (6) Nutritional deficiencies

           (7) Frontal or temporal lobe lesions

           (8) Central nervous system or systemic infections

           (9) Uncontrolled epilepsy

           (10) Other neurological conditions, such as multiple sclerosis

  10. Substance-induced persisting dementia

        a.   Dementia is related to the persisting effects of use of substances such as:

           (1) Alcohol

           (2) Inhalants

           (3) Sedatives, hypnotics, and anxiolytics

           (4) Medications, such as anticonvulsants and intrathecal methotrexate

           (5) Toxins, such as lead, mercury, carbon monoxide, organophosphate insecticides, and industrial solvents

  11. Dementia due to multiple etiologies

        a.   This diagnosis is used when the symptoms are attributed to more than one etiology.

IV. Amnestic Disorders

  A. Amnestic disorders are characterized by an inability to learn new information (short-term memory deficit) despite normal attention, and an inability to recall previously learned information (long-term memory deficit)

  B. Other symptoms include:

    1.   Disorientation to place and time (rarely to self)

    2.   Confabulation—the creation of imaginary events to fill in memory gaps

    3.   Denial that a problem exists, or acknowledgement that a problem exists, but with a lack of concern

    4.   Apathy, lack of initiative, and emotional blandness

  C. Onset may be acute or insidious, depending on the underlying pathological process.

  D. Duration and course may be quite variable and are also correlated with an extent and severity of the cause.

  E. Predisposing factors:

    1.   Amnestic disorders due to a general medical condition. Medical conditions that may be associated with amnestic disorder include:

        a.   Head trauma

        b.   Cerebrovascular disease

        c.   Cerebral neoplastic disease

        d.   Cerebral anoxia

        e.   Herpes simplex encephalitis

        f.   Poorly controlled insulin-dependant diabetes

        g.   Surgical intervention to the brain

    2.   Transient amnestic syndromes can occur from:

        a.   Epileptic seizures

        b.   Electroconvulsive therapy
        c.   Severe migraine headache
        d.   Drug overdose

    3.   Substance-induced persisting amnestic disorder. The amnestic symptoms are related to the persisting effects of the use of the following substances:
        a.   Alcohol
        b.   Sedatives, hypnotics, and anxiolytics
        c.   Medication, such as anticonvulsants and intrathecal methotrexate
        d.   Toxins, such as lead, mercury, carbon monoxide, organophosphate insecticides, and industrial solvents

V.   Application of the Nursing Process
  A.   The client history
    1.   The following areas of concern should be addressed:
        a.   Type, frequency, and severity of mood swings
        b.   Personality and behavioral changes
        c.   Catastrophic emotional reactions
        d.   Cognitive changes
        e.   Language difficulties
        f.   Orientation to person, place, time, and situation
        g.   Appropriateness of social behavior
        h.   Current and past use of medications
        i.   Current and past use of drugs and alcohol
        j.   Possible exposure to toxins
        k.   Client/family history of specific illnesses
  B.   Physical assessment
    1.   Assessment for diseases of various organ systems that can induce confusion, loss of memory, and behavioral changes
    2.   Neurological examination to assess mental status, alertness, muscle strength, reflexes, sensory perception, language skills, and coordination
    3.   Psychological tests to differentiate between dementia and pseudodementia (depression)
  C.   Diagnostic laboratory evaluations
    1.   Possible laboratory evaluations include blood and urine evaluations to test for:
        a.   Various infections
        b.   Hepatic and renal dysfunction
        c.   Diabetes or hypoglycemia
        d.   Electrolyte imbalances
        e.   Metabolic and endocrine disorders
        f.   Nutritional deficiencies
        g.   Presence of toxic substances, including alcohol and drugs
    2.   Other diagnostic evaluations may include:
        a.   Electroencephalogram
        b.   Computed tomography scan
        c.   Positron emission tomography
        d.   Magnetic resonance imaging (MRI)
        e.   Lumbar puncture to examine cerebrospinal fluid
  B.   Diagnosis/outcome identification
    1.   Common nursing diagnoses for the client with cognitive dysfunction include:
        a.   Risk for trauma
        b.   Risk for self-directed violence
        c.   Risk for violence toward others
        d.   Altered thought processes
        e.   Self-esteem disturbance
        f.   Self-care deficit

C. Planning/implementation
D. Client/family education
E. Evaluation
VI. Medical treatment modalities
  A. Delirium
    1. Determination and correction of the underlying causes.
    2. Staff should remain with client at all times to monitor behavior and provide reorientation and assurance.
    3. Room with low level of stimuli.
    4. Low-dose neuroleptics (e.g., haloperidol) to relieve agitation and aggression.
  B. Dementia
    1. Primary consideration is given to etiology, with focus on identification and resolution of potentially reversible processes.
    2. A number of pharmaceutical agents have been tried with varying degrees of success in the treatment of dementia. They include:
      a. For cognitive impairment:
        (1) Physotigmine (Antilirium)
        (2) Cyclandelate (Cyclan)
        (3) Ergoloid mesylate (Hydergine)
        (4) Tacrine (Cognex)
        (5) Donepezil (Aricept)
      b. For agitation, aggression, hallucinations, thought disturbances, and wandering:
        (1) Thiothizene (Navane)
        (2) Chlorpromazine (Thorazine)
        (3) Thioridazine (Mellaril)
        (4) Haloperidol (Haldol)
      c. For depression:
        (1) Amitriptyline (Elavil)
        (2) Desipramine (Norpramine)
        (3) Doxepin (Adapin)
        (4) Imipramine (Tofranil)
        (5) Trazodone (Desyrel)
        (6) Bupropion (Wellbutrin)
      d. For anxiety (these medications should not be used routinely or for prolonged periods):
        (1) Diazepam (Valium)
        (2) Chlordiazepoxide (Librium)
        (3) Alprazolam (Xanax)
        (4) Lorazepam (Ativan)
        (5) Oxazepam (Serax)
      e. For sleep disturbances (for short-term therapy only):
        (1) Flurazepam (Dalmane)
        (2) Temazepam (Restoril)
        (3) Triazolam (Halcion)
VII. Summary
VIII. Critical Thinking Exercise
IX. Review Questions

ANSWERS TO CRITICAL THINKING EXERCISE

1. Anxiety, confusion, disorientation, physically abusive, suspiciousness

2. Risk for trauma related to confusion and disorientation

3. Outcomes would be based on short-term goals. Because the disease is progressive, it would be unrealistic to expect resolution, so a series of step-objectives would be used. For example:

   Goal: Joe will not harm himself in his confused state.

   Outcome criteria:
   1. Joe is allowed to wander in a safe, enclosed area.
   2. Joe is able to find his room with the aid of a large sign on the door that identifies it by name.

   Goal: Joe will be able to perform self-care needs with assistance.

   Outcome criteria:
   1. Joe washes his face with supplies provided by nurse.
   2. Joe dresses himself with step-instructions from the nurse.
   3. Joe straightens up his room with direction from the nurse.

CASE STUDY FOR USE WITH STUDENT LEARNING:

Case Study: Dementia of the Alzheimer's Type

Gary received a call at work recently from the police in the small town where he lived and worked. They told him that they had picked up his father, George, age 69, whom they found wandering about 10 blocks from his home. George told the police he did not remember where he lived. George, a former banker in the small town, was well known to most of the citizens. Gary retrieved his father from the police station and took him home. He and his mother made an appointment to have George evaluated. George's wife reported to the physician that George had grown progressively more forgetful over the last few years; however, they had just been laughing it off as "old age." A physical examination and MRI were conducted, resulting with the physician's diagnosis of dementia of the Alzheimer's type. A home health nurse was assigned as case manager for George and his wife to manage the progression of his illness. Design a plan of care in the management of George's illness by the nursing case manager.

LEARNING ACTIVITY

DELIRIUM, DEMENTIA, AND AMNESTIC DISORDERS

Check whether the behaviors described on the left are characteristic of delirium, dementia, or amnestic disorder.

	Delirium	Dementia	Amnestic Disorder
1. Duration of the disorder is commonly brief.	_____	_____	_____
2. Client uses confabulation to hide cognitive deficits.	_____	_____	_____
3. Symptoms may be confused with depression.	_____	_____	_____
4. It can be caused by a series of small strokes.	_____	_____	_____
5. It is commonly reversible.	_____	_____	_____
6. Denial that a problem exists is common.	_____	_____	_____
7. Level of consciousness is affected.	_____	_____	_____
8. Reversibility occurs in only 2% to 3% of cases.	_____	_____	_____
9. Severe migraine headache can cause transient symptoms.	_____	_____	_____
10. Personality change is common.	_____	_____	_____
11. Illusions and hallucinations are common symptoms.	_____	_____	_____
12. Symptoms can occur as a result of cocaine intoxication.	_____	_____	_____
13. Symptoms can occur as a result of alcohol withdrawal.	_____	_____	_____
14. High concentrations of aluminum in the brain have been implicated in the etiology of this disorder.	_____	_____	_____
15. Transient symptoms of this disorder can occur following electroconvulsive therapy.	_____	_____	_____

CHAPTER 23. TEST QUESTIONS

Gloria visits her Aunt Naomi about twice a year. Naomi is 74-years-old and lives in a city about 300 miles away from Gloria. During her most recent visit, Gloria notices that her aunt has become quite forgetful. Two days' worth of mail are still in the mailbox, and Naomi has forgotten to have her prescription for her antihypertensive medication refilled. There is very little food in the house, and Naomi is unable to tell Gloria when or what she last ate. Gloria calls Naomi's physician, who has Naomi hospitalized for evaluation.

1. The physician diagnoses Naomi with dementia. From the information given, which of the following types of dementia does Naomi have?
    a. DAT
    • b. Vascular dementia
    c. Dementia due to head trauma
    d. Dementia due to Parkinson's disease

2. Which of the following statements is *true* about this type of dementia?
    a. It is reversible.
    b. It is characterized by plaques and tangles in the brain.
    c. It exhibits a gradual, progressive deterioration.
    • d. It exhibits a fluctuating pattern of deterioration.

3. The physician orders cyclandelate (Cyclan) for Naomi. The rationale for this order is:
    • a. To enhance circulation to the brain
    b. To elevate levels of acetylcholine in the brain
    c. To control aggressive behavior
    d. To prevent depression

4. Which of the following nursing diagnoses would be a *priority* for the nurse caring for Naomi?
    a. Altered thought processes
    b. Self-care deficit
    • c. Risk for trauma
    d. Risk for violence toward others

5. The physician tells Gloria that it is not safe for Naomi to return to live alone in her home, so arrangements are made for Naomi to move into a nursing home. Naomi becomes very depressed and withdrawn. The physician believes Naomi would benefit from an antidepressant medication. Which of the following is an example of an antidepressant that the physician may prescribe for Naomi?
    a. haloperidol (Haldol)
    b. tacrine (Cognex)
    • c. amitriptyline (Elavil)
    d. diazepam (Valium)

CHAPTER 24. SUBSTANCE-RELATED DISORDERS

CHAPTER FOCUS

The focus of this chapter is on the physical and behavioral manifestations and personal and social consequences for the individual who abuses or is dependent upon substances. Predisposing factors are discussed, and the role of the nurse in the care of these clients is emphasized.

LEARNING OBJECTIVES

After reading this chapter, the student will be able to:

1. Define *abuse, dependence, intoxication,* and *withdrawal.*
2. Discuss predisposing factors implicated in the etiology of substance-related disorders.
3. Identify symptomatology and use the information in assessment of clients with various substance-use disorders and substance-induced disorders.
4. Identify nursing diagnoses common to clients with substance-use disorders and substance-induced disorders, and select appropriate nursing interventions for each.
5. Identify topics for client and family teaching relevant to substance-use disorders and substance-induced disorders.
6. Describe relevant criteria for evaluating nursing care of clients with substance-use disorders and substance-induced disorders.
7. Discuss the issue of substance-related disorders within the profession of nursing.
8. Define codependency and identify behavioral characteristics associated with the disorder.
9. Discuss treatment of codependency.
10. Describe various modalities relevant to treatment of individuals with substance-use disorders and substance-induced disorders.

KEY TERMS

amphetamines
cannabis
opioids
phencyclidine
abuse
dependence
Wernicke's encephalopathy
Korsakoff's psychosis

esophageal varices
hepatic encephalopathy
peer assistance programs
codependence
Alcoholics Anonymous
disulfiram
substitution therapy
detoxification
ascites

CHAPTER OUTLINE/LECTURE NOTES

I. Introduction
    A. Substance-related disorders are composed of two groups:
        1. Substance-use disorders
            a. Abuse
            b. Dependence

2. Substance-induced disorders (only intoxication and withdrawal are discussed in this chapter)
   a. Intoxication
   b. Withdrawal
   c. Delirium
   d. Dementia
   e. Amnesia
   f. Psychosis
   g. Mood disorder
   h. Anxiety disorder
   i. Sexual dysfunction
   j. Sleep disorders
   B. Some illegal substances have achieved a degree of social acceptance by various subcultural groups within our society.
II. Substance-Use Disorders
   A. Substance abuse. *DSM-IV* criteria for substance abuse:
      1. Recurrent substance use resulting in a failure to fulfill major role obligations at work, school, or home
      2. Recurrent substance use in situations in which it is physically hazardous
      3. Recurrent substance-related legal problems
      4. Continued substance use despite having persistent or recurrent social or interpersonal problems caused or exacerbated by the effects of the substance
   B. Substance dependence
      1. Physical dependence is manifested by the need for increasing amounts to produce the desired effects and a syndrome of withdrawal upon cessation.
      2. Psychological dependence exists when an individual believes that use of a substance is necessary to maintain an optimal state of personal well-being, interpersonal relations, or skill performance.
      3. *DSM-IV* criteria for substance dependence include:
         a. Evidence of tolerance, as defined by either of the following:
            (1) A need for markedly increased amounts of the substance to achieve intoxication or desired effects
            (2) Markedly diminished effect with continued use of the same amount of the substance
         b. Evidence of withdrawal symptoms, as manifested by either of the following:
            (1) The characteristic withdrawal syndrome for the substance.
            (2) The same (or a closely related) substance is taken to relieve or avoid withdrawal symptoms.
         c. The substance is often taken in larger amounts or over a longer period than was intended.
         d. There is a persistent desire or unsuccessful efforts to cut down or control substance use.
         e. Much time is spent in activities necessary to obtain the substance, use the substance, or recover from its effects.
         f. Important social, occupational, or recreational activities are given up or reduced because of substance use.
         g. The substance use is continued despite knowledge of having a persistent or recurrent physical or psychological problem that is likely to have been caused or exacerbated by the substance.
III. Substance-Induced Disorders
   A. Substance intoxication. *DSM-IV* criteria include:
      1. The development of a reversible substance-specific syndrome caused by recent ingestion of (or exposure to) a substance.
      2. Clinically significant maladaptive behavior or psychological changes that are due to the effect of the substance on the central nervous system and develop during or shortly after use of the substance.
      3. The symptoms are not due to a general medical condition and are not better accounted for by another mental disorder.
   B. Substance withdrawal. *DSM-IV* criteria include:
      1. The development of a substance-specific syndrome caused by the cessation of (or reduction in) heavy and prolonged substance use.

2. The substance-specific syndrome causes clinically significant distress or impairment in social, occupational, or other important areas of functioning.
3. The symptoms are not due to a general medical condition and are not better accounted for by another mental disorder.

IV. Classes of Psychoactive Substances
    A. Alcohol
    B. Amphetamines and related substances
    C. Caffeine
    D. Cannabis
    E. Cocaine
    F. Hallucinogens
    G. Inhalants
    H. Nicotine
    I. Opioids
    J. Phencyclidine and related substances
    K. Sedatives, hypnotics, or anxiolytics

V. Predisposing Factors
    A. Biological factors
        1. Genetics. Apparent hereditary factor, particularly with alcoholism.
        2. Biochemical. Alcohol may produce morphinelike substances in the brain that are responsible for alcohol addiction.
    B. Psychological factors
        1. Developmental influences. They may relate to severe ego impairment and disturbances in the sense of self.
        2. Personality factors. Certain personality traits have been suggested to play a part in both the development and maintenance of alcohol dependence. They include impulsivity, negative self-concept, weak ego, low social conformity, neuroticism, and introversion.
    C. Sociocultural factors
        1. Social learning. Children and adolescents are more likely to use substances if they have parents who provide a model for substance use. Use of substances may also be promoted within one's peer group.
        2. Conditioning. Pleasurable effects from substance use act as a positive reinforcement for their continued use.
        3. Cultural and ethnic Influences. Some cultures are more prone to use of substances than others.

VI. The Dynamics of Substance-Related Disorders
    A. Alcohol abuse and dependence
        1. A profile of the substance
        2. Historical aspects
        3. Patterns of use/abuse
            a. Phase I. The Prealcoholic Phase
            b. Phase II. The Early Alcoholic Phase
            c. Phase III. The Crucial Phase
            d. Phase IV. The Chronic Phase
        4. Effects on the body
            a. Peripheral neuropathy
            b. Alcoholic myopathy
            c. Wernicke's encephalopathy
            d. Korsakoff's psychosis
            e. Alcoholic cardiomyopathy
            f. Esophagitis
            g. Gastritis
            h. Pancreatitis
            i. Alcoholic hepatitis
            j. Cirrhosis of the liver

        (1) Portal hypertension

        (2) Ascites

        (3) Esophageal varices

        (4) Hepatic encephalopathy

      k. Leukopenia

      l. Thrombocytopenia

      m. Sexual dysfunction

B. Alcohol intoxication

    1. Occurs at blood alcohol levels between 100 and 200 mg/dL

C. Alcohol withdrawal

    1. Occurs within 4 to 12 hours of cessation of or reduction in heavy and prolonged alcohol use

D. Sedative, hypnotic, or anxiolytic abuse and dependence

    1. A profile of the substance

        a. Barbiturates

        b. Nonbarbiturate hypnotics

        c. Antianxiety agents

    2. Historical aspects

    3. Patterns of use/abuse

    4. Effects on the body

        a. Effects on sleep and dreaming

        b. Respiratory depression

        c. Cardiovascular effects

        d. Renal function

        e. Hepatic effects

        f. Body temperature

        g. Sexual functioning

E. Sedative, hypnotic, or anxiolytic intoxication

    1. Intoxication with these central nervous system (CNS) depressants can range from disinhibition and aggressiveness to coma and death (with increasing dosages of the drug).

F. Sedative, Hypnotic, or Anxiolytic Withdrawal

    1. Onset of symptoms depends on the half-life of the drug from which the individual is withdrawing.

    2. Severe withdrawal from CNS depressants can be life threatening.

G. CNS stimulant abuse and dependence

    1. A profile of the substance

        a. Amphetamines

        b. Nonamphetamine stimulants

        c. Cocaine

        d. Caffeine

        e. Nicotine

    2. Historical aspects

    3. Patterns of use/abuse

    4. Effects on the body

        a. CNS effects

        b. Cardiovascular/pulmonary effects

        c. Gastrointestinal and renal effects

        d. Sexual functioning

H. CNS stimulant intoxication

    1. Amphetamine and cocaine intoxication produces euphoria, impaired judgment, confusion, changes in vital signs (even coma or death, depending on amount consumed).

    2. Intoxication from caffeine usually occurs following consumption in excess of 250 mg. Restlessness and insomnia are the most common symptoms.

I. CNS stimulant withdrawal

1. Withdrawal from amphetamines and cocaine may include dysphoria, fatigue, sleep disturbances, and increased appetite.
2. Withdrawal from caffeine may include headache, fatigue, anxiety, and nausea and vomiting.
3. Withdrawal from nicotine may include dysphoria, anxiety, difficulty concentrating, restlessness, and increased appetite.
J. Opioid abuse and dependence
   1. A profile of the substance
      a. Opioids of natural origin
      b. Opioid derivatives
      c. Synthetic opiatelike drugs
   2. Historical aspects
   3. Patterns of use/abuse
   4. Effects on the body
      a. CNS
      b. Gastrointestinal effects
      c. Cardiovascular effects
      d. Sexual functioning
K. Opioid intoxication
   1. Symptoms are consistent with the half-life of most opioid drugs, and usually last for several hours.
   2. Severe opioid intoxication can lead to respiratory depression, coma, and death.
L. Opioid withdrawal
   1. Symptoms occur within 6 to 24 hours after the last dose, peak within 1 to 3 days, and gradually subside over a period of 5 to 7 days (differing according to drug half-life).
   2. Symptoms include nausea, vomiting, diarrhea, abdominal cramping, sweating, fever, dysphoric mood, muscle aches, lacrimation or rhinorrhea, pupillary dilation, yawning, insomnia, and piloerection.
M. Hallucinogen abuse and dependence
   1. A profile of the substance
      a. Naturally occurring hallucinogens
         (1) Mescaline
         (2) Psilocybin and psilocin
         (3) Ololiuqui
      b. Synthetic compounds
         (1) Lysergic acid diethylamide (LSD)
         (2) Dimethyltryptamine
         (3) STP
         (4) Phencyclidine (PCP)
         (5) Designer drugs
   2. Historical aspects
   3. Patterns of use/abuse
   4. Effects on the body
N. Hallucinogen intoxication
   1. It occurs within minutes to a few hours after using the drug.
   2. Symptoms include perceptual alterations, depersonalization, derealization, tachycardia, and palpitations. Symptoms of PCP intoxication also include belligerence, assaultiveness, and may proceed to seizures or coma.
O. Cannabis abuse and dependence
   1. A profile of the substance
      a. Marijuana
      b. Hashish
   2. Historical aspects
   3. Patterns of use/abuse
   4. Effects on the body

　　　　　a.　Cardiovascular effects
　　　　　b.　Respiratory effects
　　　　　c.　Reproductive effects
　　　　　d.　CNS effects
　　　　3.　Sexual functioning
　　P.　Cannabis intoxication
　　　　1.　Symptoms include impaired motor coordination, euphoria, anxiety, a sensation of slowed time, and impaired judgment.
　　　　2.　Impairment of motor skills lasts for 8 to 12 hours.
VII.　Application of the Nursing Process
　　A.　Nurse must begin relationship development with a substance abuser by examining own attitudes and drinking habits.
　　B.　Various assessment tools are available for determining extent of the client's problem with substances:
　　　　1.　Michigan Alcoholism Screening Test
　　　　2.　CAGE Questionnaire
　　C.　Nursing diagnoses are formulated from the data gathered during the assessment phase. Outcome criteria are established for each.
　　D.　Nursing intervention for the client with substance use disorder is aimed at acceptance of use of substances as a problem, acceptance of personal responsibility for use of substances, identification of more adaptive coping strategies, and restoration of nutritional status.
　　E.　Evaluation of care is based upon achievement of the outcome criteria.
VIII.　The Impaired Nurse
　　A.　The American Nurses Association (ANA) has estimated that 6 to 8 percent of nurses use alcohol or other drugs to an extent sufficient to impair their professional performance.
　　B.　Narcotic addiction among nurses has been estimated to be at least 30 times greater than it is among the general population.
　　C.　Clues that may identify an impaired nurse:
　　　　1.　May appear happy or sad
　　　　2.　May have increased appetite or no appetite at all
　　　　3.　May be verbal and energetic, or slow thinking with impaired concentration
　　　　4.　May volunteer to work extra shifts.
　　　　5.　May leave the floor a lot or spend a lot of time in the restroom
　　　　6.　May have more accidents or unusual occurrences reported when impaired nurse is on duty
　　　　7.　More clients may complain of pain and insomnia even though many narcotic analgesics and sedatives have been documented as administered.
　　　　8.　As the impairment progresses, there may be inaccurate drug counts, increased vial breakage and drug wastage, and discrepancies in documentation.
　　　　9.　Lapses in memory may occur.
　　　　10.　Personal appearance and job performance will likely be affected.
　　D.　Peer Assistance Program was developed by the ANA in 1982.
　　　　1.　It assists impaired nurses to recognize their impairment.
　　　　2.　It helps them to obtain necessary treatment
　　　　3.　It helps them to regain accountability within their profession
　　　　4.　Contract is drawn up:
　　　　　a.　To detail method of treatment
　　　　　b.　To establish guidelines for monitoring course of treatment
　　　　5.　Participation usually lasts for a period of 2 years.
IX.　Codependency
　　A.　Defined as an exaggerated dependent pattern of learned behaviors, beliefs, and feelings that make life painful. It is a dependence on people and things outside the self, along with neglect of the self to the point of having little self-identity.
　　B.　Derives self-worth from others.
　　C.　Feels responsible for the happiness of others.

D. Denies that problems exist is common.

E. Keeps feelings in control and releases anxiety in the form of stress-related illnesses or compulsive behaviors, such as eating, spending, working, or using of substances.

F. The codependent nurse
  1. Certain characteristics associated with codependency seem to apply to some nurses, who often have a tendency to fulfill everyone's needs but their own.
    a. Caretaking. Meeting the needs of others to the point of neglecting their own.
    b. Perfectionism. Low self-esteem and fear of failure drive codependent nurses to strive for an unrealistic level of achievement.
    c. Denial. A refusal to acknowledge that any personal problems or painful issues exist.
    d. Poor communication. Codependent nurses rarely express their true feelings.

G. Treating codependence
  1. Stage I: The survival stage. Letting go of the denial that problems exist
  2. Stage II: The reidentification stage. Taking responsibility for own dysfunctional behavior
  3. Stage III. The core issues stage. Facing the fact that relationships cannot be managed by force or will
  4. Stage IV. The reintegration stage. Accepting self and willingness to change

X. Treatment Modalities for Substance-Related Disorders
  A. Alcoholics Anonymous
  B. Various support groups patterned after Alcoholics Anonymous, but for individuals with problems with other substances
  C. Pharmacotherapy
  D. Counseling
  E. Group therapy
  F. Psychopharmacology for substance intoxication and substance withdrawal

XI. Summary

XII. Critical Thinking Exercise

XIII. Review Questions

ANSWERS TO CRITICAL THINKING EXERCISE

1. Risk for self-directed violence.

2. Suicide precautions. Decrease environmental stimuli. Let her sleep as much as she wants. Provide adequate diet to restore nutrition.

3. To help recognize the correlation between taking the drugs and the problems she is having in her life.

LEARNING ACTIVITY

SYMPTOMS ASSOCIATED WITH PSYCHOACTIVE SUBSTANCES

Fill in the spaces provided with the most common examples and symptoms of substance-related disorders of which the nurse should be aware.

Drugs	Symptoms of Use	Symptoms of Intoxication	Symptoms of Withdrawal
CNS depressants Examples:			
CNS stimulants Examples:			
Opioids Examples:			
Hallucinogens Examples:			
Cannabinols Examples:			

CHAPTER 24. TEST QUESTIONS

Situation: Michael, a 47-year-old salesman, is brought to the emergency department at midnight by the police because of aggressive, uninhibited behavior, slurred speech, and impaired motor coordination. His blood alcohol level is found to be 347 mg/dL He is admitted to the alcohol and drug treatment unit for detoxification.

1. At what minimum level of alcohol in the blood is an individual considered intoxicated?
    a. 50 mg/dL
  • b. 100 mg/dL
    c. 200 mg/dL
    d. 300 mg/dL

2. Michael's wife is notified, and she reports to the admitting nurse that Michael's drinking has increased over the last several years. Michael has lately been drinking a pint of bourbon a day, mostly in the evening, but sometimes also during the day. "He usually just comes home from work and drinks until he passes out." She stated that yesterday Michael's boss told him if he did not increase his sales, he would be fired. Michael started drinking in the early afternoon and drank continuously into the night. She did not know what time he left the house. It is now 2 A.M. When might the nurse expect withdrawal symptoms to begin?
  • a. Around 4 to 6 A.M.
    b. Around 10 A.M.
    c. In 2 to 3 days
    d. Around 4 to 6 PM.

3. For what initial withdrawal symptom should the nurse be on the alert?
    a. Suicidal ideation, increased appetite
    b. Lacrimation, rhinorrhea, piloerection
  • c. Tremors, tachycardia, sweating
    d. Belligerence, assaultiveness

4. What would be the expected treatment for Michael as he withdraws from alcohol?
    a. Tricyclic antidepressants
    b. A long-acting barbiturate, such as phenobarbital
    c. Alcohol deterrent therapy, such as disulfiram
  • d. Substitution therapy with chlordiazepoxide

5. The physician also orders daily administration of thiamine for Michael. What is the rationale behind this order?
    a. To restore nutritional balance
    b. To prevent pancreatitis
    c. To prevent alcoholic hepatitis
  • d. To prevent Wernicke's encephalopathy

6. Symptoms of the correct answer to the previous question include:
    a. Peripheral neuropathy and pain
    b. Epigastric pain and nausea/vomiting
  • c. Diplopia, ataxia, somnolence
    d. Inflammation and necrosis of the liver

7. Although Michael denies that he is an alcoholic, the nurse encourages him to seek rehabilitative treatment. The nurse understands that for Michael to be successful in treatment, he must first:
    a. Identify someone to whom he can go for support
    b. Give up all his old drinking buddies
    c. Understand the dynamics of alcohol on the body
  • d. Correlate life problems to his drinking of alcohol

CHAPTER 25. SCHIZOPHRENIA AND OTHER PSYCHOTIC DISORDERS

CHAPTER FOCUS

The focus of this chapter is on nursing care of the client with psychotic disorders. Predisposing factors and symptomatology are explored, and nursing care is presented in the context of the six steps of the nursing process. Medical treatment modalities are also discussed.

LEARNING OBJECTIVES

After reading this chapter, the student will be able to:

1. Discuss the concepts of schizophrenia and related psychotic disorders.
2. Identify predisposing factors in the development of these disorders.
3. Describe various types of schizophrenia and related psychotic disorders.
4. Identify symptomatology associated with these disorders and use this information in client assessment.
5. Formulate nursing diagnoses and goals of care for clients with schizophrenia and other psychotic disorders.
6. Identify topics for clients and family teaching relevant to schizophrenia and other psychotic disorders.
7. Describe appropriate nursing interventions for behaviors associated with these disorders.
8. Describe relevant criteria for evaluating nursing care of clients with schizophrenia and related psychotic disorders.
9. Discuss various modalities relevant to treatment of schizophrenia and related psychotic disorders.

KEY TERMS

delusions
double-bind communications
paranoia
magical thinking
neologism
word salad
tangentiality
illusion
echopraxia
waxy flexibility
social skills training

hallucinations
catatonic behavior
religiosity
associative looseness
clang association
circumstantiality
perseveration
echolalia
autism
anhedonia
neuroleptic

CHAPTER OUTLINE/LECTURE NOTES

I. Introduction
   A. The word schizophrenia is derived from the Greek words "schizo" (split) and "phren" (mind).
   B. Schizophrenia is probably caused by a combination of factors, including genetic predisposition, biochemical dysfunction, and psychosocial stress.
   C. Schizophrenia requires treatment that is comprehensive and is presented in a multidisciplinary effort.
   D. Schizophrenia probably causes more lengthy hospitalizations, more chaos in family life, more exorbitant costs to individuals and governments, and more fears than any other mental illness.
II. Nature of the Disorder

A. Schizophrenia results in disturbances in thought processes, perception, and affect.
B. There is severe deterioration of social and occupational functioning.
C. Approximately 1% of the population will develop schizophrenia over the course of a lifetime.
D. The premorbid behavior of an individual with schizophrenia can be viewed in four phases.
  1. Phase 1: The schizoid personality. Indifferent, cold, and aloof, these individuals are loners. They do not enjoy close relationships with others.
  2. Phase II: The prodromal phase. In this phase, the individuals are socially withdrawn and have behavior that is peculiar or eccentric. Role functioning is impaired, personal hygiene is neglected, and disturbances exist in communication, ideation, and perception.
  3. Phase III: Schizophrenia. In the active phase of the disorder, psychotic symptoms are prominent. These include delusions; hallucinations; and impairment in work, social relations, and self-care.
  4. Phase IV. residual phase. Symptoms are similar to the prodromal phase, with flat affect and impairment in role functioning being prominent.
III. Predisposing factors
  A. Genetic influences. A growing body of knowledge indicates that genetics plays an important role in the development of schizophrenia.
  B. Biochemical influences. One theory suggests that schizophrenia may be caused by an excess of dopamine-dependent neuronal activity in the brain. Abnormalities in the neurotransmitters norepinephrine, serotonin, acetylcholine, and gamma-aminobutyric acid have also been suggested.
  C. Physiological influences. Several physiological factors have been implicated, including viral infection, brain abnormalities, and histological changes in the brain. Various physical conditions, such as epilepsy, systemic lupus erythematosus, myxedema, parkinsonism, and Wilson's disease, have also been implicated.
  D. Psychological influences. Purely psychological factors are being questioned at this time. Researchers in the last decade are focusing their studies more on schizophrenia as a brain disorder. These theories probably developed early on out of a lack of information related to a biological connection. The psychological theories include poor early mother-child relationships, dysfunctional family system, and double-bind communication.
  E. Environmental influences. Lower socioeconomic status has been linked to the development of schizophrenia. Stressful life events have been associated with the onset of schizophrenic symptoms. Responses vary according to the number and severity of life events and the degree of vulnerability to the impact of the life event.
  F. The transactional model. Schizophrenia is likely the result of a combination of biological, psychological, and environmental influences on an individual who is vulnerable to the illness.
IV. Types of schizophrenia and other psychotic disorders
  A. Disorganized schizophrenia. Chronic variety with flat or inappropriate affect. Silliness and incongruous giggling is common. Behavior is bizarre, and social interaction is impaired.
  B. Catatonic schizophrenia:
    1. Catatonic stupor—characterized by extreme psychomotor retardation. The individual is usually mute. Posturing is common.
    2. Catatonic excitement—extreme psychomotor agitation. Purposeless movements that must be curtailed to prevent injury to the client or others.
  C. Paranoid schizophrenia. Characterized by paranoid delusions. Client may be argumentative, hostile, and aggressive.
  D. Undifferentiated schizophrenia. Bizarre behavior that does not meet the criteria outlined for the other types of schizophrenia. Delusions and hallucinations are prominent.
  E. Residual schizophrenia. This category is used with the individual who has a history of at least one episode of schizophrenia with prominent psychotic symptoms. Also known as ambulatory schizophrenia, this is the stage that follows an acute episode.
  F. Schizoaffective disorder. Schizophrenic symptoms accompanied by a strong element of symptomatology associated with the mood disorders, either mania or depression.
  G. Brief psychotic disorder. Sudden onset of psychotic symptoms following a severe psychosocial stressor. Symptoms last less than 1 month, and the individual returns to the full premorbid level of functioning.

H. Schizophreniform disorder. Same symptoms as schizophrenia with the exception that the duration of the disorder has been at **least 1 month but less than 6 months.**
I. Delusional disorder. The existence of prominent, nonbizarre delusions.
    1. Erotomanic type. The individual believes that someone, usually of a higher status, is in love with him or her.
    2. Grandiose type. Irrational ideas regarding own worth, talent, knowledge, or power.
    3. Jealous type. Irrational idea that the person's sexual partner is unfaithful.
    4. Persecutory type. The individual believes he or she is being malevolently treated in some way.
    5. Somatic type. The individual has an irrational belief that he or she has some physical defect, disorder, or disease.
J. Shared psychotic disorder. A delusional system develops in a second person as a result of a close relationship with another person who already has a psychotic disorder with prominent delusions. Also called *folie à deux.*
K. Psychotic disorder due to a general medical condition. Symptoms of this disorder include prominent hallucinations and delusions that can be directly attributed to a general medical condition.
L. Substance-induced psychotic disorder. The presence of prominent hallucinations and delusions that are judged to be directly attributable to the physiological effects of a substance.
V. Application of the Nursing Process
  A. Background assessment data
    1. Content of thought
      a. Delusion—false personal beliefs
      b. Religiosity—excessive demonstration of obsession with religious ideas and behavior
      c. Paranoia—extreme suspiciousness of others
      d. Magical thinking—the idea that if one thinks something it will be true
    2. Form of thought
      a. Associative looseness—shift of ideas from one topic to another
      b. Neologisms—made-up words that have meaning only to the individual who invents them
      c. Concrete thinking—literal interpretations of the environment
      d. Clang associations—choice of words is governed by sound (often rhyming)
      e. Word salad—a group of words put together in a random fashion
      f. Circumstantiality—a delay in reaching the point of a communication because of the inclusion of unnecessary and tedious details
      g. Tangentiality—unable to get point of communication due to introduction of many new topics
      h. Mutism—inability or refusal to speak
      i. Perseveration—persistent repetition of the same word or idea in response to different questions
    3. Perception—the interpretation of stimuli through the senses
      a. Hallucinations—false sensory perceptions not associated with real external stimuli
      b. Illusions—misperceptions of real external stimuli
    4. Affect—emotional tone
      a. Inappropriate effect—emotions are incongruent with the circumstances
      b. Bland or flat—weak emotional tone
      c. Apathy—disinterest in the environment
    5. Sense of self—the uniqueness and individuality a person feels
      a. Echolalia—repeating words that are heard
      b. Echopraxia—repeating movements that are observed
      c. Identification and imitation—taking on the form of behavior one observes in another
      d. Depersonalization—feelings of unreality
    6. Volition— impairment in the ability to initiate goal-directed activity
      a. Emotional ambivalence—the coexistence of opposite emotions toward the same object
    7. Impaired interpersonal functioning and relationship to the external world
      a. Autism— the focus inward on a fantasy world, while distorting or excluding the external environment
      b. Deteriorated appearance—personal grooming and self-care activities are impaired

8. Psychomotor behavior
   a. Anergia—a deficiency of energy
   b. Waxy flexibility—passive yielding of all moveable parts of the body to any efforts made at placing them in certain positions
   c. Posturing—voluntary assumption of inappropriate or bizarre postures
   d. Pacing and rocking—pacing back and forth and rocking of the body
9. Associated features
   a. Anhedonia—inability to experience pleasure
   b. Regression—retreat to an earlier level of development
10. Positive and negative symptoms
    a. Positive symptoms reflect an excess or distortion of normal functions, such as disorganized thinking, and are thought to have a relatively good response to treatment.
    b. Negative symptoms reflect a diminuation or loss of normal functions, such as diminished emotional expression and apathy, and are less likely than the positive symptoms to respond to treatment.

B. Nursing diagnosis/outcome identification
   1. Nursing diagnoses
      a. Alteration in thought processes
      b. Sensory-perceptual alteration: auditory/visual
      c. Social isolation
      d. Risk for violence: self or others
      e. Impaired verbal communication
      f. Self-care deficit
      g. Ineffective family coping: disabling
      h. Altered health maintenance
      i. Impaired home maintenance management
   2. Outcome criteria
C. Planning/implementation
   1. Care plan for the client with schizophrenia
D. Client/family education
E. Evaluation
   1. Reassessment data on which to base the effectiveness of nursing actions

VI. Treatment Modalities for Schizophrenia and Other Psychotic Disorders
A. Psychological Treatments
   1. Individual psychotherapy. Long-term therapeutic approach; difficult because of client's impairment in interpersonal functioning.
   2. Group therapy. Some success if occurring over the long-term course of the illness; less successful in acute treatment.
   3. Behavior therapy. Chief drawback has been the inability to generalize to the community setting once the client has been discharged from the hospital.
   4. Social skills training. The use of role play to teach client appropriate eye contact, interpersonal skills, voice intonation, posture, and so forth, aimed at improvement in relationship development
B. Social treatment
   1. Milieu therapy. Best if used in conjunction with psychopharmacology
   2. Family therapy. Aimed at helping family members cope with the long-term effects of the illness
C. Organic treatment
   1. Psychopharmacology
      a. Antipsychotics. Used to decrease agitation and psychotic symptoms.
      b. Antiparkinsonian. Agents used to counteract the extrapyramidal symptoms associated with antipsychotic medications.
      c. Others. Reserpine, lithium carbonate, carbamazepine, diazepam (Valium), and propranolol have been used with mixed results.

VII. Summary
VIII. Critical Thinking Exercise
IX. Review Questions

ANSWERS TO CRITICAL THINKING EXERCISE

1. Possible command hallucinations.

2. Alteration in sensory-perception: auditory

3. Decrease Sara's anxiety and establish trust

CASE STUDY FOR USE WITH STUDENT LEARNING

Case Study: Paranoid Schizophrenia

Caroline, age 22, was diagnosed with paranoid schizophrenia at age 19. She led a relatively normal life during school-age and high school years. She left her parents at age 17 to attend a college somewhat distant to her home. She apparently had no problems during her first year, but when she returned for Thanksgiving break during her second year, her parents noticed a distancing about her. She spent a lot of time alone, was irritable, and had begun chain smoking and drinking alcohol. She failed two courses that fall and was placed on probation. When she went back to school in the spring, her former roommate refused to stay with her, saying, "She acts so crazy sometimes. She talks out of her head, and I'm afraid of her." In late February, Caroline's parents got a call from the dean of students, who related that the campus police had to be called to Caroline's room to quiet her. She had been "yelling and screaming" and no one could understand what it had been all about. She had apparently really frightened the other students in the dormitory. These bizarre behaviors continued and during spring break in March, Caroline's parents moved her home and made an appointment with a psychiatrist for an evaluation. During the assessment, Caroline's thought processes were loose, vague, and often circumstantial. She exhibited behaviors that suggested auditory hallucinations (stopping midsentence and "cocking" her head to the side as if listening); although when questioned about whether or not she heard voices, she denied it. Paranoid delusional thinking was evident. She made statements such as, "There is no one I can trust at that college. Every student in that dorm has been told to keep an eye on me. They all know I am too smart to be there, so they will do what they can to make me fail. If I pass, then everyone else fails." She also expressed somatic delusions: "I'm pregnant, you know. It will be a virgin birth. That's another reason the college kids are out to get me. They are so jealous! I am the chosen one." Since that time, she has been on several antipsychotic medications (chlorpromazine, clozapine, and risperidone), each with only minimal success, and which she would eventually quit taking altogether. She currently lives at home with her parents, who are beside themselves with concern and frustration. The psychiatrist has admitted Caroline to the hospital at this time to evaluate her behavior and to begin her on a trial of fluphenazine decanoate, which will eventually be administered only every 3 weeks by intramuscular injection, in an effort to encourage increased medication compliance on Caroline's part. Design a nursing care plan for Caroline during this hospital admission.

LEARNING ACTIVITIES

Match the behaviors on the right to the appropriate terminology listed on the left.

_____ 1. Autism

_____ 2. Mutism

_____ 3. Hallucinations

_____ 4. Persecutory delusion

_____ 5. Word salad

_____ 6. Religiosity

_____ 7. Associative looseness

_____ 8. Inappropriate affect

_____ 9. Paranoia

_____ 10. Magical thinking

_____ 11. Neologism

_____ 12. Clang association

_____ 13. Waxy flexibility

_____ 14. Regression

_____ 15. Delusion of grandeur

a. Kneels to pray in front of water fountain; prays during group therapy and during other group activities.

b. Refuses to eat food that comes on tray, stating, "They are trying to poison me."

c. "When I get out of the hospital I'm going to buy me a sprongle."

d. Does not talk.

e. Keeps arm in position nurse left it after taking blood pressure. Assumed this position for hours.

f. "When I speak, presidents and kings listen."

g. A withdrawal inward into one's own fantasy world.

h. "I'm going to the circus. Jesus is God. The police are playing for keeps."

i. "We can't close the drapes, for if we do, the sun won't shine."

j. "Test, test, this is a test. I do not jest; we get no rest."

k. Laughs when told that his or her mother has just died.

l. In response to stressful situation, begins to suck thumb and soils clothing.

m. "Get by for anyone just to answer fortune cookies."

n. "If the FBI finds me here, I'll never get out alive."

o. Stops talking in midsentence, tilts head to side, and listens.

CASE STUDY

Read the following case study and fill in the blanks with the description of the information that is underlined and numbered in the text.

Sandra was a 37-year-old woman who was picked up by the police after she ran away from her parents' home. Sandra has had a history of paranoid schizophrenia for 17 years. She has had numerous hospitalizations.

Police were called when Sandra began wandering through a local park and screaming at everyone, "I know you are possessed by the devil!" During her initial interview, she is very guarded and suspicious of the nurse (1). "I can read your mind, you know." (2)

Sandra is assigned to a room and oriented to the unit. At 5 P.M., the nurse says to Sandra, "Sandra, it's time for dinner." Sandra responds, "time for dinner; time for dinner; time for dinner." (3) The nurse notices that each time she wipes her mouth with her napkin at dinner, Sandra does the same. (4)

Sandra's mother reports that Sandra stopped taking her medicine about a month ago, stating, "When you don't have a brain, (5) you don't need a brain medicine." Shortly afterward, she became totally despondent, taking no pleasure in activities she had always found enjoyable. (6) She stayed in her room, sitting on her bed moving back and forth in a slow, rhythmic fashion. (7) Sometimes she would not even get up to go to the bathroom, instead soiling herself in an infantile manner. (8) She seemed to experience a total lack of energy for usual activities of daily living. (9) On the unit, Sandra appears disinterested in everything around her. (10) She sits alone, talking and laughing to herself. (11) At one point she hears a laugh track on TV and states, "They're laughing at me. I know they are." (12)

(1) _____paranoia_____

(2) _____

(3) _____

(4) _____

(5) _____

(6) _____

(7) _____

(8) _____

(9) _____

(10) _____

(11) _____

(12) _____

Sandra's anxiety level starts to rise. She begins to pace the floor. Her agitation increases and she finally picks up a chair and hurls it toward the nurses' station, yelling "The devil says all blondes must be annihilated!"

a.   What would be Sandra's priority nursing diagnosis?

b.   What medication would you expect the physician to order for Sandra?

c.   For what adverse effects would you be on the alert with this drug?

d.   In what developmental stage (Erikson) would you place Sandra? Why?

e.   Theoretically, in what developmental stage *should* she be?

CHAPTER 25. TEST QUESTIONS

Situation: Frankie, a 20-year-old college student, seemed "different" when he was home for Thanksgiving. His thinking was somewhat disorganized, and he was convinced that a fellow student was spreading untruths about him. After arriving home for the Christmas break, he stopped bathing and isolated himself in his room, often staying up all night, then sleeping most of the following day. He complained of voices whispering his name.

In April, Frankie's parents received a call from the dean of students at Frankie's college. He told them that Frankie had quit attending his classes. He stayed in his room all of the time and often would not let his roommate enter. He yelled accusations at his roommate and other students, believing that they were conspiring against him. Last night, he charged after his roommate with a knife in his hands. He was taken to the local hospital by police, where he was admitted to the psychiatric unit. The psychiatrist had diagnosed Frankie with paranoid schizophrenia.

1. Based on the above information, what *initial* nursing diagnosis would the nurse make?
    a. Risk for self-directed violence
    b. Sensory-perceptual alteration
    • c. Risk for violence directed toward others
    d. Altered thought processes

2. Based on background knowledge, in what stage of development would the nurse place Frankie?
    • a. Trust versus Mistrust
    b. Autonomy versus Shame and Doubt
    c. Identity versus Role Confusion
    d. Intimacy versus Isolation

3. Because of his developmental level, what must be an *initial* intervention for the nurse?
    a. Allowing Frankie to take charge of his self-care independently
    b. Putting Frankie in the first group therapy session with an opening
    c. Helping Frankie decide where he wants to go i his life from here
    • d. Helping Frankie decrease his anxiety and establish trust

4. The physician orders 100 mg chlorpromazine (Thorazine) bid and 2 mg benztropine (Cogentin) bid prn. Rationale for the chlorpromazine order is:
    a. To ensure that Frankie can get enough sleep.
    • b. To reduce psychotic symptoms.
    c. To decrease Frankie's aggressiveness.
    d. To prevent tardive dyskinesia.

5. Under what circumstances would the nurse administer a dose of prn Cogentin?
    a. When Frankie becomes aggressive
    b. When Frankie needs to be calmed down before bedtime
    • c. When Frankie exhibits tremors and shuffling gait.
    d. When Frankie complains of constipation.

6. Frankie says to the nurse, "My roommate was plotting with others to have me killed!" The most appropriate response by the nurse would be:
    • a. "I find that hard to believe, Frankie."
    b. "What would make you think such a thing?"
    c. "No one was trying to kill you, Frankie."
    d. "I might feel the same way if you came after *me* with a knife!"

7. The nurse notices that Frankie is stopping in midsentence when they are talking. He tilts his head to the side as if listening to something. The most appropriate intervention by the nurse would be:

    a. Call and report the behavior to the physician.
    b. Give Frankie a prn dose of benztropine.
    •   c. Say to Frankie, "What are the voices saying to you, Frankie?"
    d. Say to Frankie, "Well, I see you are distracted right now. We'll talk more later."

CHAPTER 26. MOOD DISORDERS

CHAPTER FOCUS

The focus of this chapter is on nursing care of the client with mood disorders (depression or mania). Predisposing factors and symptomatology are explored, and nursing care is presented in the context of the six steps of the nursing process. Medical treatment modalities are also discussed.

LEARNING OBJECTIVES

After reading this chapter, the student will be able to:

1. Recount historical perspectives of mood disorders.
2. Discuss epidemiological statistics related to mood disorders.
3. Differentiate between normal and maladaptive responses to loss.
4. Describe various types of mood disorders.
5. Identify predisposing factors in the development of mood disorders.
6. Discuss implications of depression related to developmental stage.
7. Identify symptomatology associated with mood disorders and use this information in client assessment.
8. Formulate nursing diagnoses and goals of care for clients with mood disorders.
9. Identify topics for client and family teaching relevant to mood disorders.
10. Describe appropriate nursing interventions for behaviors associated with mood disorders.
11. Describe relevant criteria for evaluating nursing care of clients with mood disorders.
12. Discuss various modalities relevant to treatment of mood disorders.

KEY TERMS

anticipatory grieving
tyramine
psychomotor retardation
bereavement overload
bipolar disorder
cognitive therapy
cyclothymic disorder
delayed grief
delirious mania
dysthymic disorder

exaggerated grief
grief
hypomania
mania
melancholia
mood
mourning
postpartum depression
prolonged grief
premenstrual dysphoric disorder

CHAPTER OUTLINE/LECTURE NOTES

I.   Introduction
     A. Depression is the oldest and most frequently described psychiatric illness.
     B. Transient symptoms are normal, healthy responses to everyday disappointments in life.
     C. Pathological depression occurs when adaptation is ineffective.
     D. Various medical treatment modalities are explored.
II. Historical Perspectives
     A. Many ancient cultures have believed in the supernatural or divine origin of depression and mania.

B. Hippocrates believed that melancholia was caused by an excess of black bile, a heavily toxic substance produced in the spleen or intestine, which affected the brain.

C. Various other theories were espoused regarding the etiology of depression. It was described as the result of obstruction of vital air circulation, excessive brooding, or helpless situations beyond the client's control.

D. Nineteenth century definitions of mania narrowed it down to a disorder of affect and action.

E. The perspectives of twentieth century theorists lend support to the notion of multiple causation in the development of mood disorders.

III. Epidemiology

A. Ten to fourteen million Americans are afflicted with some form of major affective disorder.

B. Gender. Depression is more prevalent in women than men. Bipolar disorder is roughly equal.

C. Age. Depression is more common in young women and has a tendency to decrease with age. The opposite is true with men. Studies regarding bipolar disorder suggest the median age is 18 years in men and 20 years in women.

D. Social class. There is an inverse relationship between social class and report of depressive symptoms. The opposite is true with bipolar disorder.

E. Race. No consistent relationship between race and affective disorder has been reported.

F. Marital status. Single and divorced persons are more likely to experience depression than married persons.

G. Seasonality. Affective disorders are more prevalent in the spring and in the fall.

IV. The Grief Response

A. Loss is an experience in which an individual relinquishes a connection to a valued object (animate/inanimate; a relationship or situation; or even a change or failure [real or perceived]).

B. Stages of grief
   1. Elizabeth Kubler-Ross
      a. Denial
      b. Anger
      c. Bargaining
      d. Depression
      e. Acceptance
   2. John Bowlby
      a. Numbness/protest
      b. Disequilibrium
      c. Disorganization and despair
      d. Reorganization
   3. George Engel
      a. Shock and disbelief
      b. Developing awareness
      c. Restitution
      d. Resolution of the loss
      e. Recovery

C. Length of the grief process
   1. Resolution is thought to have occurred when a bereaved individual is able to remember comfortably and realistically both pleasures and disappointments associated with that which has been lost.
   2. Several factors influence length of the grief process:
      a. Importance of the lost object as a source of support
      b. Degree of dependency on the relationship with the lost object
      c. Degree of ambivalence felt toward the lost object
      d. Number and nature of the mourner's other meaningful relationships
      e. Number and nature of previous grief experiences
      f. Age of the lost person
      g. Health of the mourner at the time of loss
      h. Degree of preparation for the loss

D. Anticipatory grief
1. The initiation and process of grieving before the significant loss actually occurs.
2. Thought to facilitate the final grief response when the loss actually occurs.
V. Maladaptive Responses to Loss
A. Types
1. Delayed or inhibited grief. The absence of evidence of grief when it ordinarily would be expected.
a. It can be considered pathological because the person does not deal with the reality of the loss.
2. Prolonged grief. This type exists when there has been no resumption of normal activities of daily living within 4 to 8 weeks of a loss.
3. Exaggerated grief response. A distorted grief reaction in which all of the symptoms associated with normal grieving are exaggerated.
a. Individual becomes fixed in the anger stage of the grief response.
b. Depressive mood disorder is a type of exaggerated grief reaction.
B. Normal versus maladaptive grieving
1. One crucial difference between normal and maladaptive grieving is the loss of self-esteem.
2. The loss of self-esteem that almost invariably occurs in depression is not present with normal grief.
VI. Types of Mood Disorders
A. Depressive disorders
1. Major depressive disorder
a. Single episode or recurrent
b. Mild, moderate, or severe
c. With psychotic features
d. With melancholic features
e. Chronic
f. With seasonal pattern
g. With postpartum onset
2. Dysthymic disorder
a. Early onset
b. Late onset
3. Premenstrual dysphoric disorder
a. Depressed mood, marked anxiety, mood swings, and decreased interest in activities during the week prior to menses and subsiding shortly after the onset of menstruation
B. Bipolar disorders
1. Bipolar I disorder
2. Bipolar II disorder
3. Cyclothymic disorder
C. Other mood disorders
1. Mood disorder due to a general medical condition
2. Substance-induced mood disorder
VII. Depressive Disorders
A. Predisposing theories
1. Biological theories
a. Genetics. Hereditary factor may be involved.
b. Biochemical influences. Deficiency of norepinephrine, serotonin, and dopamine have been implicated.
c. Neuroendocrine disturbances:
(1) Possible failure within the hypothalamic-pituitary-adrenocortical axis
(2) Possible diminished release of thyroid-stimulating hormone
d. Physiological Influences:
(1) Medication side effects
(2) Neurological disorders
(3) Electrolyte disturbances
(4) Hormonal disturbances

          (5) Nutritional deficiencies

          (6) Other physiological conditions

    2. Psychosocial theories

       a. Psychoanalytical theories

          (1) Freud—a loss is internalized and becomes directed against the ego

          (2) Klein—the result of a poor mother-infant relationship

       b. Learning theory

          (1) Learned helplessness—the individual who experiences numerous failures learns to give up trying

       c. Object-loss theory

          (1) It occurs when an individual is separated from a significant other during the first 6 months of life.

       d. Cognitive theory

          (1) Theory that cognitive distortions result in negative, defeatist attitudes that serve as the basis for depression

       e. Transactional model. Exact etiology of depression remains unclear. Evidence continues to mount in support of multiple causation.

  B. Developmental implications

    1. Childhood depression

    2. Adolescent depression

    3. Senescence

    4. Postpartum depression

  C. Application of the Nursing Process to Depressive Disorders

    1. Background assessment data

       a. Symptoms occur by degree of severity and may be described as transient, mild, moderate, or severe.

          (1) Transient depression: life's everyday disappointments that result in the "blues"

          (2) Mild depression: identified with those symptoms of normal grieving

          (3) Moderate depression: identified by those symptoms associated with dysthymic disorder

          (4) Severe depression: identified by those symptoms associated with major depressive disorder and bipolar depression

    2. Nursing diagnoses are formulated by analyzing the data gathered during the assessment phase of the nursing process. Outcome criteria are identified for each.

    3. Nursing intervention for the depressed client is aimed at:

       a. Protecting client from harming self

       b. Assisting with progression through the grief process

       c. Enhancing the client self-esteem

       d. Helping the client determine ways to take control over his or her life

       e. Assisting in confronting anger that has been turned inward on the self

       f. Ensuring that needs related to nutrition, elimination, activity, rest, and personal hygiene are met

    4. Evaluation of the effectiveness of nursing interventions is measured by fulfillment of the outcome criteria.

VIII. Bipolar Disorder (Mania)

  A. Predisposing factors

    1. Biological theories

       a. Genetics. Strong hereditary implications.

       b. Biochemical influences. Possible excess of norepinephrine and dopamine.

       c. Electrolytes. Increased intracellular sodium and calcium has been implicated.

       d. Physiological influences.

          (1) Brain lesions

          (2) Medication side effects

    2. Psychosocial theories. (Less credibility is currently given to these theories. Bipolar disorder is more commonly viewed as a brain disorder.)

a. Psychoanalytical theories. Mania is viewed as a denial of, or defense against, depression.
b. Theory of family dynamics. Views mania as the result of conditional love.
c. The transactional model. Bipolar disorder most likely occurs as the result of multiple influences.
B. Application of the Nursing Process to Bipolar Disorder (Mania)
   1. Background assessment data
      a. Symptoms may be categorized by degree of severity.
         (1) Stage I: Hypomania. Symptoms not sufficiently severe to cause marked impairment in social or occupational functioning or to require hospitalization.
         (2) Stage II: Acute mania. Marked impairment in functioning of mood, cognition and perception, and activity and behavior. Usually requires hospitalization.
         (3) Stage III: Delirious mania. A grave form of the disorder characterized by severe clouding of consciousness and representing an intensification of the symptoms associated with acute mania.
   2. Nursing diagnoses are formulated by analyzing the data gathered during the assessment phase of the nursing process. Outcome criteria are identified for each.
   3. Nursing intervention for the client experiencing a manic episode is aimed at:
      a. Protection from injury due to hyperactivity
      b. Protection from harm to self or others
      c. Restoration of nutritional status
      d. Progression toward resolution of the grief process
      e. Improvement in interactions with others
      f. Acquiring sufficient rest and sleep
   4. Evaluation of the effectiveness of the nursing interventions is measured by fulfillment of the outcome criteria.
IX. Treatment Modalities for Mood Disorders
   A. Psychological treatments
      1. Individual Psychotherapy
      2. Group Therapy
      3. Family Therapy
      4. Cognitive Therapy
   B. Organic treatments
      1. Psychopharmacology
      2. Electroconvulsive Therapy
X. Summary
XI. Critical Thinking Exercise
XII. Review Questions

ANSWERS TO CRITICAL THINKING EXERCISE

1. Protection from injury, adequate nutrition, and rest.

2. Evidence of a full manic episode.

3. Ataxia, blurred vision, persistent diarrhea, nausea and vomiting, tinnitus.

4. Lithium does not take effect for 1 to 3 weeks. The Thorazine was ordered to calm her hyperactivity until the lithium takes effect.

CASE STUDIES FOR USE WITH STUDENT LEARNING

Case Study No. 1: <u>Major Depressive Disorder</u>

Valerie, age 25, is admitted to the psychiatric unit by her psychiatrist after stating that she no longer wanted to live. She has a long history of psychiatric problems, beginning at age 15 when she swallowed a handful of aspirin and acetaminophen. Valerie's mother has a history of depression and her father is very authoritarian. He ruled Valerie and her sister with an iron hand and rarely showed affection or gave positive feedback. In college, Valerie met Bob with whom she immediately fell in love. He was very affectionate, and she felt she received some nurturing from him that she had not received from her parents. In the semester before graduation, Bob told her he was leaving to go to graduate school in another state and that he was not ready to get married at this time. Valerie became hysterical and went into a deep depression. After a few weeks she met Jack, with whom she immediately began a sexual relationship and became pregnant. Jack agreed to marry Valerie, and so they began a short, but extremely stormy, relationship. Six months after the birth of their baby boy, they began divorce proceedings, with a great deal of negative negotiations regarding custody and child support. The child is 4-years-old now, and Valerie has had several "serious" relationships since her divorce, having just broken off from the most recent one this week. Ralph told her that she is just "too intense, draining him of all his energy." She said he told her that she expects too much from their relationship—more than he has to give. She admits that she got serious really fast, but that she really believes she loves him. She says to the admitting nurse, "What's the matter with me? Why can't I have normal relationships like other people? If it weren't for my little boy, I wouldn't even be here now." Design a plan of care for Valerie's hospital stay.

Case Study No. 2: <u>Bipolar Mania</u>

Noreen, age 32, had always been described as "moody." Depending upon what was happening in her life at the time, she could be very sad and depressed, or very lighthearted and happy. During her "down" times she would feel tired, experience loss of appetite, and sleep a lot. During her "happy" times, she would party a lot, be very outgoing, and have a remarkable amount of energy. Noreen did well in college and graduated at age 26 with an MBA. Since that time, she has been employed in the administration department of a large corporation, in which she has had several promotions. Two weeks ago, management was to make the announcement of who would be filling the position of Vice President of Corporate Affairs. Noreen and a male colleague, Ted, were vying for the position. It was a choice position that Noreen desperately wanted. She became very depressed when the announcement was made that Ted had been chosen. She stayed at home in bed and slept a lot for several days. On about the fourth day, she got up feeling exhilarated and decided to go shopping. She spent over a thousand dollars on clothing. She then decided to have a party for several hundred people, having it catered and planning all the details. Tonight was the party. Noreen wore a new, very expensive dress, drank a lot of champagne, was very jovial and seductive, and bragged to everyone who would listen that she would soon be getting a new job and that the people at her old organization would be sorry they had failed to promote her. She left the party with a man she hardly knew. At 3 A.M., she was picked up by the police under the grandstand at the local baseball stadium wearing only her underclothes and high-heeled shoes and carrying a half-filled bottle of champagne. She was alone and speaking very loudly and rapidly. The police brought her to the emergency department where she was admitted to the psychiatric unit with a diagnosis of manic episode. Design an initial care plan for Noreen

LEARNING ACTIVITIES

Symptoms of Mood Disorders

Beside each of the behaviors listed below, write the letter that identifies the disorder in which the behavior is most prevalent. The first one is completed as an example.

a. Dysthymic disorder
b. Major depressive disorder
c. Transient depression
d. Cyclothymic Disorder
e. Bipolar disorder (mania)
f. Delirious mania

__c__ 1. Feeling of the "blues" in response to everyday disappointments.

_____ 2. A clouding of consciousness occurs.

_____ 3. Outlook is gloomy and pessimistic.

_____ 4. Disorder characterized by mood swings between hypomania and mild depression.

_____ 5. Feelings of total despair and hopelessness.

_____ 6. Physical movement may come to a standstill.

_____ 7. Paranoid and grandiose delusions are common.

_____ 8. Client feels at best early in the morning and continually feels worse as the day progresses.

_____ 9. Excessive interest in sexual activity.

_____ 10. Client is able to carry out thoughts of self-destructive behavior.

_____ 11. Client feels at worst early in the morning and somewhat better as the day progresses.

_____ 12. Accelerated, pressured speech.

_____ 13. Frenzied motor activity characterized by agitated, purposeless movements.

CHAPTER 26. TEST QUESTIONS

Situation: Janet, age 28, was diagnosed at age 24 with bipolar disorder. The physician prescribed lithium carbonate 300 mg tid for maintenance therapy. Janet lives at home with her parents. Her mother reports that Janet quit taking her lithium about 3 months ago, stating that she felt just fine and did not like taking the medication because it was making her gain weight. Her behavior has become more and more hyperactive. She has slept very little. She has managed to maintain her office job, but today Janet's mother got a call from Janet's boss saying that Janet had lost her temper, started yelling and cursing at the other people in the office, and walked out yelling that she did not need this job anymore. The police were called by a downtown department store when Janet became aggressive and belligerent after being confronted for shoplifting. She was taken to the emergency department (ED) of the local hospital, and her parents were notified that she had been admitted to the psychiatric unit.

1. Janet is agitated, pacing, talking loudly and abusively as if in response to an unseen person, and flailing her arms in exaggerated gestures. She is begun on lithium carbonate and haloperidol (Haldol) immediately. What is the rationale for the haloperidol order?
    a. Haloperidol cures manic symptoms.
    b. Haloperidol prevents extrapyramidal side effects.
    c. Haloperidol will ensure that she gets a good night's sleep.
    • d. Haloperidol will calm hyperactivity until the lithium takes effect.

2. At this level of her illness, the nurse caring for Janet must consider which of the following nursing diagnoses as the priority?
    • a. Risk for injury related to excessive hyperactivity.
    b. Sleep pattern disturbance related to manic hyperactivity.
    c. Alteration in nutrition, less than body requirements related to inadequate intake.
    d. Self-esteem disturbance related to embarrassment from being arrested for shoplifting.

3. Janet tells the physician that she does not want to take lithium carbonate because she has gained a lot of weight on this medication. She says that if he sends her home on this drug, she will just stop taking it again. The physician decides to change her medication in hopes that she will be more compliant. Which of the following medications might the physician choose to prescribe for Janet?
    a. Sertraline (Zoloft)
    • b. Valproic Acid (Depakote)
    c. Trazodone (Desyrel)
    d. Paroxetine (Paxil)

Janet is stabilized on her medication and the hyperactivity subsides. She is discharged from the hospital to her parents' home. She apologizes to her boss for her behavior and is rehired. However, 10 months later, because of cutbacks and downsizing, Janet is laid off. She becomes very depressed, refuses to look for another job, stays in her room, eats very little, and neglects her personal hygiene. She tells her mother, "What's the use of trying? I fail at everything I do, anyway. Nothing ever works out for me." The next morning, when Janet's mother went into check on her, she found Janet unconscious, but still breathing, with an empty bottle of sertraline (Zoloft) beside her. She called an ambulance and had Janet transported to the hospital ED. Janet was stabilized in the ED and admitted to the psychiatric unit. Her diagnosis is bipolar I disorder: current episode depressed.

4. Why does the physician give Janet this diagnosis rather than major depression?
    a. Because he does not feel she is that severely depressed
    • b. Because she has experienced a full manic episode in the past
    c. Because he needs to make a more extensive assessment before he decided
    d. Because she has no history of major depression in her family

5. What would be the *priority* nursing diagnosis for Janet at this time?
    a. Alteration in nutrition, less than body requirements, related to refusal to eat
    b. Anxiety (severe) related to threat to self-esteem
    •   c. Risk for self-directed violence related to depressed mood
    d. Dysfunctional grieving related to loss of employment

6. The physician prescribes paroxetine (Paxil) for Janet. She is encouraged to participate in unit activities and to talk about her feelings. Despite all efforts, her depression becomes profound. She is in total despair and in a vegetative state. The physician obtains consent from her parents to perform electroconvulsive therapy (ECT). What is the rationale behind this treatment for profound depression?
    a. The client is made to forget painful memories from the past and go on with his or her life.
    b. The treatment causes stimulation of the central nervous system (CNS) similar to CNS stimulant medication, thereby lifting mood.
    c. The treatment satisfies the need for punishment that severely depressed clients sometimes think they deserve.
    •   d. The treatment is thought to increase levels of norepinephrine and serotonin, resulting in mood elevation.

7. The physician orders a medication to be administered by the nurse 30 minutes prior to each ECT treatment that will decrease secretions and maintain heart rate during the convulsion. Which of the following medications would the physician prescribe for this purpose?
    a. Thiopental sodium (Pentothal)
    •   b. Atropine sulfate
    c. Succinylcholine (Anectine)
    d. Clonazepam (Klonopin)

8. Which of the following currently receives the most credibility as etiologically implicated in the development of bipolar disorder?
    •   a. Genetics and biochemical alterations
    b. Poor mother-child relationship
    c. Evidence of lesion in temporal lobe
    d. Learned helplessness within a dysfunctional family system

CHAPTER 27. ANXIETY DISORDERS

CHAPTER FOCUS

The focus of this chapter is on nursing care of the client with anxiety disorders. Predisposing factors and symptomatology are explored, and nursing care is presented in the context of the six steps of the nursing process. Medical treatment modalities are also discussed.

LEARNING OBJECTIVES

After reading this chapter, the student will be able to:

1. Differentiate among the terms *stress, anxiety,* and *fear.*
2. Discuss historical aspects and epidemiological statistics related to anxiety disorders.
3. Differentiate between normal anxiety and psychoneurotic anxiety.
4. Describe various types of anxiety disorders and identify symptomatology associated with each. Use this information in client assessment.
5. Identify predisposing factors in the development of anxiety disorders.
6. Formulate nursing diagnoses and outcome criteria for clients with anxiety disorders.
7. Describe appropriate nursing interventions for behaviors associated with anxiety disorders.
8. Identify topics for client and family teaching relevant to anxiety disorders.
9. Evaluate nursing care of clients with anxiety disorders.
10. Discuss various modalities relevant to treatment of anxiety disorders.

KEY TERMS

agoraphobia
flooding
generalized anxiety disorder
implosion therapy
panic disorder
phobias
posttraumatic stress disorder
obsessive-compulsive disorder
ritualistic behavior
specific phobia
social phobia
systematic desensitization

CHAPTER OUTLINE/LECTURE NOTES

I. Introduction
   A. Anxiety is a necessary force for survival. It is not the same as stress.
   B. Stress (or stressor) is an external pressure that is brought to bear upon the individual. Anxiety is the subjective emotional response to that stressor.
   C. Anxiety is distinguished from fear in that anxiety is an emotional process whereas fear is a cognitive one.
II. Historical Aspects

A. Anxiety was once identified by its physiological symptoms, which focused largely on the cardiovascular system.

B. Freud was the first to associate anxiety with neurotic behaviors.

C. For many years, anxiety disorders were viewed as purely psychological or purely biological in nature.

III. Epidemiological Statistics

    A. Primary anxiety disorders represent one of the most prevalent mental health problems in the United States today.

    B. Anxiety disorders are more common in women than in men.

IV. How Much Is Too Much?

    A. Anxiety is pathological if:

        1. The response is greatly disproportionate to the risk and severity of the danger of threat

        2. The response continues beyond the existence of a potential danger or threat

        3. Intellectual, social, or occupational functioning is impaired

        4. The individual suffers from a psychosomatic effect (e.g., colitis or dermatitis)

V. Application of the Nursing Process

    A. Panic disorder

        1. Background assessment data

            a. It is characterized by recurrent panic attacks, the onset of which are unpredictable, and manifested by intense apprehension, fear, or terror, often associated with feelings of impending doom and accompanied by intense physical discomfort.

                (1) Palpitations, pounding heart, or accelerated heart rate

                (2) Sweating

                (3) Trembling or shaking

                (4) Sensations of shortness of breath or smothering

                (5) Feeling of choking

                (6) Chest pain or discomfort

                (7) Nausea or abdominal distress

                (8) Feeling dizzy, unsteady, lightheaded, or faint

                (9) Derealization (feelings of unreality) or depersonalization (being detached from oneself)

                (10) Fear of losing control or going crazy

                (11) Fear of dying

                (12) Paresthesias (numbness or tingling sensations)

                (13) Chills or hot flashes

            b. With agoraphobia

                (1) When panic disorder is accompanied by agoraphobia, the individual experiences the symptoms described above, but in addition, experiences a fear of being in places or situations from which escape might be difficult or embarrassing or in which help might not be available in the event of a panic attack.

    B. Generalized anxiety disorder

        1. Background assessment data

            a. It is characterized by chronic, unrealistic, and excessive anxiety and worry. Symptoms include:

                (1) Excessive anxiety and worry about a number of events that the individual finds difficult to control

                (2) Restlessness or feeling keyed up or on edge

                (3) Being easily fatigued

                (4) Difficulty concentrating or mind "going blank"

                (5) Irritability

                (6) Muscle tension

                (7) Sleep disturbance

        2. Predisposing factors to panic and generalized anxiety disorders

            a. Psychodynamic theory. An underdeveloped ego is not able to intervene when conflict occurs between the id and the superego, producing anxiety.

b. Cognitive theory. This theory places emphasis on distorted cognition, which results in anxiety that is maintained by mistaken or dysfunctional appraisal of a situation.

c. Biological aspects

    (1) Neuroanatomical. The lower brain centers may be responsible for initiating and controlling states of physiological arousal and for the involuntary homeostatic functions.

    (2) Biochemical. Abnormal elevations of blood lactate have been noted in clients with panic disorder.

    (3) Neurochemical. Evidence exists for the involvement of the neurotransmitter norepinephrine in the etiology of panic disorder.

    (4) Medical conditions. Various medical conditions, such as acute myocardial infarction, hypoglycemia, mitral valve prolapse, and complex partial seizures, have been associated to a greater degree with individuals who suffer panic and generalized anxiety disorders than in the general population.

d. Transactional model of stress-adaptation. The etiology of panic and generalized anxiety disorders is most likely influenced by multiple factors.

3. Diagnosis/outcome identification

  a. Nursing diagnoses are formulated from the data gathered during the assessment phase.

    (1) Panic anxiety

    (2) Powerlessness

  b. Outcome criteria are used as measurement guidelines to evaluate effectiveness of nursing care.

4. Planning/implementation

  a. Nursing intervention for the client with panic or generalized anxiety disorder is aimed at relief of acute panic symptoms.

  b. The nurse also works at assisting the client to take control of own life situation and accept those situations over which he or she has no control.

5. Evaluation is based on accomplishment of previously established outcome criteria.

C. Phobias

1. Background assessment data

  a. Agoraphobia without history of panic disorder. A fear of being in places or situations from which escape might be difficult, or in which help might not be available in the event of suddenly developing a panic or limited symptom attack.

  b. Social phobia. An excessive fear of situations in which a person might do something embarrassing or be evaluated negatively by others.

  c. Specific phobia. A persistent fear of a specific object or situation, other than the fear of being unable to escape from a situation or the fear of being humiliated in social situations.

2. Predisposing factors to phobias

  a. Psychoanalytical theory. Freud believed that during the oedipal period, the child becomes frightened of the aggression he fears the same-sex parent feels for him. This fear is repressed and displaced on to something safer, which becomes the phobic stimulus.

  b. Learning theory. Learning theorists believe that fears are learned, and become conditioned responses when the individual escapes panic anxiety (a negative reinforcement) by avoiding the phobic stimulus.

  c. Cognitive theory. Cognitive theorists espouse that anxiety is the product of faulty cognitions or anxiety-inducing self-instructions.

  d. Biological aspects

    (1) Temperament. Innate fears may represent a part of the overall characteristics or tendencies with which one is born that influence how he or she responds throughout life to specific situations.

  e. Life experiences. Certain early experiences may set the stage for phobic reactions later in life.

  f. Transactional model of stress-adaptation. The etiology of phobias is most likely influenced by multiple factors.

3. Diagnosis/outcome identification

  a. Nursing diagnoses are formulated using information gathered during the assessment phase.

(1) Fear

(2) Social isolation

b. Outcome criteria are used as measurement guidelines to evaluate effectiveness of nursing care.

4. Planning/implementation

a. Nursing intervention for the client with phobias is aimed at decreasing the fear and increasing the ability to function in the presence of the phobic stimulus.

D. Obsessive-compulsive disorder (OCD)

1. Background assessment data

a. Recurrent obsessions or compulsions that are severe enough to be time consuming or to cause marked distress or significant impairment.

2. Predisposing factors to obsessive-compulsive disorder

a. Psychoanalytical theory. Individuals with this disorder have weak, underdeveloped egos. Regression to the preoedipal phase of development during times of anxiety produce the symptoms of obsessions and compulsions.

b. Learning theory. Obsessive-compulsive behavior is viewed as a conditioned response to a traumatic event. The traumatic event produces anxiety and discomfort, and the individual learns to decrease the anxiety by engaging in behaviors that provide relief.

c. Biological aspects

(1) Neuroanatomy. Abnormalities in various regions of the brain have been implicated in the neurobiology of obsessive compulsive disorder.

(2) Physiology. Some individuals with obsessive compulsive disorder exhibit nonspecific electroencephalogram changes.

(3) Biochemical. A decrease in the neurotransmitter serotonin may be influential in the etiology of obsessive-compulsive disorder.

d. Transactional model of stress-adaptation. The etiology of obsessive-compulsive disorder is most likely influenced by multiple factors.

3. Diagnosis/outcome identification

a. Nursing diagnoses are formulated from the assessment data gathered during the first phase.

(1) Ineffective individual coping

(2) Altered role performance

b. Outcome criteria are used as measurement guidelines to evaluate effectiveness of nursing care.

4. Planning/Implementation

a. Nursing intervention of the client with OCD is aimed at helping him or her maintain anxiety at a manageable level without having to resort to use of ritualistic behavior. The focus is on development of more adaptive methods of coping with anxiety.

5. Evaluation is based on accomplishment of previously established outcome criteria.

E. Posttraumatic Stress Disorder (PTSD)

1. Background assessment data

a. The development of characteristic symptoms following exposure to an extreme traumatic stressor involving a personal threat to physical integrity or to the physical integrity of others.

b. Symptoms may include a re-experiencing of the traumatic event, a sustained high level of anxiety/arousal, or general numbing of responsiveness.

2. Predisposing factors to PTSD

a. Psychosocial Theory

(1) It seeks to explain why some individuals exposed to massive trauma develop PTSD whereas others do not.

(2) Variables include characteristics that relate to the traumatic experience, the individual, and the recovery environment.

b. Learning theory. The avoidance behaviors and psychic numbing in response to a trauma are mediated by negative reinforcement (behaviors that decrease the emotional pain of the trauma).

c. Cognitive theory. This theory takes into consideration the cognitive appraisal of an event and focuses on assumptions that an individual makes about the world.

    d.   Biological aspects. It is suggested that the symptoms related to the trauma are maintained by the production of endogenous opioid peptides that are produced in the face of arousal and that result in increased feelings of comfort and control. When the stressor terminates, the individual may experience opioid withdrawal, the symptoms of which bear strong resemblance to those of PTSD.

    e.   Transactional model of stress-adaptation. The etiology of PTSD is most likely influenced by multiple factors.

  3. Diagnosis/outcome identification

    a.   Nursing diagnoses are formulated from the data collected during the assessment phase.

      (1) Posttrauma response

      (2) Dysfunctional grieving

    b.   Outcome criteria are used as measurement guidelines to evaluate effectiveness of nursing care.

  4. Planning/implementation

    a.   Nursing intervention for the client with PTSD is aimed at:

      (1) Reassurance of safety

      (2) Decrease in maladaptive symptoms (e.g., flashbacks, nightmares)

      (3) Demonstration of more adaptive coping strategies

      (4) Adaptive progression through the grief process

  5. Anxiety disorder due to a general medical condition

F. Anxiety disorder due to a general medical condition

  1. Background assessment data

    a.   The symptoms are judged to be the direct physiological consequence of a general medical condition.

    b.   Symptoms may include generalized anxiety symptoms, panic attacks, or obsessions and compulsions.

G. Substance-induced anxiety disorder

  1. Background assessment data

    a.   Prominent anxiety symptoms judged to be due to the direct physiological effects of a substance.

    b.   Symptoms may occur during substance intoxication or withdrawal and may involve prominent anxiety, panic attacks, phobias, or obsessions or compulsions.

VI. Treatment modalities for anxiety disorders

A. Individual Psychotherapy

B. Cognitive Therapy

C. Behavior Therapy

  1. Systematic Desensitization

  2. Implosion Therapy (Flooding)

D. Group/Family Therapy

E. Psychopharmacology

VII. Summary

VIII. Critical Thinking Exercises

IX. Review Questions

ANSWERS TO CRITICAL THINKING EXERCISE

1. Panic anxiety related to threat to self-concept (fear of failure).

2. Stay with her and reassure her of her safety.

3. A benzodiazepine (clonazepam, alprazolam, or lorazepam) and individual psychotherapy.

CASE STUDIES FOR USE WITH STUDENT LEARNING

Case Study No. 1: Obsessive-Compulsive Disorder

Lana, age 28, has been admitted to the psychiatric unit with a diagnosis of OCD. She has been under the care of a psychiatrist since she was 14-years-old. At that time she was diagnosed with anorexia nervosa. She was treated for that disease, stabilized, and her family underwent counseling for about a year. She had a mild recurrence of the disease during her college years but was treated on an outpatient basis. Lana reported to the admitting nurse that during the last few years she has become increasingly obsessed with neatness and cleanliness. She washes her hands many times a day and, when possible, changes her clothing several times a day. She spends an enormous amount of time doing laundry and cleaning her apartment. Her hands crack and bleed from the excessive hand washing. She takes hours to get ready to go somewhere. If the routine is interrupted in any way, she starts over from the beginning. Recently, she got up at 1:30 A.M. to start getting ready for work. She has also started to lose weight again. She has a poor body image, and although her weight is appropriate for her height, she sees herself as overweight. She tells the nurse that she knows her behavior is inappropriate, but she cannot seem to stop herself. Design a care plan for Lana.

Case Study No. 2: Posttraumatic Stress Disorder

Sarah, age 25, graduated from college with a degree in Journalism. She was thrilled to obtain a position as a reporter with a local TV station. She has been working as a production assistant for 6 months and was recently promoted to reporter. About a month ago, she received the police alert of someone about to jump off a tall building and was dispatched with a photographer to the scene. For several hours, she witnessed the scene unravel as the police tried in vain to keep the man from jumping. Sarah watched with horror as the man jumped 20 stories to his death. She had always believed that she could be objective about such events and not have them affect her personally, but since that time, she has thought about the event on a daily basis. She has flashbacks and nightmares of seeing the man fall, and lately she has been reluctant even to go to work. Her boss suggests that she seek assistance of a psychiatrist. She is admitted to the partial hospitalization program with a diagnosis of PTSD. Design a nursing plan of care for Sarah during her partial hospitalization.

LEARNING ACTIVITY

BEHAVIORS ASSOCIATED WITH ANXIETY DISORDERS

Identify with which anxiety disorder the behaviors listed are associated. The first one is completed as an example.

a. Panic disorder
b. Agoraphobia
c. Specific phobia
d. PTSD

e. Generalized anxiety disorder
f. Social phobia
g. OCD

_c_ 1. Janet becomes panicky when she gets near a dog.

____ 2. Patricia weighs and measures her food. Long after everyone else has finished eating, she is still calculating the caloric value and remeasuring the amount.

____ 3. Frances will not leave her home unless a friend or relative goes with her.

____ 4. Harold has intrusive thoughts and, sometimes, visual illusions of his platoon's invasion of a village in Vietnam.

____ 5. Sonja refuses to eat in a restaurant. She is afraid others will laugh at the way she eats.

____ 6. About once a week, without warning, Stanley's heart begins to pound, he becomes short of breath, and sometimes he experiences chest pain. The doctor has ruled out physical problems.

____ 7. Janie wants desperately to visit a foreign country with her friends, but because of her fear of needles, she has not been able to receive the required immunizations.

____ 8. Helen is a very restless person. She is always nervous and keyed up. She worries about many things over which she has no control.

____ 9. Timmie's family recently survived a tornado by taking refuge in the basement of their home. The home and all of its contents were destroyed. Timmie has nightmares about the event.

____ 10. George never volunteers to speak in class. He is afraid his classmates will laugh at what he says.

____ 11. Carl will go to church, but only if he can sit right near the door.

____ 12. When Sally sees a spider on the floor, she screams and runs out of the room.

____ 13. Every day when Wanda goes home from work, she cleans her house. She has told her friends not to call her during this time, and if anything interferes with her cleaning, she becomes very upset, and starts over from the beginning.

____ 14. Don has always been an excellent student and was valedictorian of his high school graduating class. Since starting college, he has been unusually worried about his academic performance. Lately, he has been unable to sleep, is irritable, has difficulty concentrating, and has begun experiencing nausea and vomiting due to worry that he will not do well academically.

____ 15. Last month, on her way out of the hospital after working the evening shift, Amanda was abducted by a man with a gun and taken to a remote area and raped. Since that time, she has become detached and estranged from her friends, she has difficulty sleeping, and has had problems concentrating at work.

CHAPTER 27. TEST QUESTIONS

Sharon is a 25-year-old graduate student working on a doctorate in pharmacy. She is very bright and very achievement oriented. She works very hard and pushes herself to excel. Lately, she has been very upset because she is not studying as much as she usually does, and she is afraid she will fail some of her courses. She has begun cleaning out her drawers and closets incessantly. If she notices one thing out of place, she removes the entire contents and begins to rearrange them. Many times during the ritual, she gets interrupted and starts all over again. She knows that the behavior is not normal, but she feels powerless to change. She has been admitted to the psychiatric unit with the diagnosis of obsessive-compulsive disorder.

1. After her initial assessment and introduction to the unit, Sharon goes to her room to unpack her suitcase. She begins to arrange her belongings in the drawers and closet. Forty-five minutes later, when the nurse comes to check o her, Sharon is still folding and unfolding her clothes and arranging and rearranging them in the drawers. What is the appropriate nursing intervention at this time?
   a. Explain to Sharon that she must come out of her room and join the others in the dayroom at this time.
   b. Give Sharon a task to complete, to get her mind off the ritual.
 • c. Allow Sharon as much time as she wants to perform the ritual.
   d. Take Sharon by the hand and state, "It's time to go to group therapy now."

2. The most likely reason Sharon arranges and rearranges her clothing so often is:
 • a. It relieves her anxiety.
   b. Her mother taught her to be very neat.
   c. It provides her with a feeling of control over her life.
   d. It makes her feel good about herself.

3. The physician writes an order for medication for Sharon. Which of the following is an appropriate prescription for OCD?
   a. diazepam (Valium)
 • b. fluvoxamine (Luvox)
   c. propranolol (Inderal)
   d. alprazolam (Xanax)

4. Which of the following would be an appropriate nursing intervention with Sharon?
   a. Distract Sharon with other activities whenever she tries to clean out her drawers.
   b. Report the behavior to the physician each time she begins the ritual.
   c. Lock Sharon's room so that she cannot engage in the ritualistic behavior.
 • d. Help Sharon identify what is causing the anxiety that leads to the ritualistic behavior.

5. As Sharon becomes more comfortable on the unit and begins to interact with others, what change, if any, should the nurse make in her plan of care?
 • a. Begin to set limits on the amount of time Sharon may engage in the ritual.
   b. Give negative reinforcement to the behavior by pointing out its inappropriateness.
   c. Establish firm consequences if Sharon performs the ritualistic behavior.
   d. No change should be made in the plan of care.

6. Recently, the biochemical theory of etiology of OCD has been given an increasing amount of credibility. Which neurotransmitter has been associated with this disorder?
   a. Norepinephrine
   b. Dopamine
 • c. Serotonin
   d. Acetylcholine

CHAPTER 28. SOMATOFORM AND SLEEP DISORDERS

CHAPTER FOCUS

The focus of this chapter is on nursing care of clients with somatoform and sleep disorders. Predisposing factors and symptomatology are explored, and nursing care is presented in the context of the six steps of the nursing process. Medical treatment modalities are also discussed.

LEARNING OBJECTIVES

After reading this chapter, the student will be able to:

1. Define the term *hysteria*.
2. Discuss historical aspects and epidemiological statistics related to somatoform and sleep disorders.
3. Describe various types of somatoform and sleep disorders; identify symptomatology associated with each, and use this information in client assessment.
4. Identify predisposing factors in the development of somatoform and sleep disorders.
5. Formulate nursing diagnoses and goals of care for clients with somatoform and sleep disorders.
6. Describe appropriate nursing interventions for behaviors associated with somatoform and sleep disorders.
7. Identify topics for client and family teaching relevant to somatoform and sleep disorders.
8. Evaluate the nursing care of clients with somatoform and sleep disorders.
9. Discuss various modalities relevant to treatment of somatoform and sleep disorders.

KEY TERMS

anosmia

aphonia

hypochondriasis

hysteria

la belle indifference

primary gain

pseudocyesis

insomnia

hypersomnia

narcolepsy

parasomnias

tertiary gain

somatization

secondary gain

CHAPTER OUTLINE/LECTURE NOTES

I. Introduction
    A. The somatoform disorders are characterized by physical symptoms suggesting medical disease, but no demonstrable organic pathology or known pathophysiological mechanism can be found to account for them.
    B. Somatization refers to all those mechanisms by which anxiety is translated into physical illness or bodily complaints.
    C. Disordered sleep is a problem for many people. The problem may temporarily be caused by stress or anxiety; or the cause may be physiological.
II. Somatoform Disorders
    A. Historical aspects
        1. The concept of hysteria, which is characterized by recurrent, multiple somatic complaints often described dramatically, is at least 4000-years-old, and probably originated in Egypt.

2. Witchcraft, demonology, and sorcery were associated with hysteria in the Middle Ages.
3. In the 19th century, the French physician Paul Briquet attributed the disorder to dysfunction in the nervous system.
4. Out of his work with hypnosis, Freud proposed that emotion that is not expressed can be "converted" into physical symptoms.

B. Epidemiological statistics
1. Somatoform disorders are more common in women than in men. They are more common in poorly educated persons, rural inhabitants, religious fundamentalists, and ethnic groups as well as lower socioeconomic classes.

C. Application of the nursing process to somatoform disorders
1. Somatization disorder: Background assessment data
   a. A chronic syndrome of multiple somatic symptoms that cannot be explained medically and that are associated with psychosocial distress and long-term seeking of assistance from health-care professionals.
   b. Any organ system may be affected, but common complaints involve the neurological, gastrointestinal, psychosexual, or cardiopulmonary systems.
   c. Anxiety and depression are frequently manifested, and suicidal attempts and threats are not uncommon.
   d. Predisposing factors to somatization disorder
      (1) Psychodynamic theory. Views somatoform disorders as the result of a poor mother-child relationship. When love is given conditionally, the child defends against insecurity by learning to gain affection and care through illness.
      (2) Theory of family dynamics. In dysfunctional families, when a child becomes ill, a shift in focus is made from the open conflict to the child's illness, leaving unresolved the underlying issues that the family is unable to confront in an open manner. Somatization brings some stability to the family, and positive reinforcement to the child.
      (3) Cultural and environmental factors. Various cultures deal with physical symptoms in different ways. Environmental factors may be influential when there is a lack of language sophistication required to express oneself psychologically or social restrictions against conceptualizing life difficulties in psychological terminology.
      (4) Genetic factors. No genetic link can be made to somatization disorder, although some studies have shown it is more prevalent in some families than others.
      (5) Transactional model of stress-adaptation. The etiology of somatization disorder is most likely influenced by multiple factors.
   e. Diagnosis/outcome identification
      (1) Nursing diagnoses for the client with somatization disorder include:
         (a) Ineffective individual coping
         (b) Knowledge deficit
      (2) Outcome criteria are identified for measuring effectiveness of nursing care.
   f. Planning/implementation
      (1) Nursing intervention for the client with somatization disorder is aimed at assisting the client to learn to cope with stress by means other than preoccupation with physical symptoms.
      (2) The nurse also works to help the client correlate appearance of the physical symptoms with times of stress.
   g. Evaluation is based on accomplishment of previously established outcome criteria.
2. Pain Disorder: Background assessment data
   a. The predominant disturbance in pain disorder is severe and prolonged pain that causes clinically significant distress or impairment in social, occupational, or other areas of functioning.
   b. Even when organic pathology is detected, the pain complaint may be evidenced by the correlation of a stressful situation with the onset of the symptom.
   c. The disorder may be maintained by:

(1) Primary gains—the symptom enables the client to avoid some unpleasant activity
(2) Secondary gains—the symptom promotes emotional support or attention for the client
(3) Tertiary gains—in dysfunctional families, the physical symptom may take such a position that the real issue is disregarded and remains unresolved, even though some of the conflict is relieved
d. Predisposing factors to pain disorder
(1) Psychoanalytical theory. This theory postulates that pain for some clients serves the purposes of punishment and atonement for unconscious guilt. Occurs with individuals who have been severely punished as children.
(2) Behavioral theory. In behavioral terminology, psychogenic pain is explained as a response that is learned through operant and classical conditioning. Occurs when pain behaviors are positive or negatively reinforced.
(3) Theory of family dynamics. "Pain games" may be played in families burdened by conflict. Pain may be used for manipulating and gaining the advantage in interpersonal relationships. Tertiary gain may also be influential.
(4) Neurophysiological theory. This theory postulates that the cerebral cortex and medulla are involved in inhibiting the firing of afferent pain fibers. These individuals may have decreased levels of serotonin and endorphins.
(5) Transactional model of stress-adaptation. The etiology of pain disorder is most likely influenced by multiple factors.
e. Diagnosis/outcome identification
(1) Nursing diagnoses for the client with pain disorder include:
(a) Chronic pain
(b) Social isolation
(2) Outcome criteria are identified for measuring the effectiveness of nursing care.
f. Planning/implementation
(1) Nursing intervention for the client with pain disorder is aimed at relief from pain.
(2) Emphasis is placed on learning more adaptive coping strategies for dealing with stress. Reinforcement is given at times when the client is not focusing on pain.
g. Evaluation is based on accomplishment of previously established outcome criteria.
3. Hypochondriasis: Background Assessment Data
a. Unrealistic preoccupation with fear of having a serious illness
b. Even in the presence of medical disease, the symptoms are grossly disproportionate to the degree of pathology.
c. Predisposing factors to hypochondriasis
(1) Psychodynamic theory
(a) One view suggests that hypochondriasis is an ego defense mechanism. Physical complaints are the expression of low self-esteem and feelings of worthlessness, because it is easier to feel something is wrong with the body than to feel something is wrong with the self.
(b) Another psychodynamic view explains hypochondriasis as the transformation of aggressive and hostile wishes toward others into physical complaints to others.
(c) Still other psychodynamicists have viewed hypochondriasis as a defense against guilt.
(2) Cognitive theory. Cognitive theorists view hypochondriasis as arising out of perceptual and cognitive abnormalities.
(3) Sociocultural/familial factors. Somatic complaints are often reinforced when the sick role serves to relieve the individual from the need to deal with a stressful situation, whether it occurs within society or within the family constellation.
(4) Past experience with physical illness. Personal experience of or the experience of close family members with serious or life-threatening illness can predispose an individual to hypochondriasis.
(5) Genetic Influences. Little is known about hereditary influences in hypochondriasis.

(6) Transactional model of stress/adaptation. The etiology of hypochondriasis is most likely influenced by multiple factors.

d. Diagnosis/outcome identification

(1) Nursing diagnoses for hypochondriasis include:

(a) Fear

(b) Self-esteem disturbance

(2) Outcome criteria are identified for measuring the effectiveness of nursing care.

e. Planning/implementation

(1) Nursing intervention for the client with hypochondriasis is aimed at relieving the fear of serious illness.

(2) The focus is on decreasing the preoccupation with and unrealistic interpretation of bodily signs and sensations.

(3) The nurse also works to help the client increase feelings of self-worth and resolve internalized anger.

f. Evaluation is based on accomplishment of previously established outcome criteria.

4. Conversion disorder: background assessment data

a. A loss or change in bodily functioning resulting from a psychological conflict, the bodily symptoms of which cannot be explained by any known medical disorder or pathophysiological mechanism.

b. The most obvious and "classic" conversion symptoms are those that suggest neurological disease and occur following a situation that produces extreme psychological stress for the individual.

c. The person often expresses a relative lack of concern that is out of keeping with the severity of the impairment. This lack of concern is identified as *la belle indifference* and may be a clue to the physician that the problem is psychological rather than physical.

d. Predisposing factors to conversion disorder

(1) Psychoanalytical theory. Emotions associated with a traumatic event that the individual cannot express because of moral or ethical unacceptability are "converted" into physical symptoms. The symptom is symbolic in some way of the original emotional trauma.

(2) Theory of interpersonal communication. Conversion symptoms are viewed as a type of nonverbal communication. With physical symptoms, the individual communicates that he or she (or the relationship) needs special treatment or consideration.

(3) Neurophysiological theory. This theory suggests that some clients with conversion disorder have a diminishment in central nervous system arousal.

(4) Behavioral theory. This theory suggests that conversion symptoms are learned through positive reinforcement from cultural, social, and interpersonal influences.

(5) Transitional model of stress/adaptation. The etiology of conversion disorder is most likely influenced by multiple factors.

e. Diagnosis/outcome identification

(1) Nursing diagnoses for the client with conversion disorder include:

(a) Sensory-perceptual alteration

(b) Self-care deficit

(2) Outcome criteria are identified for measuring the effectiveness of nursing care.

f. Planning/implementation

(1) Nursing intervention for the client with conversion disorder is aimed at recovery of the lost or altered function.

(2) Emphasis is given to assisting the client with activities of daily living until the function is regained. Care is given not to reinforce the physical limitation

g. Evaluation is based on accomplishment of previously established outcome criteria.

5. Body dysmorphic disorder: Background assessment data

a. This disorder is characterized by the exaggerated belief that the body is deformed or defective in some specific way.

b. Symptoms of depression and characteristics associated with obsessive-compulsive personality are common.

    c. Has been closely associated with delusional thinking, and in Europe, it is considered to be a psychosis.
    d. Predisposing factors to body dysmorphic disorder
        (1) Etiology is unknown but presumed to be psychological.
        (2) Predisposing factors may be similar to those associated with hypochondriasis or phobias.
        (3) It is most likely that multiple factors are involved in the predisposition to body dysmorphic disorder.
    e. Diagnosis/outcome identification
        (1) Nursing diagnoses for the client with body dysmorphic disorder include:
            (a) Body image disturbance
        (2) Outcome criteria are identified for measuring effectiveness of nursing care.
    f. Planning/implementation
        (1) Nursing intervention for the client with body dysmorphic disorder is aimed at development of a realistic perception of body appearance.
        (2) A focus is on resolution of repressed fears and anxieties that contribute to altered body image.
        (3) Positive reinforcement is given for accomplishments unrelated to physical appearance.
    g. Evaluation is based on accomplishment of previously established outcome criteria.
III. Sleep Disorders
    A. Background assessment data
        1. Insomnia—difficulty with initiating or maintaining sleep.
        2. Hypersomnia (somnolence)—excessive sleepiness or seeking excessive amounts of sleep.
        3. Narcolepsy: sleep attacks—the individual cannot prevent falling asleep, even in the middle of a task or a sentence.
        4. Parasomnias—unusual to undesirable behaviors that occur during sleep. Examples include:
            a. Nightmare disorder—frightening dreams that lead to awakenings from sleep and are sufficiently severe to interfere with social or occupational functioning
            b. Sleep terror disorder—abrupt arousal from sleep with a piercing scream or cry. The individual is difficult to awaken or comfort, and if wakefulness does occur, the individual is usually disoriented, expresses a sense of intense fear but cannot recall the dream episode.
            c. Sleepwalking—the performance of motor activity initiated during sleep in which the individual may leave the bed and walk about, dress, go to the bathroom, talk, scream, or even drive. Episodes may last from a few minutes to a half-hour.
        5. Sleep-wake schedule disturbances—a misalignment between sleep and wake behaviors. The normal sleep-wake schedule is disrupted from its usual circadian rhythm. Examples include shift work and airplane travel that produces "jet lag."
        6. Predisposing factors to sleep disorders
            a. Genetic or familial patterns. These are thought to play a contributing role in primary insomnia, primary hypersomnia, narcolepsy, sleep terror disorder, and sleepwalking.
            b. Medical conditions implicated in the etiology of insomnia. These include pain, sleep apnea syndrome, restless leg syndrome, use or withdrawal from substances, endocrine or metabolic disorders, infectious or other diseases, and central nervous system (CNS) lesions.
            c. Psychiatric or environmental conditions. These include anxiety, depression, environmental changes, circadian rhythm sleep disturbances, posttraumatic stress disorder, and schizophrenia.
            d. Neurological abnormalities, such as temporal lobe epilepsy, may contribute to night terrors.
            e. Extreme fatigue and sleep deprivation may contribute to episodes of sleepwalking.
        7. Diagnosis/outcome identification
            a. Nursing diagnoses for the client with sleep disorders include:
                (1) Sleep pattern disturbance
                (2) Risk for injury
            b. Outcome criteria are identified for measuring the effectiveness of nursing are.
        8. Planning/implementation

a. Nursing intervention for the client with a sleep disorder is aimed at determining the cause of the disturbance and performing actions that promote sleep and rest for the client.

IV. Treatment Modalities
    A. Somatoform disorders
        1. Individual psychotherapy
        2. Group psychotherapy
        3. Behavior therapy
        4. Psychopharmacology
    B. Sleep Disorders
        1. Relaxation therapy
        2. Biofeedback
        3. Psychopharmacology
        4. Phototherapy
V. Summary
VI. Critical Thinking Exercise
VII. Review Questions

ANSWERS TO CRITICAL THINKING EXERCISE

1. His physical safety.

2. Siderails up. Bed in low position. Night light on. Furniture out of harm's way. Attach bell to bed in position that would cause it to ring if he tried to get out of bed. Frequent checks.

3. Encourage him to talk about stressors in his life. Possible family therapy to discuss family situation. Possible tricyclic antidepressant or low-dose benzodiazepine therapy at bedtime.

CASE STUDIES TO USE WITH STUDENT LEARNING

Case Study No. 1: Somatization Disorder

Lois's psychiatrist has admitted her to the psychiatric unit with a diagnosis of somatization disorder. Lois is 38-years-old and has been seeing a psychiatrist off and on since she was 16-years-old, when the family was deserted by her father. Lois was the oldest of five children. At that time, Lois was admitted to the hospital by the family physician for "abdominal pain." No physical etiology was found and the physician told Lois's mother that Lois suffered from "nervous stomach." Over the years, she has been either treated on an outpatient basis or hospitalized for chest pain, abdominal pain, backaches, food intolerances, and fatigue. She has had a hysterectomy and a thyroidectomy. She is insisting at this time that she has a problem with her stomach that the doctor is not finding. She is very depressed and tells the nurse, "I can't stand all this pain. I just can't understand why the doctor can't find my problem. I know I'm depressed, but that's not causing my stomach pain. They need to keep looking for it." The psychiatrist keeps reassuring Lois that no pathophysiology exists for her pain. Design a care plan for Lois.

Case Study No. 2: Conversion Disorder

Carol has always been very shy. Her parents had been concerned about this when Carol was a child and had tried to bring her out of her shyness by involving her with other children, but they were not successful. Carol preferred to be alone and seemed to be perfectly contented to do so. When Carol was in college, she took courses that she could study in solitude. The courses that required public participation often sent Carol into feelings of panic. She visited the student health center and the counseling center at the college. The student health center would provide her with medication to help her through anxious times, and the counseling center would try to help her with coping strategies to get through the anxiety. When she graduated from college, Carol got a job in the research and development department of a pharmaceutical company. It was the perfect job for Carol. She was able to do her research without many interactions with others. However, in the last year-and-a-half, the new supervisor has decided that every 6 months, each member of the research department staff will present work individually to the board of trustees at its semiannual meetings. Carol panicked the first time she heard this, but with the help of some antianxiety medication, she made it through the first presentation. When it was time for her second presentation, she woke up the morning of the meeting and was unable to speak. She presented herself at the emergency department (ED), and her boss was notified of her hospitalization. She was released when nothing physiological could be found. Today is the day of Carol's scheduled presentation. She has again awakened with the inability to make a sound. She has presented herself to the ED and does not appear to be very concerned about the problem. The admitting ED physician cannot find an organic reason for her aphonia. A psychiatrist is notified, and Carol is admitted to the psychiatric unit with a diagnosis of conversion disorder, aphonia. Design a care plan for Carol.

LEARNING ACTIVITY

BEHAVIORS ASSOCIATED WITH SOMATOFORM DISORDERS

Identify with which somatoform disorder the behaviors listed is associated. List the primary nursing diagnosis for each.

  a. Somatization disorder
  b. Pain disorder
  c. Hypochondriasis
  d. Conversion disorder
  e. Body dysmorphic disorder

_____ 1. Nancy fell on the ice last winter and injured her elbow. She complains that she has had pain ever since, even though x-rays reveal the elbow has healed appropriately.
Nursing diagnosis: _____

_____ 2. Virginia has some freckles across her nose and cheeks. She visits dermatologists regularly trying to find one who will "get rid of these huge spots on my skin."
Nursing diagnosis: _____

_____ 3. Franklin is assigned to secure a contract for his company. The boss tells Franklin, "If we don't get this contract, the company may have to fold." When Franklin wakes up on the morning of the negotiations, he is unable to see. The physician has ruled out organic pathology.
Nursing diagnosis: _____

_____ 4. Sarah has had what she calls a "delicate stomach" for years. She has sought out many physicians with complaints of nausea and vomiting, abdominal pain, bloating, and diarrhea. No organic pathology can be detected.
Nursing diagnosis: _____

_____ 5. John's father died of a massive myocardial infarction when John (now age 34) was 15-years-old. The two of them were playing basketball at the time. Since then, John becomes panicky when he feels his heart beating faster than usual. He takes his pulse several times a day and seeks out a physical examination from his physician several times a year.
Nursing diagnosis: _____

CHAPTER 28. TEST QUESTIONS

1. Louise has just moved to a new city and sees her new primary care practitioner (PCP) for the first time because of gastrointestinal distress. When she takes Louise's history, the PCP suspects some type of somatoform disorder. What is the *next step* necessary to confirm a diagnosis in this category?
   - a. Gastrointestinal workup
   - • b. Thorough physical examination
   - c. Review of old medical records
   - d. Referral to a psychiatrist

2. The PCP diagnoses Louise with somatization disorder. Which of the following data enables the physician to distinguish between hypochondriasis and somatization disorder in arriving at a diagnosis for Louise?
   - a. Pain
   - b. Gender distribution
   - • c. Persistent fear
   - d. Impaired functioning

3. Tyler, a 25-year-old law school graduate who has worked in his first job with a private law firm for a year, makes an appointment with his PCP because of weakness in his right hand and arm that he discovered when he awoke yesterday morning. He delayed making the appointment because he thought he "slept on it wrong," but it has not improved. He is unable to hold a pen or use his computer. He plays racquetball twice a week and last played 4 days ago, but he denies recent injury. Other extremities are normal, and he shows no other evidence of neurological impairment. Tyler says he enjoys the challenge of his job and has gotten used to the hectic pace and stress. He is scheduled to take the bar examination in 10 days for the second time, but he seems philosophical about his inability to use his hand. Which of these data, taken together, form the basis for a diagnosis of conversion disorder?
   1. Sudden onset
   2. The specific functional loss
   3. Negative neurological findings
   4. Upcoming bar examination
   5. Philosophical attitude
      - a. 1 & 2
      - b. 3 only
      - c. 4 only
      - • d. All of the above

4. The psychodynamic theory underlying Tyler's symptoms is
   - a. Relief from despair
   - b. Repression of anger
   - • c. Unconscious resolution of conflict
   - d. Cognitive deficit

5. Tommy, age 9, has begun sleepwalking, and his parents are afraid for his safety. He has begun getting up and wandering around outside their house in the middle of the night. Which of the following interventions might the practitioner prescribe for Tommy?
   - • a. low-dose alprazolam (Xanax) and bell on side of bed
   - b. methylphenidate (Ritalin) and biofeedback
   - c. temazepam (Restoril) and relaxation therapy
   - d. sertraline (Zoloft) and phototherapy

6. Edith, a 69-year-old widow, is very troubled by increasing difficulty sleeping well at night. She wakes frequently during the night, and feels tired when she wakes early in the morning. What is the outcome that *best* indicates that treatment of Edith's sleep disorder is successful?
   - a. Is compliant with medications
   - b. Has not experienced injury
   - c. Verbalizes understanding of the sleep disorder
   - • d. Reports increased sense of well-being and feeling rested

CHAPTER 29. DISSOCIATIVE DISORDERS

CHAPTER FOCUS

The focus of this chapter is on nursing care of clients with dissociative disorders. Predisposing factors and symptomatology are explored, and nursing care is presented in the context of the six steps of the nursing process. Medical treatment modalities are also discussed.

LEARNING OBJECTIVES

After reading this chapter, the student will be able to:

1. Discuss historical aspects and epidemiological statistics related to dissociative disorders.
2. Describe various types of dissociative disorders and identify symptomatology associated with each; use this information in client assessment.
3. Identify predisposing factors in the development of dissociative disorders.
4. Formulate nursing diagnoses and goals of care for clients with dissociative disorders.
5. Describe appropriate nursing interventions for clients with dissociative disorders.
6. Identify topics for client and family teaching relevant to dissociative disorders.
7. Evaluate nursing care of clients with dissociative disorders.
8. Discuss various modalities relevant to treatment of dissociative disorders.

KEY TERMS

abreaction
amnesia
association
   directed
   free
continuous amnesia
depersonalization
derealization
fugue
generalized amnesia
hypnosis
integration
localized amnesia
selected amnesia
systematized amnesia

CHAPTER OUTLINE/LECTURE NOTES

I.   Introduction
    A. The essential feature of dissociative disorders is a disturbance or alteration in the normally integrative functions of identity, memory, consciousness, or perception of the environment.
    B. Dissociative responses occur when anxiety becomes overwhelming and a disorganization of the personality ensues.
    C. Four types of dissociative disorders include dissociative amnesia, dissociative fugue, dissociative identity disorder, and depersonalization disorder.

II.   Historical Aspects
    A. The concept of dissociation was first formulated during the 19th century.
    B. Freud viewed dissociation as a type of repression, an active defense mechanism utilized in the removal of threatening or unacceptable mental contents from conscious awareness.
III. Epidemiological Statistics
    A. Dissociative syndromes are statistically quite rare.
    B. Dissociative amnesia and dissociative fugue are both rare, but occur most often under conditions of war or during natural disasters, or other severe psychosocial stress.
    C. The incidence of dissociative identity disorder is now known, but does occur more often in women than in men. It most commonly begins in childhood, but symptoms do not appear until adolescence or early adulthood.
    D. The prevalence of severe depersonalization disorder is unknown. Single brief episodes appear to be common in young adulthood, particularly in time of severe stress.
IV.   Application of the Nursing Process
    A. Dissociative Amnesia: Background Assessment Data
        1. Defined as a sudden inability to recall important personal information that is too extensive to be explained by ordinary forgetfulness, and which is not due to the direct effects of substance use or a general medical condition.
        2. Five types of disturbance in recall:
            a. Localized amnesia. The inability to recall all incidents associated with the traumatic event for a specific time period following the event (usually a few hours to a few days).
            b. Selective amnesia. The inability to recall only certain incidents associated with a traumatic event for a specific time period following the event.
            c. Generalized amnesia. The inability to recall anything that has happened during the individual's entire lifetime, including personal identity.
            d. Continuous amnesia. The inability to recall events occurring after a specific time up to and including the present.
            e. Systematized amnesia. The individual cannot remember events that relate to a specific category of information, such as one's family, or to one particular person or event.
        3. Predisposing Factors to Dissociative Amnesia
            a. Psychodynamic Theory. Freud described amnesia as the result of repression of distressing mental contents from conscious awareness.
            b. Behavioral Theory. Suggests that dissociative amnesia may be the result of learning and reinforced by primary and secondary gains for the individual.
            c. Biological Theory. Some efforts have been made to explain dissociative amnesia on the basis of neurophysiological dysfunction, although current data are inadequate and lacking in credibility.
            d. Transactional Model of Stress/Adaptation. The etiology of dissociative amnesia is most likely influenced by multiple factors.
        4. Diagnosis/Outcome Identification
            a. Nursing diagnoses for the client with dissociative amnesia include:
                (1) Altered thought processes
                (2) Powerlessness
            b. Outcome criteria are identified for measuring the effectiveness of nursing care.
        5. Planning/Implementation
            a. Nursing intervention for the client with dissociative amnesia is aimed at ability to recall lost mental contents.
            b. The nurse also works at assisting the client to deal more appropriately with severe anxiety.
        6. Evaluation is based on accomplishment of previously established outcome criteria.
    B. Dissociative Fugue: Background Assessment Data
        1. The characteristic feature of dissociative fugue is a sudden, unexpected travel away from home or customary workplace.
        2. An individual in a fugue state is unable to recall personal identity, and assumption of a new identity is common.
        3. Predisposing Factors to Dissociative Fugue

a. Psychodynamic Theory, Behavioral Theory, and possible Biological Theory. Same as dissociative amnesia.
b. Theory of Family Dynamics. Unsatisfactory parent/child relationship, with subsequent internalization of loss, has been implicated in the etiology of dissociative fugue. Unfulfilled separation anxiety, a defect in personality development, and unmet dependence needs may also be related to dysfunctional family dynamics.
c. Transactional Model of Stress/Adaptation. The etiology of dissociative fugue is most likely influenced by multiple factors.
4. Diagnosis/Outcome Identification
a. Nursing diagnoses for the client with dissociative fugue include:
(1) Risk for violence directed toward others
(2) Ineffective individual coping
b. Outcome criteria are identified for measuring the effectiveness of nursing care.
5. Planning/Implementation
a. Nursing intervention for the client with dissociative fugue is aimed at protection of client and others from uncontrolled aggression.
b. The nurse also works at assisting the client to deal more appropriately with severe anxiety.
6. Evaluation is based on accomplishment of previously established outcome criteria.
C. Dissociative Identity Disorder: Background Assessment Data
1. Characterized by the existence of two or more personalities within a single individual.
2. The transition from one personality to another is usually sudden, often dramatic, and usually precipitated by stress.
3. Predisposing Factors to Dissociative Identity Disorder
a. Biological Theories.
(1) Genetics. Dissociative identity disorder is more common in first degree biological relatives of people with the disorder than in the general population.
(2) Organic. Various studies have suggested a possible link to certain neurological alterations (e.g., temporal lobe epilepsy, severe migraine headaches, and cerebral cortical damage) and dissociative identity disorder.
b. Psychological Influences. A growing body of evidence points to the etiology of DID as a set of traumatic experiences that overwhelms the individual's capacity to cope by any means other than dissociation. These experiences usually take the form of severe physical, sexual or psychological abuse by a parent or significant other in the child's life.
c. Theory of Family Dynamics. A dysfunctional family system, with at least one caretaker who exhibits severe psychopathology, has been implicated as an etiology of DID.
d. Transactional Model of Stress/Adaptation. The etiology of dissociative identity disorder is most likely influences by multiple factors.
4. Diagnosis/Outcome Identification
a. Nursing diagnoses for the individual with dissociative identity disorder include:
(1) Risk for self-directed violence
(2) Personal identity disturbance
b. Outcome criteria are identified for measuring the effectiveness of nursing care.
5. Planning/Implementation
a. Nursing intervention for the client with dissociative identity disorder is aimed at protection from self-directed violence.
b. The nurse also works at assisting the client to understand the reasons for existence of various personalities and the importance of eventual integration of the personalities into one.
6. Evaluation is based on accomplishment of previously established outcome criteria.
D. Depersonalization Disorder: Background Assessment Data
1. Characterized by a temporary change in the quality of self-awareness, which often takes the form of feelings of unreality, changes in body image, feelings of detachment from the environment, or a sense of observing oneself from outside the body.
2. Depersonalization is defined as a disturbance in the perception of oneself.
3. Derealization is described as an alteration in the perception of the external environment.

4. Symptoms of depersonalization disorder are often accompanied by anxiety, dizziness, fear of going insane, depression, obsessive thoughts, somatic complaints, and a disturbance in the subjective sense of time.
5. Predisposing Factors to Depersonalization Disorder
   a. Physiological Theories. Suggest that the phenomenon of depersonalization has a neurophysiological basis, such as brain tumor or epilepsy.
   b. Psychodynamic Theories. Place emphasis on psychic conflict and disturbances of ego structure in the predisposition to depersonalization disorder.
   c. Transactional Model of Stress/Adaptation. The etiology of depersonalization disorder is most likely influences by multiple factors.
6. Diagnosis/Outcome Identification
   a. Nursing diagnoses for the client with depersonalization disorder include
      (1) Sensory-perceptual alteration (visual or kinesthetic)
      (2) Anxiety (severe to panic)
   b. Outcome criteria are identified for measuring the effectiveness of nursing care.
7. Planning/Implementation
   a. Nursing intervention for the client with depersonalization disorder is aimed at promoting accurate perception of self and the environment.
   b. The nurse also works at assisting the client to respond more adaptively to severe anxiety.
8. Evaluation is based on accomplishment of previously established outcome criteria.

V. Treatment Modalities
   A. Dissociative Amnesia
      1. Most cases resolve spontaneously.
      2. Refractory conditions may require intravenous administration of amobarbital in the retrieval of lost memories.
      3. Supportive psychotherapy may also be useful.
      4. Hypnosis has been used successfully.
   B. Dissociative Fugue
      1. Recovery is usually rapid, spontaneous, and complete.
      2. Supportive are may be required.
      3. Refractory conditions may require encouragement, persuasion, or directed association, either alone, or in combination with hypnosis or amobarbital administration.
   C. Dissociative Identity Disorder
      1. Integration is considered desirable, but in some cases a reasonable degree of conflict-free collaboration among the personalities is all that can be achieved.
      2. Long-term psychotherapy, with the use of abreaction, has been successful.
      3. Hypnosis is usually used in the process of integration.
   D. Depersonalization Disorder
      1. No particular therapy has proven widely successful.
      2. Pharmacotherapy with dextroamphetamines or amobarbital has been tried with inconclusive results.
      3. Benzodiazepines provide symptomatic relief if anxiety is an important element of the clinical condition.
      4. Some clinicians believe long-term psychoanalysis may be helpful for clients with intrapsychic conflict.

VI. Summary
VII. Critical Thinking Exercise
VIII. Review Questions

ANSWERS TO CRITICAL THINKING EXERCISE

1.   Reassurance of his safety and security.

2.   Encourage him to discuss the stressful life situation that preceded the fugue state and his feelings associated with his life situation.

3.   To develop more adaptive coping strategies.

CASE STUDY FOR USE WITH STUDENT LEARNING

Case Study: Dissociative Identity Disorder

Sandy, age 32, is a newly admitted client on the psychiatric unit, having been transferred from the emergency department where she was stabilized after swallowing a variety of medications. Sandy has been a psychiatric client of Dr. M's for many years. She was first diagnosed as having Atypical Depression. Later, she was given the diagnosis of Borderline Personality Disorder. She has experienced many episodes of self-mutilation and attempted suicide. Five years ago, she was placed in state-supported long-term psychiatric care, where it was discovered that she has multiple personalities. Her history, childhood history, which was only retrieved through use of hypnosis and amobarbital interviews, revealed severe physical and sexual abuse by both her mother and her father, who are now both deceased. Eleven personalities have come forth, 3 children, 3 adolescents, and 5 adults. Two are male. Since the discovery of these personalities, she has continued to work with Dr. M in am attempt at integration. The work has been long and progress is slow. Dr. M's psychiatric history on Sandy states that the continuum of behavioral personalities range from dependent to aggressive. The suicidal personality, Ann, emerged yesterday and swallowed the pills. When Sandy is introduced to the admitting nurse on the psychiatric unit, she responds, "Don't call me Sandy!" I'm not Sandy! And I'm not that wimpy Ann, either!" How should the nurse respond? Design a nursing plan of care for Sandy.

LEARNING ACTIVITY

BEHAVIORS ASSOCIATED WITH DISSOCIATIVE DISORDERS

Identify with which dissociative disorder the behaviors listed are associated.

a. Localized amnesia
b. Selective amnesia
c. Generalized amnesia
d. Continuous amnesia

e. Dissociative fugue
f. Dissociative Identity Disorder
g. Depersonalization Disorder

_____ 1. A young man is brought into the emergency department by the police. He does not know who he is or anything at all about his life.

_____ 2. A young man is brought into the emergency department by the police. He gives his identity and home address (which is several hundred miles away) to the admissions clerk. He tells the nurse he is very frightened, for he doesn't know when or how he came to be in this place.

_____ 3. Sandra is a clerk in an all-night convenience store. Three nights ago, the store was robbed at gunpoint, and Sandra was locked in a storage compartment for several hours until the manager was contacted by passersby who reported the robbery. She has been unable to recall the incident until just today, when details began to emerge. She is now able to report the entire event to the authorities.

_____ 4. Sam is a salesman for a leading manufacturing company. His job requires that he make presentations for large corporations who are considering Sam's company's product. Sam is up for promotion, and realizes that the outcomes of these presentations will weight heavily on whether or not he gets the promotion. Lately, he has been worried that he is going insane. Each time he is about to make a presentation, his thinking becomes "foggy," his body feels without life, and he describes the feeling as being somewhat "anesthetized." These episodes sometimes last for hours, and are beginning to interfere with his performance.

_____ 5. Melody's husband complained of severe chest pain. Melody called the ambulance and accompanied her husband to the hospital. He died in the emergency department of a massive myocardial infarction. With the help of family and friends, Melody made arrangements for the memorial service and the burial. Now that it is all over, Melody is able to remember only certain aspects about the time since her husband first experienced the severe pain. She remembers the doctor telling her her husband was dead, but she cannot remember attending the funeral service.

_____ 6. Margaret explains to the nurse that during the last year, she has periods of time for which she cannot account. She has been attending college, and she finds pages of notes in her notebook that she cannot recall writing. Her roommate recently recounted an incident that took place when they were supposedly out together, for which Margaret has no recall. Most recently she has been hospitalized when her roommate found her unconscious in their room with an empty bottle of sleeping pills beside her. She tells the nurse she has no memory of taking the pills.

_____ 7. Kelly was involved in an automobile accident in which her best friend was killed. Kelly remembers nothing about the accident, nor does she remember anything that has occurred since the accident.

CHAPTER 29. TEST QUESTIONS

1. Tracy is a 27-year-old woman who, after being diagnosed as having major depression, borderline personality disorder, and antisocial personality disorder in previous contacts with the mental health care system, has recently been diagnosed with DID. She has been hospitalized because one of her personalities attempted suicide. What is the *primary* consideration in planning care for Tracy?
   - • a. Safety
     b. Establishing trust
     c. Awareness of all personalities
     d. Recognition of events that trigger transition between personalities

2. The primary nursing diagnosis for Tracy during this hospitalization is
     a. Personal identity disturbance
     b. Sensory-perceptual alteration
     c. Altered thought processes
   - • d. Risk for self-directed violence

3. Anxiety is involved in understanding the problem of dissociative amnesia. The defense mechanism used in this psychogenic process is:
     a. Suppression
     b. Denial
   - • c. Repression
     d. Rationalization

4. Bill C. has been diagnosed with a dissociative disorder that is identified as a fugue state. Which of the following behaviors best illustrates this diagnosis?
     a. Seeking privacy in his office.
     b. Driving a long distance to visit a friend.
   - • c. Sudden unexpected travel away from home.
     d. Taking a vacation to a place he would not usually go.

5. Bill's unusual activity (from question #4) may have occurred in response to which of the following?
     a. Severe psychological stress
     b. Excessive alcohol use
     c. Psychogenic amnesia
   - • d. a or b

6. Which of the following is an example of systematized amnesia?
     a. George has no memory of his entire lifetime, including his personal identity.
   - • b. AnnMarie knows she was beaten by her mother as a child, but cannot remember the details of any of the beatings.
     c. Nancy, who was driving the car in which her best friend was killed, cannot recall the accident or events since the accident.
     d. Sarah, whose home was destroyed in a tornado, only remembers hearing the tornado hit, the ambulance siren, and waking up in the hospital.

CHAPTER 30. SEXUAL AND GENDER IDENTITY DISORDERS

CHAPTER FOCUS

The focus of this chapter is on nursing care of clients with sexual or gender identity disorders. Predisposing factors and symptomatology are explored, and nursing care is presented in the context of the six steps of the nursing process. Medical treatment modalities are also discussed.

LEARNING OBJECTIVES

After reading this chapter, the student will be able to:

1.   Describe developmental processes associated with human sexuality.
2.   Discuss historical and epidemiological aspects of paraphilias and sexual dysfunction disorders.
3.   Identify various types of paraphilias, sexual dysfunction disorders, and gender identity disorders.
4.   Discuss predisposing factors associated with the etiology of paraphilias, sexual dysfunction disorders, and gender identity disorders.
5.   Describe the physiology of the human sexual response.
6.   Conduct a sexual history.
7.   Formulate nursing diagnoses and goals of care for clients with sexual and gender identity disorders.
8.   Identify appropriate nursing interventions for clients with sexual and gender identity disorders.
9.   Identify topics for client/family education relevant to sexual disorders.
10. Evaluate nursing care of clients with sexual and gender identity disorders.
11. Describe various treatment modalities for clients with sexual and gender identity disorders.
12. Discuss variations in sexual orientation.
13. Identify various types of sexually transmitted diseases and discuss the consequences of each.

KEY TERMS

anorgasmia
dyspareunia
exhibitionism
fetishism
frotteurism
gonorrhea
homosexuality
lesbianism
masochism
orgasm
paraphilia

pedophilia
premature ejaculation
retarded ejaculation
sadism
sensate focus
syphilis
transsexualism
transvestic fetishism
vaginismus
voyeurism

CHAPTER OUTLINE/LECTURE NOTES

I.   Introduction
     A.   Sexuality is a basic need and an aspect of humanness that cannot be separated from life events.
     B.   Although not all nurses need to be educated as sex therapists, they can readily integrate information on sexuality in the care they give by focusing on preventive, therapeutic, and educational interventions to assist individuals attain, regain, or maintain sexual wellness.
II. Development of Human Sexuality

A. Birth Through Age 12
   1. By age 2 or 2-1/2, children know what gender they are.
   2. By age 4 or 5, children engage in heterosexual play.
   3. Late childhood and preadolescence may be characterized by homosexual play.
   4. Ages 10 to 12 are preoccupied with pubertal changes and the beginnings of romantic interest in the opposite gender.
B. Adolescence
   1. Adolescents relate to sexual issues such as how to deal with new or more powerful sexual feelings, whether to participate in various types of sexual behavior, how to recognize love, how to prevent unwanted pregnancy, and how to define age-appropriate sex roles.
C. Adulthood. This period begins at approximately 20 years of age and continues to age 65.
   1. Marital Sex. Choosing a marital partner or developing a sexual relationship with another individual is one of the major tasks in the early years of this life cycle stage.
   2. Extramarital Sex. Approximately 20-30% of all married men have extramarital sex at some time in their lives, compared with about 15-20% of all women.
   3. Sex and Single Person. Attitudes about sexual intimacy vary greatly from individual to individual. Some enjoy their freedom and independence while others are desperately seeking an intimate relationship.
   4. The Middle Years--46 to 55. Hormonal changes occurring during this period produce changes in sexual activity for both men and women.
III. Sexual Disorders
A. Paraphilias. A term used to identify repetitive or preferred sexual fantasies or behaviors that involve preference for use of nonhuman object, repetitive sexual activity with humans involving real or simulated suffering or humiliation, and repetitive sexual activity with nonconsenting partners.
   1. Historical Aspects
      a. At certain times in history, various sexual behaviors have been, and still are, condemned by certain social and religious sanctions.
   2. Epidemiological Statistics
      a. Most paraphiliacs are men, and more than 10 percent of these individuals develop the onset of their paraphilic arousal prior to age 18.
   3. Types of Paraphilias
      a. Exhibitionism: characterized by recurrent, intense, sexual urges, behaviors, or sexually arousing fantasies involving the exposure of one's genitals to an unsuspecting stranger.
      b. Fetishism: involves recurrent, intense, sexual urges or behaviors or sexually arousing fantasies involving the use of nonliving objects (e.g., bras, underpants, stockings).
      c. Frotteurism: the recurrent preoccupation with intense sexual urges or fantasies involving touching or rubbing against a nonconsenting person.
      d. Pedophilia: recurrent sexual urges, behaviors or sexually arousing fantasies involving sexual activity with a prepubescent child.
      e. Sexual Masochism: recurrent, intense, sexual urges, behaviors, or sexually arousing fantasies involving the act (real, not simulated) of being humiliated, beaten, bound, or otherwise made to suffer.
      f. Sexual Sadism: recurrent, intense, sexual urges, behaviors, or sexually arousing fantasies involving acts (real, not simulated) in which the psychological or physical suffering (including humiliation) of the victim is sexually exciting.
      g. Voyeurism: recurrent, intense, sexual urges, behaviors, or sexually arousing fantasies involving the act of observing unsuspecting people, usually strangers, who are either naked, in the process of disrobing, or engaging in sexual activity.
   4. Predisposing Factors to Paraphilias
      a. Biological Factors. Various studies have implicated several organic factors in the etiology of paraphilias. These include abnormalities in the limbic system and the temporal lobe. Abnormal levels of androgens have also been implicated.
      b. Psychoanalytical Theory. Suggests that a paraphiliac is one who has failed the normal developmental process toward heterosexual adjustment. This occurs when the individual fails

to resolve the oepidal crisis and either identifies with the parent of the opposite gender or selects an inappropriate object for libido cathexis.

    c.   Behavioral Theory. The behavioral model hypothesizes that whether or not an individual engages in paraphiliac behavior depends on the type of reinforcement he receives following the behavior. The initial act may be committed for various reasons (e.g., modeling the paraphilic behavior of others; mimicking sexual behavior depicted in the media). But once the initial act has been committed, a conscious evaluation of the behavior occurs, and a choice is made of whether or not to repeat it.

    d.   Transactional Model of Stress/Adaptation. It is most likely that the etiology of paraphilias is influenced by multiple factors.

    5.   Treatment Modalities

        a.   Biological Treatment. The focus of this treatment is on blocking or decreasing the level of circulating androgens.

        b.   Psychoanalytical Therapy. With this type of therapy, the client is assisted to identify unresolved conflicts and traumas from early childhood, thus resolving the anxiety that prevents him or her from forming appropriate sexual relationships.

        c.   Behavioral Therapy. Aversion techniques, such as the use of electric shock and chemical induction of nausea and vomiting, usually in combination with exposure to photographs depicting the undesired behavior, have been used to modify undesirable paraphilic behavior.

    6.   Role of the Nurse

        a.   Nursing may best become involved in the primary prevention process.

        b.   The focus of primary prevention in sexual disorders is to intervene in home life or other facets of childhood in an effort to prevent problems from developing.

        c.   An additional concern of primary prevention is to assist in the development of adaptive coping strategies to deal with stressful life situations.

B.   Sexual Dysfunctions

    1.   Usually occur as a problem in one of the following phases of the sexual response cycle:

        a.   Phase I: Desire

        b.   Phase II: Excitement

        c.   Phase III: Orgasm

        d.   Phase IV: Resolution

    2.   Historical and Epidemiological Aspects Related to Sexual Dysfunction

        a.   Concurrent with the cultural changes occurring during the sexual revolution of the 1960s and 1970s came an increase in scientific research into sexual physiology and sexual dysfunctions.

        b.   Masters and Johnson pioneered this work with their studies on human sexual response and the treatment of sexual dysfunctions.

    3.   Types of Sexual Dysfunction

        a.   Sexual Desire Disorders

            (1) Hypoactive Sexual Desire Disorder. Persistent or recurrent deficiency or absence of sexual fantasies and desire for sexual activity.

            (2) Sexual Aversion Disorder. Persistent or recurrent extreme aversion to, and avoidance of, all or almost all genital sexual contact with a sexual partner.

        b.   Sexual Arousal Disorders

            (1) Female Sexual Arousal Disorder. Failure to attain or maintain the lubrication-swelling response, or experience a subjective sense of sexual excitement and pleasure in a female during sexual activity.

            (2) Male Erectile Disorder. Persistent or recurrent inability to attain, or maintain until completion of the sexual activity, an adequate erection.

        c.   Orgasmic Disorders

            (1) Female Orgasmic Disorder (Anorgasmia). The recurrent and persistent inhibition of the female orgasm, as manifested by the absence or delay of orgasm following a period of sexual excitement judged adequate in intensity and duration to produce such a response.

            (2) Male Orgasmic Disorder (Retarded Ejaculation). Persistent or recurrent delay in, or absence of, orgasm following a normal sexual excitement phase during sexual activity that

the clinician, taking into account the person's age, judges to be adequate in focus, intensity, and duration.

(3) Premature Ejaculation. Persistent or recurrent ejaculation with minimal sexual stimulation or before, upon, or shortly after penetration and before the person wishes it.

d. Sexual Pain Disorders
(1) Dyspareunia. Recurrent or persistent genital pain in either a male or female before, during or after sexual intercourse, that is not associated with vaginismus or with lack of lubrication.
(2) Vaginismus. An involuntary constriction of the outer one-third of the vagina that prevents penile insertion and intercourse.

e. Sexual Dysfunction Due to a General Medical Condition and Substance-Induced Sexual Dysfunction
(1) With these disorders, the sexual dysfunction is judged to be caused by the direct physiological effects of a general medical condition or use of a substance.

4. Predisposing Factors to Sexual Dysfunctions
a. Biological Factors. Suggestive evidence exists of a relationship between serum testosterone and hypoactive sexual desire disorder in men and increased libido in women. Certain medications, such as antihypertensives, antipsychotics, antidepressants, anxiolytics, and anticonvulsants may also be implicated in the etiology of hypoactive sexual desire disorder. Erectile disorders in men may be affected by arteriosclerosis and diabetes. In women, consumption of alcohol, as well as certain medications, have been shown to affect a woman's ability to have orgasms. Various organic factors have also been associated with painful intercourse in both men and women.

b. Psychosocial Factors. A number of psychosocial factors have been associated with sexual desire disorders, as well as with virtually all the sexual disorders. A few of these factors include religious orthodoxy, secret sexual deviations, fear of pregnancy, childhood sexual abuse, rape, fears, anxiety, and depression.

c. Transactional Model of Stress/Adaptation. The etiology of sexual disorders is most likely influenced by multiple factors.

IV. Application of the Nursing Process
A. Assessment. A tool for gathering a sexual history is included. Additional information should be gathered for the clients who have medical or surgical conditions that may affect their sexuality; clients with infertility problems, sexually transmitted disease, or complaints of sexual inadequacy; clients who are pregnancy, or present with gynecologic problems; those seeking information on abortion or family planning; and individuals in premarital, marital, or psychiatric counseling.

B. Diagnosis/Outcome Identification
1. Nursing diagnoses for clients experiencing sexual dysfunction include:
   a. Sexual dysfunction
   b. Altered sexuality patterns
2. Outcome criteria are identified for measuring the effectiveness of nursing care.

C. Planning/Implementation
1. Nursing intervention for the client with sexual disorders is aimed at assisting the individual to gain or regain the aspect of his or her sexuality that is desired.
2. The nurse must remain nonjudgmental and ensure that personal feelings, attitudes, and values have been clarified and do not interfere with acceptance of the client.

D. Evaluation is based on accomplishment of previously established outcome criteria.

V. Treatment Modalities. Various sexual dysfunctions and some treatment modalities that have been tried are listed here.
A. Hypoactive Sexual Desire Disorder
1. Testosterone
2. Cognitive Therapy
3. Behavioral Therapy
4. Marital Therapy
B. Sexual Aversion Disorder
1. Systematic Desensitization

    2. Antidepressant Medications
  C. Female Sexual Arousal Disorder
    1. Sensate Focus Exercises
  D. Male Erectile Disorder
    1. Sensate Focus Exercises
    2. Group Therapy
    3. Hypnotherapy
    4. Systematic Desensitization
    5. Testosterone
    6. Sildenafil (Viagra)
    7. Penile implantation
  E. Female Orgasmic Disorder
    1. Sensate Focus Exercises
    2. Directed Masturbation
  F. Premature Ejaculation
    1. Senate Focus Exercises
    2. "Squeeze" Technique
  G. Dyspareunia
    1. Physical and Gynecological Examination
    2. Systematic Desensitization
  H. Vaginismus
    1. Education of the woman and her partner regarding the anatomy and physiology of the disorder
    2. Systematic desensitization with dilators of graduated sizes
VI. Gender Identity Disorders
  A. Gender identity is the sense of knowledge to which sex one belongs, that is, the awareness of one's masculinity or femininity.
  B. Gender identity disorders occur when there is an incongruence between anatomical sex and gender identity.
  C. Predisposing Factors
    1. Biological Influences. Possible link to congenital adrenal hyperplasia.
    2. Family Dynamics. May be influenced by parents who encourage strong interests in opposite-gender activities and weak reinforcement of normative gender-role behavior.
    3. Psychoanalytical Theory. Suggests that gender identity problems begin during the struggle with the oepidal conflict, which interferes with the child's loving of the opposite-gender parent and identifying with the same-gender parent, and ultimately with normal gender identity.
VII. Application of the Nursing Process
  A. Background Assessment Data (Symptomatology)
    1. Gender Identity Disorder in Children
      a. Repeatedly stated desire to be, or insistence that he or she is, the other sex.
      b. In boys, preference for cross-dressing or simulating female attire; in girls, insistence on wearing only stereotypical masculine clothing.
      c. Strong and persistent preferences for cross-sex roles in make-believe play or persistent fantasies of being the other sex.
      d. Intense desire to participate in the stereotypical games and pastimes of the other sex.
      e. Strong preference for playmates of the other sex.
    2. Gender Identity Disorder in Adolescents and Adults
      a. Symptomatic manifestations include a stated desire to be the other sex, frequent passing as the other sex, a desire to live or be treated as the other sex, or the conviction that he or she has the typical feelings and reactions of the other sex.
  B. Diagnosis/Outcome Identification
    1. Nursing diagnoses for the client with gender identity disorder include:
      a. Personal identity disturbance
      b. Impaired social interaction
      c. Self-esteem disturbance
  C. Planning/Implementation

1. Nursing intervention for the client with gender identity disorder is aimed at enhancing culturally appropriate same-sex behaviors, but not necessarily to extinguish all coexisting opposite-sex behaviors.
2. Emphasis is also given to improvement in social interactions and enhancement of positive self-esteem.
   D. Evaluation is based on accomplishment of previously established outcome criteria.
VIII. Variations in Sexual Orientation
   A. Homosexuality. The lifestyle that expresses a sexual preference for individuals of the same gender. This is only seen by the psychiatric community as a problem when the individual experiences "persistent and marked distress about his or her sexual orientation."
   1. Predisposing Factors
      a. Biological Theories. It has been suggested that a genetic tendency for homosexuality may be inherited, or that a decreased level of testosterone may be influential. Neither hypothesis has been substantiated.
      b. Psychosocial Theories.
         (1) Freud suggested a possible fixation in the stage of development where homosexual tendencies are common.
         (2) Bieber and coworkers suggested a dysfunctional family pattern as an etiological influence in the development of male homosexuality. The mother was described as dominant, overprotective, possessive, and seductive in her interactions with her son. The father was found to be passive, distant, and covertly or overtly hostile, and was openly devalued and dominated by the mother.
         (3) These theories of family dynamics have been disputed by some clinicians who believe that parents have very little influence on the outcome of their children's sexual-partner orientation.
   2. Special Concerns
      a. Sexually transmitted diseases, in particular, AIDS
      b. Discovery of their sexual orientation
      c. Fear of being rejected by parents and significant others
      d. Discrimination within society
   B. Transsexualism. A disorder of gender identity or gender dysphoria (unhappiness or dissatisfaction with one's gender) of the most extreme variety. An individual, despite having the anatomical characteristics of a given gender, has the self-perception of being of the opposite gender.
   1. Predisposing Factors
      a. Biological Theories. There has been some speculation that gender-disordered individuals may be exposed to inappropriate hormones during the prenatal period, which can result in a genetic female having male genitals, or a genetic male having female genitals. Evidence is inconclusive.
      b. Psychosocial Theories.
         (1) Extensive, pervasive childhood femininity in a boy or childhood masculinity in a girl increases the likelihood of transsexualism.
         (2) Repeated cross-dressing of a young child.
         (3) Lack of separation/individuation of a boy from his mother.
   2. Special Concerns
      a. Extensive psychological testing prior to surgical intervention.
      b. Hormonal treatment initiated during this period.
      c. Both men and women continue to receive maintenance hormone therapy following surgery.
   C. Bisexuality. An individual who is not exclusively heterosexual or homosexual, but engages in sexual activity with members of both genders.
   1. Predisposing Factors
      a. Little research exists on the etiology of bisexuality.
      b. Freud believed that all humans are inherently bisexual.
      c. Riddle suggests that gender identity (determining whether one is male or female) seems to be established during the preschool years.

        d.   Sexual identity (determining whether one is heterosexual or homosexual or both) most likely continues to evolve throughout one's lifetime.

IX.   Sexually Transmitted Diseases

    A. Sexually Transmitted Diseases (STDs) are a group of disease syndromes that can be transmitted sexually irrespective of whether the disease has genital pathologic manifestations. They may be transmitted from one person to another through heterosexual or homosexual, anal, oral, or genital contact.

    B. Sexually transmitted diseases are at epidemic levels in the United States.

    C. The nurse's first responsibility in STD control is to educate clients who may develop or have a sexually transmitted infection.

    D. Prevention of STD's is the ideal goal, but early detection and appropriate treatment continue to be considered a realistic objective.

    E. Information regarding the following types of STDs is presented:

        1. Gonorrhea

        2. Syphilis

        3. Chlamydial Infection

        4. Genital Herpes

        5. Genital Warts

        6. Hepatitis B

        7. Acquired Immunodeficiency Syndrome (AIDS)

X.   Summary

XI.   Critical Thinking Exercise

XII.   Review Questions

ANSWERS TO CRITICAL THINKING EXERCISE

1. Sexual dysfunction related to unresolved sexual issues from her own teen years evidenced by loss of sexual desire.

2. Encourage her to talk about the incident from her adolescence. Encourage her to talk about her relationship with her husband. Explore her fears of having sex with her husband with the teenagers in the house. Help her problem solve ways to overcome these fears (e.g., a lock on their bedroom door). Take a medication history to ensure lack of sexual desire is not related to a substance. Suggest they spend regular time alone (away from the house if necessary). Help her problem solve ways to accomplish this. Help her to understand that she and her husband need not return to the level of sexual interaction in which they participated early in their marriage.

3. To resume sexual activity with her husband at a level of participation that is satisfactory to both. (This may mean that her husband will have to compromise his level of sexual desire. If they are unable to resolve their differences, the nurse may need to make a referral to a sex therapist who specializes in this type of problem.)

LEARNING ACTIVITY

VALUES CLARIFICATION

Answer the following questions. Move into small groups and analyze and discuss your answers.

1.   As a child, when was the first time you discussed sex? With whom?

2.   As an adolescent, when was the first time you began to notice a change in your body? Were you proud of it? Did you want to change it in any way?

3.   Did your parents talk to you outright about sex? If not, what was the underlying message?

4.   Did you make an active decision to become sexually active, or did it happen spontaneously? Has "safe sex" become an important consideration?

5.   What are your feelings about sex between elderly individuals?

6.   Describe your tolerance of homosexuality as an alternate sexual orientation.

7.   Describe your tolerance of a homosexual man as your fifth grade son's teacher.

8.   You discover your 10-year-old sister and her two playmates playing "doctor" in the garage. What is your response?

In your opinion,

9.   Should a married woman, who has a satisfactory sexual relationship with her husband, masturbate with a vibrator?

10.   Do most parents give their daughters as much sexual freedom as they do their sons? Should they?

11.   Do parents who give contraceptives to their adolescents present a message that having sex is okay?

12.   Are individuals who have sex change operations freaks?

13.   Does pornography lead to sexual crimes?

14.   Are oral and anal sex deviant behaviors?

15.   Do you ever have the right to refuse treatment to an AIDS client?

CHAPTER 30. TEST QUESTIONS

1. Tom and Susan are seeking treatment at the sex therapy clinic. They have been married for 3 years. Susan was a virgin when they married. She admits that she has never really enjoyed sex, but lately has developed an aversion to it. They have not had sexual intercourse for about 5 months. Sexual history reveals that Susan grew up in a family who were very closed about sexual issues, and with the implication that sex was sinful and dirty. The physician would most likely assign which of the following diagnoses to Susan?
    a. Dyspareunia
    b. Vaginismus
    c. Anorgasmia
 • d. Sexual aversion disorder

2. The most appropriate nursing diagnosis for Susan would be:
    a. Pain related to vaginal constriction.
 • b. Sexual dysfunction related to negative teachings about sex.
    c. Altered sexuality patterns related to lack of desire for sex.
    d. Self-esteem disturbance related to inability to please her husband sexually.

3. Which of the following interventions by the nurse may initiate treatment for Tom and Susan?
 • a. An explanation of the diagnosis
    b. Initiating sensate focus exercises
    c. Initiating directed masturbation training
    d. Teaching the "squeeze" technique

4. The sex therapist assigned to the case would likely choose which of the following therapies for Susan?
    a. Sensate focus exercises
 • b. Systematic Desensitization
    c. Hypnotherapy
    d. Gradual dilation of the vagina

5. Additional therapy may include:
    a. Minor tranquilizers
    b. Group therapy
 • c. Tricyclic Antidepressant
    d. Injections of testosterone

CHAPTER 31. EATING DISORDERS

CHAPTER FOCUS

The focus of this chapter is on nursing care of clients with eating disorders. Predisposing factors and symptomatology are explored, and nursing care is presented in the context of the six steps of the nursing process. Medical treatment modalities are also discussed.

LEARNING OBJECTIVES

After reading this chapter, the student will be able to:

1. Identify and differentiate among the various eating disorders.
2. Discuss epidemiological statistics related to eating disorders.
3. Describe symptomatology associated with anorexia nervosa, bulimia nervosa, and obesity, and use the information in client assessment.
4. Identify predisposing factors in the development of eating disorders.
5. Formulate nursing diagnoses and goals of care for clients with eating disorders.
6. Describe appropriate interventions for behaviors associated with eating disorders.
7. Identify topics for client and family teaching relevant to eating disorders.
8. Evaluate the nursing care of clients with eating disorders.
9. Discuss various modalities relevant to treatment of eating disorders.

KEY TERMS

amenorrhea
binging
purging
body image
emaciated
anorexia
obesity
anorexigenics

CHAPTER OUTLINE/LECTURE NOTES

I. Introduction
   A. The hypothalamus contains the appetite regulation center within the brain. It regulates the body's ability to recognize when it is hungry and when it has been sated.
   B. Eating behaviors are influenced by society and culture.
   C. Historically, society and culture also have influenced what is considered desirable in the female body.
II. Epidemiological Factors
   A. The incidence rate of anorexia nervosa among young women in the United States is approximately 14 per 100,000 population.
   B. Anorexia nervosa occurs predominantly in females aged 12 to 30 years.
   C. Bulimia nervosa is more prevalent than anorexia nervosa. Estimates range from 1 percent to 3 percent of young women.
   D. Onset of bulimia nervosa occurs in late adolescence or early adulthood, with a mean age of onset of 18 years.

E. Obesity has been defined as body mass index of 30 or above.

F. Estimates show that 24% of adult males and 27% of adult females in the U.S. today suffer from obesity.

III. Application of the Nursing Process

    A. Background Assessment Data (Symptomatology)

        1. Anorexia Nervosa

            a. Characterized by a morbid fear of obesity.

            b. Symptoms include gross distortion of body image, preoccupation with food, and refusal to eat.

            c. Weight loss is extreme, usually more than 15% of expected weight.

            d. Other symptoms include hypothermia, bradycardia, hypotension, edema, lanugo, and a variety of metabolic changes.

            e. Amenorrhea is typical, and may even precede significant weight loss.

            f. There may be an obsession with food.

            g. Feelings of anxiety and depression are common.

        2. Bulimia Nervosa

            a. Bulimia is the episodic, uncontrolled, compulsive, rapid ingestion of large quantities of food over a short period of time (binging), followed by inappropriate compensatory behaviors to rid the body of the excess calories (self-induced vomiting, or the misuse of laxatives, diuretics, or enemas).

            b. Fasting or excessive exercise may also occur.

            c. Most bulimics are within a normal weight range, some slightly underweight, some slightly overweight.

            d. Excessive vomiting and laxative/diuretic abuse may lead to problems with dehydration and electrolyte imbalance.

            e. Depression, anxiety, and substance abuse are not uncommon.

        3. Predisposing Factors to Anorexia Nervosa and Bulimia Nervosa

            a. Biological Influences

                (1) Genetics. A hereditary predisposition to eating disorders has been hypothesized. Anorexia nervosa is more common among sisters and mothers of those with the disorder than among the general population.

                (2) Neuroendocrine Abnormalities. Some speculation has occurred regarding a primary hypothalamic dysfunction in anorexia nervosa. The neurotransmitters serotonin and norepinephrine may be involved in the predisposition to bulimia nervosa, while high levels of endogenous opioids may be associated with anorexia nervosa.

            b. Psychodynamic Influences

                (1) Psychodynamic theory suggests that eating disorders result from very early and profound disturbances in mother-infant interactions, resulting in retarded ego development and an unfulfilled sense of separation-individuation.

                (2) Elements of Power and Control. Power and control may become the overriding elements in the family of the client with an eating disorder. Parental criticism promotes an increase in obsessive and perfectionistic behavior on the part of the child, who continues to seek love, approval, and recognition. Ambivalence toward the parents develops, and distorted eating patterns may represent a rebellion against the parents--a way to gain control.

        4. Obesity

            a. A body mass index (weight in kilograms divided by height in meters squared) of 30 is considered obesity.

            b. At this level, weight alone can contribute to increases in morbidity and mortality.

            c. Obese people are at higher risk for hyperlipidemia, diabetes mellitus, osteoarthritis, angina, and respiratory insufficiency.

        5. Predisposing Factors to Obesity

            a. Biological Influences

                (1) Genetics. Eight percent of children born of two overweight parents will also be overweight. Twin studies have also supported a hereditary factors.

                (2) Physiological Factors

                    (a) Lesions in the appetite and satiety centers of the hypothalamus

                    (b) Hypothyroidism

               (c) Decreased insulin production

               (d) Increased cortisone production

          (3) Lifestyle Factors

               (a) Increased caloric intake

               (b) Sedentary lifestyle

     b. Psychosocial Influences

        (1) Unresolved dependency needs

        (2) Fixation in the oral stage of psychosexual development

     c. Transactional Model of Stress/Adaptation

        (1) The etiology of eating disorders is most likely influenced by multiple factors.

B. Diagnosis/Outcome Identification

  1. Nursing Diagnoses for the client with eating disorders include:

     a. Altered nutrition: less than body requirements

     b. Fluid volume deficit (risk for or actual)

     c. Ineffective denial

     d. Altered nutrition: more than body requirements

     e. Body image/Self-esteem disturbance

     f. Anxiety (moderate to severe)

  2. Outcome criteria are identified for measuring the effectiveness of nursing care.

C. Planning/Implementation

  1. Nursing care of the client with an eating disorder is aimed at restoring nutritional balance.

  2. Emphasis is also placed on helping the client gain control over life situation in ways other than inappropriate eating behaviors.

  3. Self-esteem and positive self-image are promoted in ways that relate to aspects other than appearance.

D. Evaluation is based on accomplishment of previously established outcome criteria.

IV. Treatment Modalities

  A. Behavior Modification

  B. Individual Therapy

  C. Family Therapy

  D. Psychopharmacology

V. Summary

VI. Critical Thinking Exercise

VII. Review Questions

ANSWERS TO CRITICAL THINKING EXERCISE

1. Restoring her nutritional condition.

2. A program of behavior modification, with privileges based on weight gain.

3. The door to her bathroom will need to be kept locked for at least one hour following meals. However, she will still need to be watched carefully, as she may go into other clients' bathrooms to purge herself.

CASE STUDY FOR USE WITH STUDENT LEARNING

Case Study: Bulimia Nervosa

Abby, age 29, was married and the mother of a 5-year-old girl. Her husband, Tom, was a rising young executive in a prominent business firm. Abby did not work outside the home, and Tom had expectations about how he expected Abby to care for their daughter and their home. Abby had grown up as the only child of a professional couple who had high expectations of her. Feeling unable to measure up to their expectations, Abby had developed anorexia nervosa during her sophomore year in high school, and the family had spent several years in family therapy. Abby went to college in a distant city. During these years, she did not go home often. She joined a sorority, but often felt as though she did not quite fit in with these young women. She felt very flattered when Tom began to pay attention to her during her junior year in college. But she continued to feel anxious and insecure, and during these periods of anxiety, Abby would resort to maladaptive eating patterns to cope. During this time, however, the eating behavior more often took the form of binging. She would eat whole boxes of cookies, cakes, or candy, followed by periods of intense depression. In order to keep from gaining weight, she would self-induce vomiting, or take massive doses of laxatives. She exercises excessively. She managed to keep her weight within normal limits, while hiding her behavior from her boyfriend and classmates. Once she and Tom were married, some of the anxiety subsided, and she relied less on the maladaptive eating behaviors. However, lately, she has been called upon by her husband to entertain business associates, which has created a great deal of anxiety for Abby. Tom tells her exactly how he expects things to be and also tells her how much her appearance and behavior affects how these business associates will view them. She feels a great deal of pressure from Tom to be "the perfect wife," and just doesn't feel she can measure up. She has begun to binge and purge daily. Last night, she was binging after Tom and their daughter had gone to bed. Tom heard her vomiting in their bathroom. He got up to investigate, and found her leaning over the toilet, in which he noted a large amount of blood. He took her to the emergency room where she was treated for a bleeding esophageal varicosity. She was stabilized and admitted to the psychiatric unit. Diagnosis: Bulimia Nervosa. Design a care plan for Abby.

LEARNING ACTIVITY

Check the eating disorder to which the symptoms in the left-hand column apply. Some may apply to more than one disorder. The first is completed as an example.

Symptoms	Anorexia Nervosa	Bulimia Nervosa	Obesity
1. Depression	X	X	
2. Amenorrhea			
3. Risk of diabetes mellitus			
4. Erosion of tooth enamel			
5. Preoccupation with food			
6. Self-induced vomiting			
7. Fixed in oral stage of development			
8. Is markedly underweight			
9. Weight is close to normal			
10. Is markedly overweight			
11. Abuse of substances is not uncommon			
12. May be related to hypothyroidism			
13. May be related to issues of control			
14. Genetics may play a role in the cause			
15. Takes in enormous amounts of food without gaining weight			

CHAPTER 31. TEST QUESTIONS

Situation: Stephanie, age 23, calls the eating disorders clinic for an appointment. She tells the nurse who does the assessment interview that she was hospitalized and diagnosed with anorexia nervosa when she was 14 years old. Since that time, she has seen a therapist periodically when she feels her anxiety is increasing and the fear of eating starts to take hold. She recently graduated from college and moved to this city, where she began a new job as a production assistant at a local TV station. She is nervous about starting the new job, and wants to "do a perfect job, so I can move up quickly to a more challenging position." She tells the nurse that she has been taking laxatives every day, and some days after eating, she will self-induce vomiting. She knows this is not good, but feels powerless to stop. She is 5'6" tall and weights 105 lb.

1. What other physical manifestations might the nurse expect to find upon assessment?
   - a. High blood pressure, fever
   - • b. Low blood pressure, low temperature
   - c. Slow heart rate, fever
   - d. Fast heart rate, low blood pressure

2. The *primary* nursing diagnosis on which the nurse will base her plan of care is:
   - a. Ineffective denial
   - b. Body image disturbance
   - c. Self-esteem disturbance
   - • d. Altered nutrition, less than body requirements

3. What other therapy might the physician prescribe?
   - • a. Fluoxetine (Prozac)
   - b. Diazepam (Valium)
   - c. Fenfluramine (Pondimin)
   - d. Meprobamate (Equanil)

Situation: Betty, a 38-year-old woman, is also being followed in the eating disorders clinic. Betty is 5'4" and weighs 250 pounds. When she first came to the clinic two years ago, she weighed 347 pounds. Her diagnosis at that time was Morbid Obesity. The dietitian put her on a 1500 calorie/day diet and the physician at the clinic prescribed fenfluramine and phentermine, the "fen-fen" drugs that were so popular at that time. Since then, fenfluramine has been taken off the market because it caused pulmonary hypertension in a number of individuals. Betty says to the nurse, "I don't know what to do! I know I can't lose weight without those drugs. That's the only reason I lost any at all. And I've already gained some back since I quit taking them!"

4. Fenfluramine and phentermine are part of which of the following classifications of drugs?
   - a. Antidepressants
   - • b. Anorexigenics
   - c. Antianxiety
   - d. Anticonvulsants

5. The nurse explains to Betty that the physician may be able to prescribe another medication to help her lose weight. Which of the following might the nurse expect the physician to prescribe?
   - a. Diazepam (Valium)
   - b. Dexfenfluramine (Redux)
   - • c. Sibutramine (Meridia)
   - d. Pemoine (Cylert)

6. The nurse tells Betty that she will lose weight even without medication if she just sticks to her diet and adds some exercise to her routine. What would be the most appropriate exercise for the nurse to suggest for Betty?
   - a. Low-impact aerobics 3 times a week
   - b. Jogging 1/2 mile twice a week
   - c. Swimming at the YWCA 30 minutes/day
   - • d. Walking around her neighborhood for 20 minutes/day (weather permitting)

CHAPTER 32. ADJUSTMENT AND IMPULSE CONTROL DISORDERS

CHAPTER FOCUS

The focus of this chapter is on nursing care of clients with adjustment and impulse control disorders. Predisposing factors and symptomatology are explored, and nursing care is presented in the context of the six steps of the nursing process. Medical treatment modalities are also discussed.

LEARNING OBJECTIVES

After reading this chapter, the student will be able to:

1. Discuss historical aspects and epidemiological statistics related to adjustment and impulse control disorders.
2. Describe various types of adjustment and impulse control disorders and identify symptomatology associated with each; use this information in client assessment.
3. Identify predisposing factors in the development of adjustment and impulse control disorders.
4. Formulate nursing diagnoses and goals of care for clients with adjustment and impulse control disorders.
5. Describe appropriate nursing interventions for behaviors associated with adjustment and impulse control disorders.
6. Identify topics for client and family teaching relevant to adjustment and impulse control disorders.
7. Evaluate nursing care of clients with adjustment and impulse control disorders.
8. Discuss various modalities relevant to treatment of adjustment and impulse control disorders.

KEY TERMS

adjustment disorder
Gamblers Anonymous
kleptomania
pathological gambling
pyromania
trichotillomania

CHAPTER OUTLINE/LECTURE NOTES

I.   Introduction
     A. Adjustment disorders are precipitated by an identifiable psychosocial stressor, and impulse disorders are often modulated directly by the severity of psychosocial stressors.
     B. Behaviors may include:
         1. Impairment in an individual's usual social and occupational functioning
         2. Compulsive acts that may be harmful to the person or others
II. Historical and Epidemiological Factors
     A. Historically, clients with symptoms identified by adjustment or impulse control disorders were classified as having personality disturbances.
     B. The original impulse control disorders date back to the 19th century and included alcoholism, firesetting, homicide, and kleptomania.
     C. Adjustment disorders are quite common. Some studies indicate that adjustment disorder is the most frequent diagnosis given.
III. Application of the Nursing Process
     A. Adjustment Disorders: Background Assessment Data

1. An adjustment disorder is characterized by a maladaptive reaction to an identifiable psychosocial stressor that occurs within three months after onset of the stressor and has persisted for no longer than six months after onset of the stressor.
2. Categories are distinguished by the predominant features of the maladaptive response.
    a. Adjustment Disorder with Anxiety. This category denotes a maladaptive response to a psychosocial stressor in which the predominant manifestation is anxiety.
    b. Adjustment Disorder with Depressed Mood. This category (the most common) is one of predominant mood disturbance, although less pronounced than that of major depression.
    c. Adjustment Disorder with Disturbance of Conduct. Characterized by conduct in which there is violation of the rights of others or of major age-appropriate societal norms and rules.
    d. Adjustment Disorder with Mixed Disturbance of Emotions and Conduct. Predominant features of this category include mood disturbances and emotional disturbances, as well as conduct in which there is violation of the rights of others or of major age-appropriate societal norms and rules.
    e. Adjustment Disorder Unspecified. This subtype is used when the maladaptive reaction is not consistent with any of the other categories.
3. Predisposing Factors to Adjustment Disorders
    a. Biological Theory. The presence of chronic disorders, such as organic mental disorder or mental retardation, is thought to limit the general adaptive capacity of an individual.
    b. Psychosocial Theories
        (1) Some proponents of psychoanalytic theory view adjustment disorder as a maladaptive response to stress that is caused by early childhood trauma, increased dependency, and retarded ego development.
        (2) Other psychosocial theories describe a predisposition to adjustment disorder as an inability to complete the grieving process in response to a painful life change, due to a type of "psychic overload."
    c. Transactional Model of Stress/Adaptation. The way in which certain individuals respond to various types of stressors depends upon the type of stressor, the situational context in which the stressor occurs, and intrapersonal factors. The transactional model takes into consideration the interaction between the individual and his or her internal and external environment.
4. Diagnosis/Outcome Identification
    a. Nursing diagnoses for the client with an adjustment disorder may include:
        (1) Dysfunctional grieving
        (2) Impaired adjustment
    b. Outcome criteria are identified for measuring the effectiveness of nursing care.
5. Planning/Implementation
    a. Nursing intervention for the client with adjustment disorder is aimed at assisting the individual to progress toward resolution of grief that has been generated in response to real or perceived losses.
    b. If the adjustment disorder is in response to a change in health status, the nurse assists the client to accept the change and make required life style modifications in order to function as independently as possible.
6. Evaluation is based on accomplishment of previously established outcome criteria.
B. Impulse Control Disorders: Background Assessment Data
    1. The essential features of impulse control disorders include:
        a. Failure to resist an impulse, drive, or temptation to perform some act that is harmful to the person or others.
        b. An increasing sense of tension or arousal before committing the act.
        c. An experience of either pleasure, gratification, or relief at the time of committing the act.
    2. Five categories of impulse control disorders are described:
        a. Intermittent explosive disorder. Characterized by a loss of control of a violent or aggressive impulse that culminates in serious assaultive acts or destruction of property.
            (1) Predisposing factors to intermittent explosive disorder include:
                (a) Biological Influences. Genetically, the disorder is more common in first degree biological relatives of people with the disorder than in the general population.

Physiologically, any central nervous system insult may predispose to the general clinical syndrome.

      (b) Psychosocial Influences. Individuals with intermittent explosive disorder often have very strong identification with assaultive parental figures.

  b. Kleptomania. Characterized by recurrent failure to resist impulses to steal items not needed for personal use or their monetary value.

    (1) Predisposing factors to kleptomania.

      (a) Biological Influences. Brain disease and mental retardation are known on occasion to be associated with profitless stealing.

      (b) Psychosocial Influences. Some kleptomaniacs report childhood memories of abandonment (real or imagined) and a sense of lovelessness and deprivation.

  c. Pathological Gambling. A chronic and progressive failure to resist impulses to gamble, and gambling behavior that compromises, disrupts, or damages personal, family, or vocational pursuits.

    (1) Predisposing factors to pathological gambling.

      (a) Biological Influences. Genetically, the fathers of men with the disorder and the mothers of women with the disorder are more likely to have the disorder than is the population at large. Physiologically, various neurophysiological dysfunctions have been associated with pathological gambling behaviors.

      (b) Psychosocial Influences. Possible contributors include: loss of a parent before age 15 to death, separation, divorce, or desertion; inappropriate parental discipline; exposure to gambling activities as an adolescent; a high family value placed on material and financial symbols; and a lack of family emphasis on saving, planning, and budgeting. The psychoanalytical view suggests that a punitive superego fosters the gambler's inherent need for punishment, which is then achieved through losing, and is required for psychic equilibrium.

  d. Pyromania. The inability to resist the impulse to set fires.

    (1) Predisposing factors to pyromania.

      (a) Biological Influences. Physiological factors that may contribute include mental retardation, dementia, epilepsy, minimal brain dysfunction, and learning disabilities.

      (b) Psychosocial Influences. Psychoanalytical issues associated with impulsive firesetting include an association between firesetting and sexual gratification; concerns about inferiority, impotence, and annihilation; and unconscious anger toward a parent figure.

  e. Trichotillomania. The recurrent pulling out of one's own hair that results in noticeable hair loss.

    (1) Predisposing factors to trichotillomania.

      (a) Biological Influences. May be present as a major symptom in mental retardation, obsessive-compulsive disorder, schizophrenia, borderline personality disorder, and depression.

      (b) Psychosocial Influences. Factors that have been considered include disturbances in mother-child relationships, fear of abandonment, and recent object loss. Another view associates the disorder with early emotional deprivation.

3. Transactional Model of Stress/Adaptation. The etiology of impulse control disorders is most likely influenced by multiple factors.

4. Diagnosis/Outcome Identification

  a. Nursing diagnoses for clients with impulse control disorders include:

    (1) Risk for violence directed toward others

    (2) Ineffective individual coping

5. Planning/Implementation

  a. Nursing intervention for the client with impulse control disorder is aimed at protection of the client and others from harm associated with aggressive impulses and assaultive behavior.

  b. The nurse also assists the client to learn to delay gratification and to develop more adaptive strategies for coping with stress.

6. Evaluation is based on accomplishment of previously established outcome criteria.

IV. Treatment Modalities
    A. Adjustment Disorders
        1. The major goals of therapy include:
            a. To relieve symptoms associated with a stressor.
            b. To enhance coping with stressors that cannot be reduced or removed
            c. To establish support systems that maximize adaptation
        2. Types of therapy
            a. Individual psychotherapy
            b. Family therapy
            c. Behavioral therapy
            d. Self-help groups
            e. Crisis Intervention
            f. Psychopharmacology
    B. Impulse Control Disorders
        1. Intermittent Explosive Disorder
            a. Group/family therapy
            b. Psychopharmacology
        2. Kleptomania
            a. Insight-oriented psychodynamic psychotherapy
            b. Behavior therapy
        3. Pathological Gambling
            a. Behavior therapy
            b. Psychopharmacology
            c. Gamblers Anonymous
        4. Pryomania
            a. Aversive therapy
            b. Behavior therapy
        5. Trichotillomania
            a. Behavior therapy
            b. Individual psychotherapy
            c. Psychopharmacology
V. Summary
VI. Critical Thinking Exercise
VII. Review Questions

ANSWERS TO CRITICAL THINKING EXERCISE

1. Impaired adjustment related to loss of right breast.

2. STGs: a. Alice will be able to look at the scar.
        b. Alice will express feelings regarding loss of breast.
        c. Alice will talk to the Reach to Recovery representative.

    LTG: Alice will adjust to the loss of her breast and demonstrate acceptance of her new body image.

3. Encourage exploration of feelings (particularly anger) at loss and progression of the grief process.

CASE STUDY FOR USE WITH STUDENT LEARNING

Case Study: Adjustment Disorder with Mixed Anxiety and Depressed Mood

Nancy is 16 years old. She started dating last year, and was looking forward to her prom at the end of this, her junior, year in high school. About 6 months ago, Nancy began to lose weight, even though it seemed she was eating more. She complained to her Mom about always feeling thirsty. Nancy's mom took her to their family physician, who diagnosed Nancy with Insulin Dependent Diabetes Mellitus (IDDM). Nancy was shocked and angry when she learned that she would have to check her blood sugar level and give herself insulin injections daily. "No!! I won't do it! No one else I know does that!! No one will want to have anything to do with me. They'll think I'm a freak!!" Since that time Nancy and her Mom have a constant battle to provide the necessary care that Nancy requires in the management of her diabetes. Nancy's grades have fallen in school. She spends long hours alone locked up in her room. Her close friends report that she "doesn't act like she likes us anymore." She skipped school last week for the first time. Her family found her in a bar with a 22-year-old man whom she said was going to help her find a job in a distant city. The family physician referred Nancy and her family to a psychiatrist. The psychiatrist admitted Nancy to the psychiatric unit with elopement precautions and a diagnosis of Adjustment Disorder with Mixed Anxiety and Depressed Mood. Design an initial nursing plan of care for Nancy.

LEARNING ACTIVITY

CASE STUDY

Read the following case study and answer the questions that follow.

Nancy is 30 years old. She has never been married. She is a top salesperson in a major pharmaceutical company. She has an active social life, with many friends. She has had serious relationships with several men in the past, but has no significant relationship at this time. Three months ago, in a routine physical exam, the physician discovered a lump in Nancy's right breast. It was biopsied and found to be malignant. Because of the location, size, and likely metastasis to adjacent lymph nodes, Nancy chose, with the recommendation of her physician, to have a modified radical mastectomy. Since the surgery, her physical condition has progressed unremarkably. However, her mental condition has deteriorated progressively. She is sad, tired, and has trouble sleeping and concentrating. She has been unable to return to her job. She is referred to a psychiatrist, and admitted to the hospital with a diagnosis of Adjustment Disorder with Depressed Mood. She tells the nurse, "No man will ever want to have anything to do with me because of the way I look. My personal life is over."

1. Identify relevant assessment data from the information given.

2. What are the two priority nursing diagnoses for Nancy?

3. Describe some nursing interventions for assisting Nancy with the two nursing diagnoses identified.

4. Describe relevant outcome criteria for evaluating nursing care for Nancy.

CHAPTER 32. TEST QUESTIONS

Situation: Tommy T., age 6, has just been admitted to the child psychiatric unit. His parents report that until the last 6 months Tommy has never presented a problem for them. However, since his baby sister was born 6 months ago, they have been unable to control his behavior. Normally a very bright and outgoing student, Tommy's teachers report that he is bullying other students, and this week he threw a rock at a classmate, causing a laceration on the other child's forehead. At home, when he cannot have his way, Tommy resorts to temper tantrums, and yesterday swung his fists at his Mom for not allowing him to ride his bike after dinner. This morning, Mr. and Mrs. T. became fearful when they heard the baby screaming and coughing, and found Tommy flinging baby powder all over the baby and the nursery. The physician has assigned the diagnosis of Adjustment Disorder with Mixed Disturbance of Emotions and Conduct. The following questions relate to Tommy.

1. The primary nursing diagnosis for Tommy would be:
    - • a. Dysfunctional grieving related to perceived loss of parental love.
      b. Impaired adjustment related to birth of baby sister.
      c. Ineffective individual coping related to loss of only-child status.
      d. Risk for violence directed at others related to anger at birth of sister.

2. The category of Adjustment Disorder with Mixed Disturbance of Emotions and Conduct identifies the individual who:
      a. Expresses symptoms that reveal a panic level of anxiety.
      b. Expresses feelings of suicidal ideation.
    - • c. Violates the rights of others to feel better.
      d. Exhibits severe social isolation and withdrawal.

3. The most likely treatment modality for Tommy would be:
      a. Family therapy.
      b. Group therapy.
      c. Behavior therapy.
    - • d. Individual psychotherapy.

4. Related to the correct answer in question #3, the focus of therapy with Tommy would be:
      a. To treat the dysfunctional family system.
      b. To allow input from his peer group in an effort to gain insight.
      c. To keep him from hurting others.
    - • d. To focus on his anger at baby's birth and fear of parental abandonment.

5. Tommy's predisposition to adjustment disorder is *most* likely related to which of the following?
      a. Mental retardation
    - • b. Temperamental characteristics at birth that promote vulnerability
      c. Retarded superego development
      d. Presence of psychiatric illness

The following questions relate to impulse control disorders.

6. What is the identifying dysfunction in all impulse control disorders?
    - • a. Disinhibition
      b. Thought disorder
      c. Mood disorder
      d. Loss of memory

7. Which of the following impulse control disorders has the strongest genetic predisposing factor?
      a. Kleptomania
      b. Pyromania

- c. Pathological gambling
  d. Trichotillomania

8. Psychosocial factors that are observed in many kleptomaniacs include which of the following?
   a. Stealing is due to a conduct disorder.
   - b. Feelings of being neglected, injured, or unwanted occur.
   c. Intense pleasure, gratification, and relief occur during the event.
   d. The degree of aggressiveness in an episode is out of proportion to the stressor.

CHAPTER 33. PSYCHOLOGICAL FACTORS AFFECTING MEDICAL CONDITION

CHAPTER FOCUS

The focus of this chapter is on nursing care of clients with medical conditions, the initiation or exacerbation of which is associated with psychological factors. Predisposing factors and symptomatology are explored, and nursing care is presented in the context of the six steps of the nursing process. Medical treatment modalities are also discussed.

LEARNING OBJECTIVES

After reading this chapter, the student will be able to:

1. Differentiate between somatoform and psychophysiological disorders.
2. Identify various types of psychophysiological disorders.
3. Discuss historical and epidemiological statistics related to various psychophysiological disorders.
4. Describe symptomatology associated with various psychophysiological disorders and use this data in client assessment.
5. Identify various predisposing factors to psychophysiological disorders.
6. Formulate nursing diagnoses and goals of care for clients with various psychophysiological disorders.
7. Describe appropriate nursing interventions for behaviors associated with various psychophysiological disorders.
8. Identify topics for client and family teaching relevant to psychophysiological disorders.
9. Evaluate the nursing care of clients with psychophysiological disorders.
10. Discuss various modalities relevant to treatment of psychophysiological disorders.

KEY TERMS

autoimmune
cachexia
carcinogens
essential hypertension
migraine personality
psychophysiological
type A personality
type B personality
type C personality

CHAPTER OUTLINE/LECTURE NOTES

I.   Introduction
     A. In psychophysiological responses, evidence exists of either demonstrable organic pathology or a known pathophysiological process. No such organic involvement can be identified in somatoform disorders.
     B. Virtually any organic disorder can be considered psychophysiological in nature.
II. Historical Aspects
     A. Historically, mind and body have been viewed as two distinct entities, each subject to different laws of causality.
     B. Medical research shows that a change is occurring. Research associated with biological functioning is being expanded to include also the psychological and social determinants of health and disease.

III. Application of the Nursing Process
A. Types of Psychophysiological Disorders: Background Assessment Data
1. Asthma
a. A syndrome of airflow limitation characterized by increased responsiveness of the tracheobronchial tree to various stimuli and manifested by airway smooth muscle contraction, hypersecretion of mucus, and inflammation.
b. Affects approximately 10 million adults and children in the U.S.
c. Signs and symptoms: episodes of bronchial constriction resulting in dyspnea, wheezing, productive cough, restlessness, and eosinophilia.
d. Predisposing Factors
(1) Biological Influences
(a) hereditary factors
(b) Allergies
(2) Psychosocial Influences
(a) Personality profile: excessive dependency needs
2. Cancer
a. A malignant neoplasm in which the basic structure and activity of the cells have become deranged, usually because of changes in the DNA.
b. Cancer is the second leading cause of death in the U.S. today.
c. Seven warning signs of cancer:
(1) A change in bowel or bladder habits
(2) A sore that does not heal
(3) Unusual bleeding or discharge
(4) A thickening or lump in the breast or elsewhere
(5) Indigestion or difficulty in swallowing
(6) An obvious change in a wart or mole
(7) A nagging cough or hoarseness
d. Predisposing Factors
(1) Biological Influences
(a) Familial pattern: possible hereditary link
(b) Continuous irritation
(c) Exposure to carcinogens
(d) Viruses
(2) Psychosocial Influences
(a) Type C personality
(b) Lack of close relationship with one or both parents
(c) Lack of opportunity for self-gratification
3. Coronary Heart Disease
a. Myocardial impairment caused by an imbalance between coronary blood flow and myocardial oxygen requirements caused by changes in the coronary circulation. It is the leading cause of death in the U.S.
b. Signs and symptoms: anginal pain includes sensations of strangling, aching, squeezing, pressing, expanding, choking, burning, constriction, indigestion, tightness, and heaviness. Pain associated with MI is similar, but lasts longer than 15 to 30 minutes.
c. Predisposing Factors
(1) Biological Influences
(a) Hereditary factors
(b) High serum lipoproteins
(c) Lifestyle habits: cigarette smoking, obesity, sedentary lifestyle
(2) Psychosocial Influences
(a) Type A personality
4. Peptic Ulcer
a. An erosion of the mucosal wall in the esophagus, stomach, duodenum, or jejunum.
b. More common in men than in women. Affects up to 10 percent of the general population.

    c. The characteristic clinical manifestation is pain, usually experienced in the upper abdomen near the midline, and may radiate to the back, sternum, or lower abdomen.
    d. Predisposing Factors
        (1) Biological Influences
            (a) Hereditary factors.
            (b) Environmental factors: cigarette smoking, aspirin, alcohol, steroids, and nonsteroidal anti-inflammatory drugs.
        (2) Psychosocial Influences
            (a) Unfulfilled dependency needs
5. Essential Hypertension
    a. The persistent elevation of blood pressure for which there is no apparent cause or associated underlying disease.
    b. It is the major cause of cerebrovascular accident, cardiac disease, and renal failure.
    c. Twenty percent of the adult population in the U.S. are hypertensive (blood pressure 140/90). Half of the people with hypertension do not know they have it. The disorder is more common in men than in women, and twice as prevalent in the black population as it is in the white population.
    d. Signs and symptoms: Most commonly hypertension produces no symptoms. When they do occur, they may include headache, vertigo, flushed face, spontaneous nosebleed, or blurred vision.
    e. Predisposing Factors
        (1) Biological Factors
            (a) Hereditary factors
            (b) Possible imbalance of circulating vasoconstrictors and vasodilators
            (c) Increased sympathetic nervous system activity resulting in increased vasoconstriction
            (d) Impairment in sodium and water excretion
        (2) Psychosocial Influences
            (a) Repressed anger
6. Migraine Headache
    a. A vascular event in which pain arises from the scalp, its blood vessels, and muscles; from the dura mater and its venous sinuses; and from the blood vessels at the base of the brain.
    b. Approximately 5 percent of the population suffer from migraine headaches. They are more common in women than in men.
    c. Signs and symptoms: The headache usually consists of pain on one side of the head. As it intensifies, the pain may spread to the other side as well. Nausea, vomiting, mental cloudiness, total body achiness, abdominal pain, chills, and cold hands and feet commonly accompany the headache. It may or may not be preceded by an aura.
    d. Predisposing Factors
        (1) Biological Influences
            (a) Hereditary factors
            (b) Periods of hormonal change
            (c) Certain foods, beverages, and drugs
            (d) Physical exertion
            (e) Other factors: cigarette smoking, bright lights, weather changes, high elevations, oral contraceptives, altered sleep patterns, and skipping meals.
        (2) Psychosocial Influences
            (a) Migraine personality
7. Rheumatoid Arthritis
    a. A disease characterized by chronic musculoskeletal pain caused by inflammatory disease of the joints. It is a systematic disease and may also be manifested by lesions of the major organs of the body.
    b. Rheumatoid arthritis affects 1 to 3 percent of the population in the U.S. It is more prevalent in women than in men by about 3 to 1.

c. Signs and symptoms: Joint inflammation that precedes systemic symptoms of fatigue, malaise, anorexia, weight loss, low-grade fever, myalgias, and parasthesias. Joint involvement is usually characterized by swelling, pain, redness, warmth, and tenderness.

d. Predisposing Factors
   (1) Biological Influences
       (a) Hereditary factors
       (b) Possible dysfunctional immune mechanism
   (2) Psychosocial Influences
       (a) Suppression of anger and hostility

8. Ulcerative Colitis
   a. A chronic mucosal inflammatory disease of the colon, usually associated with bloody diarrhea.
   b. Incidence of the disease is approximately 5 to 7 per 100,000 population.
   c. Signs and symptoms: The mucosa of the colon and rectum become inflamed, with diffuse areas of bleeding. Diarrhea is the predominant symptom, and may or may not be accompanied by abdominal cramping. Generalized manifestations include fever, anorexia, weight loss, nausea and vomiting.
   d. Predisposing Factors
      (1) Biological Influences
          (a) Hereditary factors
          (b) Possible dysfunctional immune mechanism
      (2) Psychosocial Influences
          (a) Obsessive-compulsive personality
          (b) Suppression of anger and hostility

B. Transactional Model of Stress/Adaptation
   1. The etiology of psychophysiological disorders is most likely influenced by multiple factors.

C. Diagnosis/Outcome Identification
   1. Nursing diagnoses for clients with psychophysiological disorders may relate to symptoms of the specific disorder. Nursing diagnoses common to the general category include:
      a. Ineffective individual coping
      b. Knowledge deficit
      c. Self-esteem disturbance
      d. Altered role performance
   2. Outcome criteria are identified for measuring the effectiveness of nursing care.

D. Planning/Implementation
   1. Nursing intervention for the client with psychophysiological disorders is determined by the type of disorder with which the client presents.
   2. Emphasis is also given to helping the individual understand the correlation between emotional problems and exacerbation of the illness. The individual receives assistance in developing more adaptive coping strategies.

E. Evaluation is based on accomplishment of previously established outcome criteria.

IV. Treatment Modalities
   A. Asthma
      1. Pharmacotherapy
      2. Individual psychotherapy
   B. Cancer
      1. Surgery
      2. Radiation Therapy
      3. Chemotherapy
      4. Autogenic relaxation and mental imagery
      5. Individual psychotherapy
   C. Coronary Heart Disease
      1. Surgery
      2. Angioplasty
      3. Pharmacotherapy
      4. Behavior modification

ANSWERS TO CRITICAL THINKING EXERCISE

1. Pain of duodenal ulcer related to stress from her job evidenced by verbal complaints of pain.

2. a. Administer the medication prescribed by the physician.
    b. Teach her to keep some food in her stomach, as pain is worse when the stomach is empty.
    c. Encourage her not to smoke or drink alcohol.
    d. Teach relaxation exercises.
    e. Encourage her to talk about her feelings associated with the stress she is experiencing on her job and with the lawsuit.
    f. Help her to understand that she needs to find satisfying experiences in which to engage *outside of her work*.
    g. Help her to see herself as a worthwhile person for reasons other than those associated with her work.

3. Melinda will develop adaptive coping strategies to deal with stressful situations and will experience healing of her ulcer.

LEARNING ACTIVITY

Fill in the blocks with information related to biological and psychosocial influences associated with each of the psychophysiological disorders listed. The first one is completed as an example.

Psychophysiological Disorders	Biological Influences	Psychosocial Influences
Asthma	Difficulty breathing, wheezing, produc-tive cough. Bronchial constriction. Diaphoretic and anxious. May be hereditary. Allergies may also play a role.	Characterized by excessive dependency needs, particularly on the mother figure.
Cancer		
Coronary Heart Disease		
Peptic Ulcer		
Migraine Headache		
Hypertension		
Rheumatoid Arthritis		
Ulcerative Colitis		

CHAPTER 33. TEST QUESTIONS

1. Which of the following psychosocial influences has been correlated with the predisposition to asthma?
    a. Unresolved Oedipus complex
    b. Underdeveloped ego
    c. punitive superego
    • d. unresolved dependence on the mother

2. Type C personality characteristics include all of the following except:
    a. Exhibits a calm, placid exterior.
    b. Puts others' needs before their own.
    • c. Has a strong competitive drive.
    d. Holds resentment toward others for perceived "wrongs."

3. Friedman and Rosenman identified two major character traits common to individuals with Type A personality. They are:
    • a. Excessive competitive drive and chronic sense of time urgency.
    b. Unmet dependency needs and low self-esteem.
    c. Chronic depression and tendency toward self-pity.
    d. Self-sacrificing and perfectionistic.

4. Which of the following statements is true about Type B personality?
    a. Their personalities are the exact opposite of Type A's.
    • b. They lack the need for competition and comparison as to Type A's.
    c. They are usually less successful than Type A's.
    d. They do not perform as well under pressure as Type A's.

5. Which of the following has *not* been implicated in the etiology of peptic ulcer disease?
    a. Genetics
    b. Cigarette smoking
    • c. Allergies
    d. Unfulfilled dependency needs

6. The individual with essential hypertension is thought to:
    • a. Suppress anger and hostility.
    b. Fear social interactions with others.
    c. Project feelings onto the environment.
    d. Deny responsibility for own behavior.

7. The "migraine personality" includes which of the following sets of characteristics?
    • a. Compulsive, perfectionistic, and somewhat inflexible.
    b. Excessively ambitious, easily aroused hostility, and highly competitive.
    c. Highly extroverted, impulsive, and expresses anger inappropriately.
    d. Chronic feelings of depression and despair, and has a tendency toward self-pity.

8. The individual who suffers from migraine headaches is thought to have:
    • a. Repressed anger.
    b. Suppressed anxiety.
    c. Unresolved dependency needs.
    d. Displaced aggression.

9. The individual with ulcerative colitis has been found to have which of the following types of personality characteristics?
    a. Passive-aggressive
    • b. Obsessive-compulsive
    c. Antisocial-suspicious
    d. Hostile-aggressive

10. Individuals with ulcerative colitis and rheumatoid arthritis share which of the following personality characteristics?
    a. Highly negativistic
    b. Strongly independent
    c. Excessively introverted
    • d. Unable to express anger directly

CHAPTER 34. PERSONALITY DISORDERS

CHAPTER FOCUS

The focus of this chapter is on nursing care of clients with personality disorders. Predisposing factors and symptomatology are explored, and nursing care is presented in the context of the six steps of the nursing process. Medical treatment modalities are also discussed.

LEARNING OBJECTIVES

After reading this chapter, the student will be able to:

1. Define personality.
2. Compare stages of personality development according to Sullivan, Erikson, and Mahler.
3. Identify various types of personality disorders.
4. Discuss historical and epidemiological statistics related to various personality disorders.
5. Describe symptomatology associated with borderline personality disorder and antisocial personality disorder, and use these data in client assessment.
6. Identify predisposing factors to borderline personality disorder and antisocial personality disorder.
7. Formulate nursing diagnoses and goals of care for clients with borderline personality disorder and antisocial personality disorder.
8. Describe appropriate nursing interventions for behaviors associated with borderline personality disorder and antisocial personality disorder.
9. Evaluate nursing care of clients with borderline personality disorder and antisocial personality disorder.
10. Discuss various modalities relevant to treatment of personality disorders.

KEY TERMS

histrionic
narcissism
object constancy
passive-aggressive
personality
schizoid
schizotypal
splitting

CHAPTER OUTLINE/LECTURE NOTES

I. Introduction
   A. Personality is a person's characteristic totality of emotional and behavioral traits apparent in ordinary life, a totality that is usually stable and predictable.
   B. Personality traits are enduring patterns of perceiving, relating to, and thinking about the environment and oneself that are exhibited in a wide range of social and personal contexts.
   C. Personality disorders occur when these traits become inflexible and maladaptive and cause either significant functional impairment or subjective distress.
II. Historical Aspects

A. The first recognition that personality disorders, apart from psychosis, were cause for their own special concern was in 1801, with the recognition that an individual can behave irrationally even when the powers of intellect are intact.

B. Personality disorders have been categorized into three clusters, according to the type of behavior observed.

   1. Cluster A: behaviors that are described as odd or eccentric.
      a. Paranoid personality disorder
      b. Schizoid personality disorder
      c. Schizotypal personality disorder
   2. Cluster B: behaviors that are described as dramatic, emotional, or erratic
      a. Antisocial personality disorder
      b. Borderline personality disorder
      c. Histrionic personality disorder
      d. Narcissistic personality disorder
   3. Cluster C: behaviors that are described as anxious or fearful
      a. Avoidant personality disorder
      b. Dependent personality disorder
      c. Obsessive-compulsive personality disorder

III. Types of Personality Disorders

A. Paranoid Personality Disorder
   1. Definition and Epidemiological Statistics
      a. A pattern of behavior, beginning by early adulthood and present in a variety of contexts, of pervasive distrust and suspiciousness of others such that their motives are interpreted as malevolent.
      b. The disorder is more common in men than in women.
   2. Clinical Picture
      a. They are constantly on guard, hypervigilant, and ready for any real or imagined threat. They trust no one, and are constantly testing the honesty of others.
      b. They are insensitive to the feelings of others but are themselves extremely oversensitive and tend to misinterpret even minute cues within the environment, magnifying and distorting them into thoughts of trickery and deception.
   3. Predisposing Factors
      a. Possible genetic link
      b. Subject to early parental antagonism and aggression

B. Schizoid Personality Disorder
   1. Definition and Epidemiological Statistics
      a. Characterized primarily by a profound defect in the ability to form personal relationships or to respond to others in any meaningful, emotional way
      b. Prevalence within the general population has been estimated at between 3 and 7.5 percent, and diagnosis occurs more frequently in men.
   2. Clinical Picture
      a. They are indifferent to others, aloof, detached, and unresponsive to praise, criticism, or any other feelings expressed by others.
      b. They have no close friends and prefer to be alone. In the presence of others, they appear shy, anxious, or uneasy.
   3. Predisposing Factors
      a. Possible hereditary factor
      b. Childhood has been characterized as bleak, cold, unempathetic, and notably lacking in nurturing.

C. Schizotypal Personality Disorder
   1. Definition and Epidemiological Statistics
      a. A graver form of the pathologically less severe schizoid personality pattern.
      b. Recent studies indicate that approximately 3 percent of the population have this disorder.
   2. Clinical Picture

       a.   Schizotypals are aloof and isolated and behave in a bland and apathetic manner.

       b.   Symptoms include magical thinking, ideas of reference, illusions, depersonalization, superstitiousness, bizarre speech, delusions, hallucinations, and withdrawal into the self.

   3.   Predisposing Factors

       a.   Possible hereditary factor

       b.   Possible physiological influence, such as anatomic deficits or neurochemical dysfunctions within certain areas of the brain.

       c.   Early family dynamics characterized by indifference, impassivity, or formality, leading to a pattern of discomfort with personal affection and closeness.

D.   Antisocial Personality Disorder

   1.   Definition and Epidemiological Statistics

       a.   A pattern of socially irresponsible, exploitative, and guiltless behavior, evident in the tendency to fail to conform to the law, to sustain consistent employment, to exploit and manipulate others for personal gain, to deceive, and to fail to develop stable relationships.

       b.   Prevalence estimates in the U.S. range from 3 percent in men to less than 1 percent in women.

   2.   Clinical Picture and Predisposing Factors

       a.   Presented later in this outline.

E.   Borderline Personality Disorder

   1.   Definition and Epidemiological Statistics

       a.   Characterized by a pattern of intense and chaotic relationships, with affective instability, fluctuating and extreme attitudes regarding other people, impulsivity, directly and indirectly self-destructive behavior, and lack of a clear or certain sense of identity, life plan, or values.

       b.   Prevalence estimates range from 2 percent to 4 percent of the population.

   2.   Clinical Picture and Predisposing Factors

F.   Histrionic Personality Disorder

   1.   Definition and Epidemiological Statistics

       a.   Characterized by colorful, dramatic, and extroverted behavior in excitable, emotional persons.

       b.   Prevalence is thought to be about 2.2 percent, and it is twice as common in women than in men.

   2.   Clinical Picture

       a.   They are self-dramatizing, attention-seeking, overly gregarious, seductive, manipulative, exhibitionistic, shallow, frivolous, labile, vain, and demanding.

       b.   Highly distractible, difficulty paying attention to detail, easily influenced by others, difficulty forming close relationships, and may complain of physical symptoms.

   3.   Predisposing Factors

       a.   Possible ease of sympathetic arousal, adrenal hyperactivity, and neurochemical imbalances.

       b.   Possible hereditary factor

       c.   Learned behavior patterns

       d.   Biogenetically determined temperament

G.   Narcissistic Personality Disorder

   1.   Definition and Epidemiological Statistics

       a.   Characterized by an exaggerated sense of self-worth.

       b.   The disorder is more common in men than in women.

   2.   Clinical Picture

       a.   They are overly self-centered and exploit others in an effort to fulfill their own desires.

       b.   Mood, which is often grounded in grandiosity, is usually optimistic, relaxed, cheerful, and carefree. Mood can easily change because of fragile self-esteem.

   3.   Predisposing Factors

       a.   Family dynamics may have fostered feelings of omnipotence and grandiosity through total indulgence of the child.

       b.   Possible unfulfilled dependency needs.

H.   Avoidant Personality Disorder

   1.   Definition and Epidemiological Statistics

       a.   Characterized by extreme sensitivity to rejection, and social withdrawal.

        b. Prevalence is between 0.5 percent and 1 percent, and is equally common in men and women.
    2. Clinical Picture
        a. They are awkward and uncomfortable in social situations. They desire to have close relationships, but cannot help believing that such will result in pain and disillusionment.
        b. They may be perceived by others as timid, withdrawn, or perhaps cold and strange.
        c. They are often lonely, and express feelings of being unwanted. They view others as critical, betraying, and humiliating.
    3. Predisposing Factors
        a. Possible hereditary influence
        b. Parental rejection and criticism
I. Dependent Personality Disorder
    1. Definition and Epidemiological Statistics
        a. A pervasive and excessive need to be taken care of that leads to submissive and clinging behavior and fears of separation.
        b. The disorder is relatively common within the population. It is more common among women than men, and more common in the youngest children of a family than the older ones.
    2. Clinical Picture
        a. They have a notable lack of self-confidence that is often apparent in their posture, voice, and mannerisms. They are typically passive and acquiescent to the desires of others.
        b. They avoid positions of responsibility and become anxious when forced into them.
        c. They have low self-worth and are easily hurt by criticism and disapproval.
    3. Predisposing Factors
        a. Possible hereditary influence
        b. Stimulation and nurturance are experienced exclusively from one source, and a singular attachment is made by the infant to the exclusion of all others.
J. Obsessive-Compulsive Personality Disorders
    1. Definition and Epidemiological Statistics
        a. Characterized by inflexibility about the way in which things must be done, and a devotion to productivity at the exclusion of personal pleasure.
        b. The disorder is relatively common and occurs more often in men than in women. Within the family constellation, it appears to be most common in oldest children.
    2. Clinical Picture
        a. They are especially concerned with matters of organization and efficiency, and tend to be rigid and unbending about rules and procedures.
        b. Social behavior tends to be polite and formal.
        c. They are very "rank conscious." They can be very ingratiating with authority figures, but quite autocratic and condemnatory with subordinates.
        d. On the surface, these individuals appear to be very calm and controlled, while underneath this exterior lies a great deal of ambivalence, conflict, and hostility.
    3. Predisposing Factors
        a. Overcontrol by parents, with notable lack of positive reinforcement for acceptable behavior and frequent punishment for undesirable behavior.
K. Passive-Aggressive Personality Disorder
    1. Definition and Epidemiological Statistics
        a. A pervasive pattern of negativistic attitudes and passive resistance to demands for adequate performance in social and occupational situations.
        b. No statistics are available, but it appears to be a relatively common syndrome.
    2. Clinical Picture
        a. They are passively resistant to authority, demands, obligations, and responsibilities by such behaviors as dawdling, procrastination, and "forgetting."
        b. They tend to be complaining, irritable, whining, argumentative, scornful, critical, discontented, disillusioned, and disgruntled.
        c. They do not acknowledge or express their anger directly, preferring instead to express it through resistant and negativistic behavior.

3. Predisposing Factors
   a. Contradictory parental attitudes and inconsistent training methods.
IV. Application of the Nursing Process
   A. Borderline Personality Disorder
      1. Background Personality Disorder
         a. Designated as "borderline" because of the tendency of these clients to fall on the border between neuroses and psychoses.
         b. A pervasive pattern of instability of interpersonal relationships, self-image, and affects, and marked impulsivity beginning by early adulthood and present in a variety of contexts.
         c. They are most strikingly identified by the intensity and instability of their affect and behavior.
         d. Common behaviors include:
            (1) Chronic depression
            (2) Inability to be alone
            (3) Clinging and distancing behaviors
            (4) Splitting
            (5) Manipulation
            (6) Self-destructive behaviors
            (7) Impulsivity
         e. Predisposing Factors: According to Margaret Mahler's Theory of Object Relations, the individual with borderline personality disorder becomes fixed in the rapprochement phase of development (16 to 24 months). The child fails to achieve the task of autonomy.
      2. Diagnosis/Outcome Intervention
         a. Nursing diagnoses for the client with borderline personality disorder may include:
            (1) Risk for self-mutilation
            (2) Dysfunctional grieving
            (3) Impaired social interaction
            (4) Personal identity disturbance
            (5) Anxiety (severe to panic)
            (6) self-esteem disturbance
         b. Outcome criteria are identified for measuring the effectiveness of nursing care.
      3. Planning/Implementation
         a. Nursing intervention for the client with borderline personality disorder is aimed at protection of the client from self-mutilation.
         b. The nurse also seeks to assist the client to advance in the development of personality by confronting his or her true source of internalized anger.
      4. Evaluation is based on accomplishment of previously established outcome criteria.
   B. Antisocial Personality Disorder
      1. Background Assessment Data
         a. Sometimes called sociopathic or psychopathic behavior.
         b. Usually only seen in clinical settings when they are admitted by court order for psychological evaluation.
         c. Most frequently encountered in prisons, jails, and rehabilitation services.
         d. Common behaviors include:
            (1) Exploitation and manipulation of others for personal gain
            (2) Belligerent and argumentative
            (3) Lacks remorse
            (4) Unable to delay gratification
            (5) Low tolerance for frustration
            (6) Inconsistent work or academic performance
            (7) Failure to conform to societal norms
            (8) Impulsive and reckless
            (9) Inability to function as a responsible parent
            (10) Inability to form lasting monogamous relationship
         e. Predisposing Factors

    (1) Possible genetic influence

    (2) Having a sociopathic or alcoholic father

    (3) Behavior disorder as a child

    (4) Parental deprivation during the first 5 years of life

    (5) Inconsistent parenting

    (6) History of severe physical abuse

    (7) Extreme poverty

  2. Diagnosis/Outcome Identification

    a. Nursing diagnoses for the client with antisocial personality disorder may include:

     (1) Risk for violence toward others

     (2) Defensive coping

     (3) Self-esteem disturbance

     (4) Impaired social interaction

     (5) Knowledge deficit

    b. Outcome criteria are identified for measuring the effectiveness of nursing care.

  3. Planning/Implementation

    a. Nursing intervention for the client with antisocial personality disorder is aimed at protection of others from the client's aggression and hostility.

    b. The nurse also seeks to assist the client to delay gratification by setting limits on unacceptable behavior.

  4. Evaluation is based on accomplishment of previously established outcome criteria.

V. Treatment Modalities for Clients with Personality Disorders

 A. Interpersonal psychotherapy

 B. Psychoanalytical psychotherapy

 C. Milieu or group therapy

 D. Cognitive/behavioral therapy

 E. Psychopharmacology

VI. Summary

VII. Critical Thinking Exercise

VIII. Review Questions

ANSWERS TO CRITICAL THINKING EXERCISE

1.   Even though the nurse believes Lana's declaration is untrue, she must proceed as though it is. Lana will undergo institutional procedures for overdose management with Desyrel (usually includes emesis or gastric lavage, activated charcoal, IV fluids, monitoring of vital signs, and ECG).

2.   Risk for self-directed violence related to fears of abandonment.

3.   Ensure that Lana is assigned various nurses to care for her (and not always the same one to which she may "cling"). Maintain consistency of care. That is, be sure that ALL nurses follow established limits and consequences with Lana and that Lana is not allowed to manipulate some nurses into violating the limits without consequences. This is Lana's way of splitting.

CASE STUDY FOR USE WITH STUDENT LEARNING

Case Study: Borderline Personality Disorder

Nancy, age 23, has just been hospitalized after she reported to her college roommate, Carol, that she had swallowed a bottle of aspirin. She has been stabilized in the ER and has been admitted to the psychiatric unit. This is Nancy's 3rd hospitalization for similar behavior since age 15. Nancy reports that her parents were divorced when she was 3 years old. She has not seen her father since that time. She lived with her mother until she was 6 years old, then her mother left her with her grandmother and went to "seek fame and fortune" in Hollywood. She sees her mother rarely. Nancy's roommate tells the admitting nurse that Nancy has been a "nervous" person ever since she has known her. "She has mood swings, and the smallest things will set her off. Once when she was particularly 'down,' I walked in on her sitting on her bed. It looked like she was cutting her arm with a razor blade. When I confronted her about it, she denied it. But I saw the blood. It really freaked me out!" Nancy's boyfriend recently broke up with her. Nancy has had a succession of boyfriends since high school. All of her relationships are very intense, and she becomes hysterical and then despondent when a boy breaks off his relationship with her. Her previous hospitalizations have been in response to these breakups. Physical exam is unremarkable except for visible scars on the underside of both upper arms. Diagnosis: Axis I: Major Depression; Axis II: Borderline Personality Disorder.

LEARNING ACTIVITY

Match the personality disorder listed on the left that is most commonly associated with the behaviors described on the right.

_____ 1. Paranoid personality disorder

_____ 2. Schizoid personality disorder

_____ 3. Schizotypal personality disorder

_____ 4. Antisocial personality disorder

_____ 5. Borderline personality disorder

_____ 6. Histrionic personality disorder

_____ 7. Narcissistic personality disorder

_____ 8. Avoidant personality disorder

_____ 9. Dependent personality disorder

_____ 10. Obsessive-compulsive disorder

_____ 11. Passive-aggressive personality disorder

a. Shows no remorse for exploitation and manipulation of others.

b. Accepts a job he does not want to do, then does a poor job and delays past the deadline.

c. Believes she is entitled to special privileges others do not deserve.

d. They are suspicious of all others with whom they come in contact.

e. Swallows a bottle of pills after therapist leaves on vacation.

f. Believes he has a "sixth sense," and can know what others are thinking.

g. Allows others to make all her important decisions for her.

h. Refuses to enter into a relationship due to fear of rejection.

i. Demonstrates highly emotional and overly dramatic behaviors.

j. Has a lifelong pattern of social withdrawal.

k. Believes everyone must follow the rules and that the rules can be "bent" for no one . . . ever.

CHAPTER 34. TEST QUESTIONS

Situation: Claudia is a 27-year-old woman who has been married and divorced four times. She is admitted to the Psychiatric Unit with a diagnosis of Borderline Personality Disorder.

1.   Which of the following behavior patterns best describes someone with borderline personality disorder?
-     a. Social isolation
-     b. Suspiciousness of others
-     c. Belligerent and argumentative
- •   d. Emotional instability

2.   As Nancy starts to leave the unit at the end of her shift, Claudia runs up to her, puts her arms around her, and yells, "Please don't go! You're the only one who understands me. If you go, I won't have anyone!" This is an example of what type of behavior common to individuals with borderline personality disorder?
-     a. Splitting
-     b. Manipulation
- •   c. Clinging
-     d. Impulsivity

3.   Which of the following nursing interventions is appropriate to help prevent the behavior described in the previous question?
-     a. Put Claudia on room restriction each time it happens.
-     b. Ignore such behaviors so that they will be extinguished for lack of reinforcement.
-     c. Secure a verbal contract with Claudia that she will discontinue this type of behavior.
- •   d. Ensure that various staff members are rotated to work with Claudia while she is in the hospital.

Situation: Joe is a client of the Psychiatric Day Treatment Program. He has been referred by his probation officer for treatment after an arrest for DUI (driving under the influence of substances). Joe has a history of many arrests for assault, grand larceny, and other serious crimes, and has served two prison sentences. His diagnosis is Antisocial Personality Disorder.

4.   Which of the following quotes is Joe's most probable comment on his past behavior?
- •   a. "It's not my fault."
-     b. "I'm too ashamed to talk about it."
-     c. "I just don't remember doing it."
-     d. "I'm really sorry about all the people I've hurt."

5.   When he arrives on the unit for the day's activities, Joe says to the nurse, "Wow, you look great today! I'm so glad you're on duty today. You're the best nurse who works here, you know." This comment of Joe's is an example of what type of behavior commonly associated with Antisocial Personality Disorder?
-     a. Impulsivity
- •   b. Manipulation
-     c. Exploitation of others
-     d. Inability to delay gratification

6.   Which of the following therapies is considered *best* for the client with Antisocial Personality Disorder?
- •   a. Milieu Therapy
-     b. Family Therapy
-     c. Individual Psychotherapy
-     d. Pharmacological Therapy

7.   Looking at the slightly bleeding paper cut she has just received, Linda screams "Somebody help me, quick!! I'm bleeding. Call 911! Hurry!" This response may reflect behavior associated with which personality disorder?

      a.   Schizoid
      b.   Obsessive-Compulsive
•   c.   Histrionic
      d.   Paranoid

8.   John had an extra calendar of the new year and left it on Andrew's desk as a gift. Andrew thinks, "I wonder what he wants from me?" This thought by Andrew may be associated with which personality disorder?
      a.   Schizotypal
      b.   Narcissistic
      c.   Avoidant
•   d.   Paranoid

9.   Fred works long hours at his job as a research analyst. He then goes home where he lives alone. He has no friends, and seldom speaks to others. This behavior is reflective of which personality disorder?
      a.   Paranoid
•   b.   Schizoid
      c.   Passive-Aggressive
      d.   Avoidant

10.   When a new graduate nurse comes up with a plan and shows Thelma how everyone can be guaranteed every other weekend off, Thelma responds, "We can't make these kinds of changes! Who do you think you are? We've always done it this way, and we will continue to do it this way!" Thelma's statement reflects behavior associated with which personality disorder?
      a.   Dependent
      b.   Histrionic
      c.   Passive-Aggressive
•   d.   Obsessive-Compulsive

CHAPTER 35. THE AGING INDIVIDUAL

CHAPTER FOCUS

The focus of this chapter is on nursing care of the aging individual. Various theories of aging and symptomatology associated with the normal aging process are presented. Special concerns of the elderly are discussed. Nursing care is described in the context of the six steps of the nursing process.

LEARNING OBJECTIVES

After reading this chapter, the student will be able to:

1.   Discuss societal perspectives on aging.
2.   Describe an epidemiological profile of aging in the United States.
3.   Discuss various theories of aging.
4.   Describe aspects of the normal aging process:
      a.   Biological
      b.   Psychological
      c.   Sociocultural
      d.   Sexual
5.   Discuss retirement as a special concern to the aging individual.
6.   Explain personal and sociological perspectives of long-term care of the aging individual.
7.   Describe the problem of elder abuse as it exists in today's society.
8.   Discuss the implications of the increasing number of suicides among the elderly population.
9.   Apply the steps of the nursing process to the care of aging individuals.

KEY TERMS

attachment
bereavement overload
disengagement
geriatrics
gerontology
geropsychiatry
"granny-bashing"
"granny-dumping"
long-term memory
Medicaid
Medicare
menopause
osteoporosis
short-term memory
reminiscence therapy

CHAPTER OUTLINE/LECTURE NOTES

I.   Introduction
      A.   Growing old is not popular in the youth-oriented American culture.

B. Sixty-six million "baby boomers" will reach their 65th birthdays by the year 2030, placing more emphasis on the needs of an aging population.

II. How Old is *Old?*
A. Our prehistoric ancestors probably had a life span of 40 years, with average life span around 18 years.
B. The average life expectancy for a child born in the U.S. today is about 76 years.
C. Myths and stereotypes affect the way in which elderly people are treated in our culture.
D. Whether one is considered "old" must be self-determined, based on variables such as attitude, mental health, physical health, and degree of independence.

III. Epidemiological Statistics
A. Population
    1. In 1996, Americans 65 years of age or older numbered 33.9 million, representing 12.8% of the population.
    2. By 2030, this number is projected at 70.2 million, or 20% of the population.
B. Marital Status
    1. In 1996, 76% of men and 43% of women 65 or over were married.
    2. There were five times as many widows as widowers.
C. Living Arrangements
    1. The majority of individuals age 65 or over live alone, with a spouse, or with relatives.
D. Economic Status
    1. About 3.4 million persons age 65 or over were below the poverty level in 1996.
E. Employment
    1. Individuals age 65 or over constituted 2.7% of the U.S. labor force in 1996.
F. Health Status
    1. The number of days in which usual activities are restricted because of illness or injury increases with age.
    2. Emotional and mental illnesses also increase over the life cycle.

IV. Theories of Aging
A. Biological Theories
    1. The exhaustion theory
    2. The accumulation theory
    3. The biological programming theory
    4. The error theory
    5. The cross-linkage or eversion theory
    6. The immunological theory
    7. The "aging clock" theory
    8. The free radical theory
B. Psychosocial Theories
    1. The activity theory of aging
    2. Continuity theory
C. Personality Theories
    1. Mature men
    2. Rocking chair
    3. Armored men
    4. Angry men
    5. Self-haters

V. The Normal Aging Process
A. Biological Aspects of Aging. Changes are observed in:
    1. Skin
    2. Cardiovascular system
    3. Respiratory system
    4. Musculoskeletal system
    5. Gastrointestinal system
    6. Endocrine system
    7. Genitourinary system

8. Immune system
9. Nervous system
10. Sensory systems
B. Psychological Aspects of Aging
   1. Memory functioning
   2. Intellectual functioning
   3. Learning ability
   4. Adaptation to the tasks of aging
      a. Loss and grief
      b. Attachment and disengagement
      c. Maintenance of self-identity
      d. Dealing with death
   3. Psychiatric disorders in later life
C. Sociocultural Aspects of Aging
   1. The elderly in virtually all cultures share some basic needs and interests:
      a. To live as long as possible or at least until life's satisfactions no longer compensate for its privations.
      b. To get some release from the necessity of wearisome exertion at humdrum tasks and to have protection from too great exposure to physical hazards.
      c. To safeguard or even strengthen any prerogatives acquired in midlife, such as skills, possessions, rights, authority, and prestige.
      d. To remain active participants in the affairs of life in either operational or supervisory roles, any sharing in group interests being preferred to idleness and indifference.
      e. To withdraw from life when necessity requires it, as timely, honorably, and comfortably as possible.
   2. In some cultures, the aged are the most powerful, the most engaged, and the most respected members of the society. This has not been the case in the American culture.
D. Sexual Aspects of Aging
   1. Americans have grown up in a society that has liberated sexual expression for all other age groups, but still retains certain Victorian standards regarding sexual expression by the elderly.
   2. Cultural stereotypes play a large part in the misperception many people hold regarding sexuality of the aged.
   3. Physical changes associated with sexuality
      a. Changes in the female
      b. Changes in the male
   4. Sexual behavior in the elderly
VI. Special Concerns of the Elderly
A. Retirement
   1. Social implications
   2. Economical implications
B. Long-Term Care
   1. Potential need for services are predicted by the following factors:
      a. Age. The 65+ population is often viewed as one of the important long-term care target groups.
      b. Health. The requirement for ongoing assistance from another human being is a consideration.
      c. Mental health status. Symptoms that would render the individual incapable of meeting the demands of daily living independently place him or her at risk.
      d. Socioeconomical and demographic factors. Lower socioeconomic status, being Caucasian, and being female are considered risk factors for long-term care.
      e. Marital status, living arrangement, and the informal support network. Living alone without resources for home care and few or no relatives living nearby to provide informal care are factors of high risk for institutionalization.
   2. Attitudinal Factors
      a. Old persons in general are opposed to the use of institutions. Many view them as "places to go to die."

251

C. Elder Abuse
   1. It has been estimated that 10 percent of individuals over age 65 are the victims of abuse or neglect.
   2. The abuser is most often a relative who lives with the elderly person and is likely to be the assigned caregiver.
   3. Factors that Contribute to Abuse
      a. Longer life
      b. Dependency
      c. Stress
      d. Learned violence
   4. Identifying Elder Abuse
D. Suicide
   1. Persons over 65 years of age represent a disproportionate high percentage of individuals who commit suicide.
   2. Seventeen percent of all suicides are committed by this age group, and suicide is now one of the to 10 causes of death among the elderly.
   3. The group at highest risk appears to be white men who are recently bereaved, living alone, experiencing anxiety due to financial instability, and with undertreated mood disorders.
VII. Application of the Nursing Process
   A. Assessment. Assessment of the elderly must consider the possible biological, psychological, sociocultural, and sexual changes that occur in the normal aging process.
      1. Age alone does not preclude that these changes have occurred, and each client must be assessed as a unique individual.
   B. Diagnosis/Outcome Identification
      1. Nursing diagnoses that relate to physiological changes in the aging individual may include any or all of the following:
         a. Risk for trauma
         b. Hypothermia
         c. Decreased cardiac output
         d. Ineffective breathing pattern
         e. Risk for aspiration
         f. Impaired physical ability
         g. Altered nutrition, less than body requirements
         h. Constipation
         i. Stress incontinence
         j. Urinary retention
         k. Sensory-perceptual alteration
         l. Sleep pattern disturbance
         m. Pain
         n. Self-care deficit
         o. Risk for impaired skin integrity
      2. Psychosocially related nursing diagnoses that may be a consideration include:
         a. Altered thought processes
         b. Dysfunctional grieving
         c. Risk for self-directed violence
         d. Powerlessness
         e. Self-esteem disturbance
         f. Fear
         g. Body image disturbance
         h. Altered sexuality patterns
         i. Sexual dysfunction
         j. Social isolation
         k. Risk for trauma (elder abuse)
         l. Caregiver role strain
      3. Outcome criteria are identified for measuring the effectiveness of nursing care.

C. Planning/Implementation
    1. Nursing care of the aging individual is aimed at protection from injury due to age-related physical changes or altered thought processes related to cerebral changes.
    2. The nurse is also concerned with preservation of dignity and self-esteem in an individual who may have come to be dependent upon others for his or her survival.
    3. Assistance is provided with self-care deficits while encouraging independence to the best of his or her ability.
    4. Reminiscence therapy is encouraged.
D. Evaluation is based on accomplishment of previously established outcome criteria.
VIII. Summary
IX. Critical Thinking Exercise
X. Review Questions

ANSWERS TO CRITICAL THINKING EXERCISE

1. Dysfunctional grieving related to loss of husband/home/independence.

2. a. Mrs. M. will begin progression through grief process by discussing her feelings about her losses.
   b. Mrs. M. will eat sufficient food to begin gaining weight.

3. Her loss of independence.

LEARNING ACTIVITY

Case Study.   Read the following case study and answer the questions that follow.

Seventy-seven-year-old Angie had been a widow for 20 years. She was fiercely independent, and had run her small farm with minimal assistance since her husband died. In the last few years, her children had noticed that Angie had become increasingly forgetful. First she began forgetting the birthdays of her children and grandchildren, which was highly unlike her. Recently, she forgot that she was supposed to visit her son and his family, and failed to show up at the designated time. Last week when her daughter visited, she found a tea kettle on the stove that had burned dry when Angie forget she had started it. Yesterday, her daughter received a call from Angie's nearest neighbor who found Angie wandering around in his field unprotected from the cold. At Angie's children's request the family physician admits Angie to the hospital, where she is placed on the geropsychiatric unit.

1. Identify relevant assessment data from the information given.

2. What are the two priority nursing diagnoses for Angie?

3. Describe some nursing interventions for assisting Angie with the two nursing diagnoses identified.

4. Describe relevant outcome criteria for evaluating nursing care for Angie.

CHAPTER 35. TEST QUESTIONS

Situation: As Eleanor, age 79, became increasingly unable to fulfill her self-care needs, her children, who lived in a distant city, agreed it would be best for her to move to a nursing home near them. The following questions pertain to Eleanor.

1. Eleanor became depressed when she knew she would have to sell her home that she had lived in for more than 50 years. The physician prescribed an antidepressant for Eleanor. Which of the following physiological changes in the elderly may require special consideration when prescribing psychotropic medications for them?
   - a. Changes in cortical and intellectual functioning.
   - b. Changes in cardiac and respiratory functioning.
   - • c. Changes in liver and kidney functioning.
   - d. Changes in endocrine and immune functioning.

2. Eleanor does not respond to the antidepressant medication and becomes more depressed. She tells the nurse, "I don't want to live here. I would rather die than live here." After hearing Eleanor make this statement, the nurse would be expected to add which of the following nursing diagnoses to Eleanor's care plan?
   - a. Risk for self-mutilation
   - • b. Risk for self-directed violence
   - c. Risk for violence toward others
   - d. Risk for injury

3. When Eleanor does not respond to the antidepressant medication, the physician considers another therapy. Which of the following is he likely to choose?
   - • a. Electroconvulsive therapy
   - b. Neuroleptic therapy
   - c. An antiparkinsonian agent
   - d. Anxiolytic therapy

4. Eleanor begins to show improvement and the physician orders additional therapy for her. Which of the following therapies is most likely to help alleviate depression in Eleanor?
   - a. Behavior therapy
   - b. Group therapy
   - c. Orientation therapy
   - • d. Reminiscence therapy

5. Which of the following nursing interventions would help Eleanor be as independent as possible in her self-care activities?
   - a. Assign a variety of caregivers so that one person doesn't become used to doing everything for Eleanor.
   - b. Allow Eleanor a specified amount of time to complete ADLs, then finish them for her.
   - c. Tell her at the beginning of each day what is expected of her that day.
   - • d. Allow ADLs to follow her home routine as closely as possible.

CHAPTER 36. THE INDIVIDUAL WITH HIV DISEASE

CHAPTER FOCUS

The focus of this chapter is on nursing care of the individual with HIV disease. Predisposing factors and symptomatology associated with the disease are explored, and nursing care is presented in the context of the six steps of the nursing process. Various treatment modalities are also discussed.

LEARNING OBJECTIVES

After reading this chapter, the student will be able to:

1. Discuss the human immunodeficiency virus (HIV) as the causative agent in the development of acquired immunodeficiency syndrome (AIDS).
2. Describe the pathophysiology incurred by the HIV.
3. Discuss historical perspectives associated with AIDS.
4. Relate epidemiological statistics associated with AIDS.
5. Identify predisposing factors to AIDS.
6. Describe symptomatology associated with HIV infection and AIDS and use this data in client assessment.
7. Formulate nursing diagnoses and goals of care for clients with AIDS.
8. Describe appropriate nursing interventions for clients with AIDS.
9. Identify topics for client and family teaching relevant to HIV disease.
10. Evaluate nursing care of clients with AIDS.
11. Discuss various modalities relevant to treatment of clients with AIDS.

KEY TERMS

acquired immunodeficiency syndrome
HIV wasting syndrome
hospice
human immunodeficiency virus
Kaposi's sarcoma
opportunistic infection
persistent generalized lymphadenopathy
pneumocystic pneumonia
seroconversion
T4 lymphocytes
standard precautions
transmission-based precautions
HIV-associated dementia

CHAPTER OUTLINE/LECTURE NOTES

I. Introduction
   A. Acquired immune deficiency syndrome (AIDS) was first recognized as a lethal clinical syndrome in 1981.
   B. It has grown to epidemic proportions and is the number one health priority in the U.S. today.
   C. The human immunodeficiency virus (HIV) is the etiological agent that produces the immunosuppression resulting in AIDS.

D. Since January 1993, the CDC has defined AIDS as immunosuppression indicated by a T4 lymphocyte count of less than 200/mm³.

II. Pathophysiology Incurred by the HIV Virus
   A. Normal Immune Response
      1. Cells responsible for nonspecific immune reactions include neutrophils, monocytes, and macrophages.
      2. Specific immune mechanisms are divided into two major types:
         a. The cellular response (controlled by the T lymphocytes, or T cells).
         b. The humoral response (controlled by the B lymphocytes, or B cells).
   B. The Immune Response to HIV
      1. The HIV affects the T4 lymphocytes, thereby destroying the very cells the body needs to direct an attack on the virus.
      2. Normal T4 count is $600^{-1200 \, mm3}$.
      3. It is not uncommon for someone with advanced HIV disease to present with a T4 count below 10 mm³.

III. Historical Aspects
   A. First described in the CDC's Mortality Weekly Report of June 5, 1981.
   B. First identified in homosexual and bisexual men in California and New York.
   C. Soon began appearing in heterosexual IV drug users and hemophiliacs.
   D. May have origin in Africa with a virus called simian T-cell leukemia virus found in monkeys and apes.
   E. Appears now in virtually every major country in the world.

IV. Epidemiological Statistics
   A. As of 1998, there were estimated to be 30 million cases of HIV infection worldwide.
   B. The largest number of cases are reported to be in Sub-Saharan Africa and South and Southeast Asia.
   C. In the U.S., the disease has been reported in all 50 states and the District of Columbia.
   D. The highest number of cases are found in New York, Florida, and California, and lowest in North Dakota and South Dakota.

V. Predisposing Factors
   A. The etiological agent associated with AIDS is the HIV.
   B. Routes of transmission include sexual, bloodborne, and perinatal transmission.
      1. Sexual transmission
         a. Heterosexual transmission
         b. Homosexual transmission
      2. Bloodborne transmission
         a. Transfusion with blood products
         b. Transmission by needles infected with HIV-1
            (1) IV drug users
            (2) Accidental needle sticks by health care workers
      3. Perinatal transmission
         a. Transplacental
         b. Exposure to maternal blood and vaginal secretions during delivery
         c. Through breastfeeding
      4. Other possible modes of transmission

VI. Application of the Nursing Process
   A. Background Assessment Data
      1. Early-Stage HIV Disease (1000 to 500 T4 cells/mm³).
         a. Acute HIV Infection. A characteristic syndrome of symptoms that occurs from 6 days to 6 weeks following exposure to the virus. May include fever, myalgia, malaise, lymphadenopathy, sore throat, anorexia, nausea and vomiting, headaches, photophobia, skin rash, and diarrhea.
         b. Asymptomatic Infection. Following the acute infection individuals progress to an asymptomatic stage. They may remain in this stage for 10 or more years.
      2. Middle-Stage HIV Disease (500 to 200 T4 cells/mm³).

a. Persistent Generalized Lymphadenopathy. Follows the asymptomatic period. Lymph nodes in neck, armpit, and groin areas remain swollen for months, with no other signs of related infectious disease.

b. Other symptoms of middle-stage HIV disease: fever, night sweats, chronic diarrhea, fatigue, minor oral infections, and headache.

3. Late-Stage HIV Disease (200 or less T4 cells/mm^3).

a. HIV Wasting Syndrome. Symptoms are associated with nutrient malabsorption enterocolitis or intestinal injury related to an opportunistic infection. Weight loss of more than 10 percent of baseline is common. Large volume diarrhea, fever, and weakness accompany the syndrome.

b. Opportunistic Infections. A defining characteristic of AIDS.

c. AIDS-Related Malignancies. Common in the immunocompromised state produced by the HIV.

    (1) Kaposi's sarcoma

    (2) Non-Hodgkin's lymphoma

d. Altered Mental Status

    (1) Delirium

    (2) Depressive syndromes

    (3) HIV-associated dementia (HAD)

4. Psychosocial Implications of HIV/AIDS

5. Psychiatric Disorders Common in Clients with HIV Infections

a. Anxiety disorders

b. Major depression

c. Mania

d. Dementia and delirium

B. Diagnosis/Outcome Identification

1. Nursing diagnoses for the client with HIV/AIDS may include:

a. Altered protection

b. Altered family processes

c. Knowledge deficit

d. Altered thought processes

e. Risk for self-directed violence

f. Impaired adjustment

2. Outcome criteria are identified for measuring the effectiveness of nursing care.

C. Planning/Implementation

1. Nursing intervention for the client with HIV/AIDS is aimed at maximizing client safety and comfort.

2. The nurse is also concerned with assisting the family to deal with the newly-acquired diagnosis for their loved one.

3. Client and family education related to protection of the client and others from infection is also an important aspect of nursing care.

D. Evaluation is based on accomplishment of previously established outcome criteria.

VII. Treatment Modalities

A. Pharmacology

1. Antiretroviral therapy

a. Nucleoside reverse transcriptase inhibitors (HRTIs)

b. Non-nucleoside reverse transcriptase inhibitors (NNRTIs)

c. Protease inhibitors

2. Other chemotherapeutic agents

3. Psychotropic medications

B. Universal Isolation Precautions

C. Hospice Care

1. Interdisciplinary team

2. Pain and symptom management

3. Emotional support

ANSWERS TO CRITICAL THINKING EXERCISE

1.   Does George have thoughts of suicide? A plan? Means?

2.   a.   Risk for self-directed violence related to depressed mood.
     b.   Impaired adjustment related to new diagnosis of HIV disease.

3.   a.   Protection from self-harm.
     b.   Education about his illness.
     c.   Encourage exploration of his fears.

LEARNING ACTIVITY

ACQUIRED IMMUNE DEFICIENCY SYNDROME

Identify the following key terms associated with acquired immune deficiency syndrome with the descriptions listed below. The first one is completed as an example.

a. HIV-associated dementia
b. opportunistic infections
c. azidothymidine (AZT)
d. human immunodeficiency virus
e. Kaposi's sarcoma
f. seroconversion
g. T4 lymphocytes

h. acute HIV infection
i. asymptomatic infection
j. universal isolation precautions
k. persistent generalized lymphadenopathy (PGL)
l. hospice
m. HIV wasting syndrome

__i__ 1. Period of time following acute HIV infection in which the individual experiences no symptoms. May last 10 years or more.

_____ 2. A syndrome that includes fever, excessive weight loss, and chronic diarrhea.

_____ 3. A type of malignancy common to AIDS clients in which tumor-type lesions may form on any body surface or in the viscera.

_____ 4. The time at which antibodies to the HIV virus may be detected in the blood.

_____ 5. An organization that dedicates itself to the provision of palliative and supportive care during the final stages of illness and during bereavement.

_____ 6. The most widely used antiviral agent in the treatment of HIV infection.

_____ 7. The controlling element of the cellular immune response, which is the major target of the HIV.

_____ 8. The etiological agent that produces the immunosuppression of acquired immune deficiency syndrome.

_____ 9. Infections with any organism that occur because of the altered physiological state of the host.

_____ 10. A syndrome of swollen lymph nodes in the neck, armpit, and groin areas that remain swollen for months with no other signs of a related infectious disease.

_____ 11. Guidelines published by the CDC for prevention of HIV transmission in a health care setting.

_____ 12. A syndrome of pathological changes in cognition, behavior, and motor ability that become more severe with progression of HIV disease.

_____ 13. A characteristic syndrome of symptoms that occur from 6 days to 6 weeks following exposure to the virus.

CHAPTER 36. TEST QUESTIONS

Situation: Tessa, a 27-year-old mother of three children, is admitted to a dual diagnosis program for clients with mental illness and substance abuse. Tessa has been HIV positive for 5 years. She was infected with the HIV by contaminated needles used to inject heroin IV. Her husband recently died from AIDS. Her diagnoses are Major Depression, Alcohol Dependence, and Opioid Dependence, in remission.

1. Which of the following data is *most* useful to determine Tessa's stage of HIV disease?
   - • a. T4 cell count
   - b. Hemoglobin and hematocrit
   - c. Date of seroconversion
   - d. Presence of opportunistic infection

2. Tessa is found to be in early-stage HIV disease. She states, "I don't need to be treated for AIDS. I've never had any symptoms." The nurse's response is based on the knowledge that:
   - a. Tessa is most likely in denial about her illness.
   - b. Tessa is lying about having no symptoms.
   - c. The physician will likely prescribe an antiviral medication for her.
   - • d. Individuals in early-stage disease may not have symptoms for many years.

3. Tessa says to the nurse, "I'm so afraid my kids are going to get the disease from me." In order to help Tessa prevent this from happening, which of the following should she be instructed to do?
   - a. Wear a face mask when preparing their food.
   - • b. When hands are chapped or cut, wear protective gloves when preparing their food.
   - c. Do not kiss them on the lips or face.
   - d. All family members should use disposable dishes and utensils from which to eat.

4. Tessa improves and is discharged from the hospital. She continues to be followed for her HIV disease by her family physician and remains symptom-free for 3 years. During one visit, her physician notices an enlarged lymph node in her armpit and one in the groin. Tessa's temperature is 100.9. The physician suspects that Tessa has progressed to middle-stage HIV disease. He orders a lymphocyte count. If his suspicion is correct, what would he expect the blood test to show?
   - a. A T4 count between 700 and 800 mm^3
   - b. A T4 count between 500 and 600 mm^3
   - • c. A T4 count between 200 and 500 mm^3
   - d. A T4 count below 200 mm^3

5. As the disease continues to progress, Tessa's mother moves in to be with her and her children. Hospice is entitled to help provide care for Tessa. Which of the following statements is true about hospice?
   - • a. They are on-call to families on a 24-hour basis.
   - b. Hospice services to Tessa's family will be discontinued upon her death.
   - c. Hospice will ensure that Tessa is hospitalized at the time of her death.
   - d. Hospice is staffed solely with volunteers.

CHAPTER 37. PROBLEMS RELATED TO ABUSE OR NEGLECT

CHAPTER FOCUS

The focus of this chapter is on nursing care of clients experiencing problems related to abuse or neglect. Predisposing factors and symptomatology are explored, and nursing care is presented in the context of the six steps of the nursing process. Various treatment modalities are also discussed.

LEARNING OBJECTIVES

After reading this chapter, the student will be able to:

1. Discuss historical perspectives associated with spouse abuse, child abuse, and sexual assault.
2. Describe epidemiological statistics associated with spouse abuse, child abuse, and sexual assault.
3. Discuss characteristics of victims and victimizers.
4. Identify predisposing factors to abusive behaviors.
5. Describe physical and psychological effects on the victim of spouse abuse, child abuse, and sexual assault.
6. Identify nursing diagnoses, goals of care, and appropriate nursing interventions for care of victims of spouse abuse, child abuse, and sexual assault.
7. Evaluate nursing care of victims of spouse abuse, child abuse, and sexual assault.
8. Discuss various modalities relevant to treatment of victims of abuse.

KEY TERMS

battering
child sexual abuse
compounded rape reaction
controlled response pattern
cycle of battering
date rape
emotional injury
emotional neglect
expressed response pattern
incest
marital rape
physical neglect
rape
safe house or shelter
sexual exploitation of a child
silent rape reaction
statutory rape

CHAPTER OUTLINE/LECTURE NOTES

I. Introduction
   A. Abuse is the maltreatment of one person by another.
   B. More injuries are attributed to battering than to all rapes, muggings, and automobile accidents combined.
   C. An increase in the incidence of child abuse has been documented.

D. Rape is thought to be vastly underreported.

II. Historical Perspectives

    A. Spouse and child abuse arrived in the U.S. with the Puritans. Women and children were viewed as personal property of men.

    B. The notion of women as subordinate and subservient to men, as well as that of "spare the rod and spoil the child," was supported by the Bible.

    C. Not until the second half of the twentieth century has legal protection been available for victims of abuse.

III. Predisposing Factors

    A. Biological Theories

        1. Neurophysiological Influences. Areas of the brain which have been implicated in both the facilitation and inhibition of aggressive impulses include the temporal lobe, the limbic system, and the amygdaloid nucleus.

        2. Biochemical Influences. Certain neurotransmitters, including norepinephrine, dopamine, and serotonin, have been implicated in the regulation of aggressive impulses.

        3. Genetic Influences. A possible hereditary factor may be involved. The genetic karyotype XYY has also been implicated.

        4. Disorders of the Brain. Aggressive and violent behavior has been correlated with organic brain syndromes, brain tumors, brain trauma, encephalitis, and temporal lobe epilepsy.

    B. Psychological Theories

        1. Psychodynamic Theory. Unmet needs for satisfaction and security result in an underdeveloped ego and a poor self-concept. Aggression and violence supply the individual with a dose of power and prestige that increases self-esteem.

        2. Learning Theory. Children learn to behave by imitating their role models. Individuals who were abused as children or whose parents disciplined with physical punishment are more likely to behave in an abusive manner as adults.

    C. Sociocultural Theories

        1. Societal Influences. Aggressive behavior is primarily a product of one's culture and social structure. The American culture was founded upon a general acceptance of violence as a means of solving problems.

        2. Societal influences also contribute to violence when individuals realize that their needs and desires are not being met relative to other persons.

IV. Application of the Nursing Process: Background Assessment Data

    A. Spouse Abuse

        1. Battering may be defined as repeated physical and/or sexual assault of an intimate partner within a context of coercive control. Approximately 95% of the victims are women.

        2. Profile of the Victim. Battered women represent all age, racial, religious, cultural, educational, and socioeconomic groups. They often have low self-esteem. They may be without adequate support systems. Many grew up in abusive homes.

        3. Profile of the Victimizer. Men who batter are generally characterized as persons with low self-esteem, pathologically jealous, presenting a "dual personality," exhibiting limited coping ability and severe stress reactions. The spouse is viewed as a personal possession.

        4. A Cycle of Battering. Three distinct phases:

            a. Phase I. The Tension-Building Phase

            b. Phase II. The Acute Battering Incident

            c. Phase III. Calm, Loving, Respite (Honeymoon) Phase

        5. Why Does She Stay? The most frequent response to this question is that they fear for their life or the lives of their children. Other reasons given include a lack of support network for leaving, religious beliefs, and a lack of financial independence to support herself and her children.

    B. Child Abuse

        1. Physical Injury. Any nonaccidental physical injury, caused by the parent or caregiver.

            a. Physical signs.

            b. Behavioral signs.

2. Emotional Injury. A pattern of behavior on the part of the parent or caretaker that results in serious impairment of the child's social, emotional, or intellectual functioning.
    a. Behavioral indicators.
3. Neglect.
    a. Physical Neglect. Refers to the failure on the part of the parent or caregiver to provide for that child's basic needs, such as food, clothing, shelter, medical/dental care, and supervision.
        (1) Physical and behavioral indicators.
    b. Emotional Neglect. Refers to a chronic failure by the parent or caretaker to provide the child with the hope, love, and support necessary for the development of a sound, healthy personality.
        (1) Behavioral indicators.
4. Sexual Abuse of a Child.
    a. Sexual Abuse of Child. Defined as "employment, use, persuasion, inducement, enticement, or coercion of any child to engage in, or assist any other person to engage in, any sexually explicit conduct or any simulation of such conduct for the purpose of producing any visual depiction of such conduct; or rape, and in cases of caretaker or inter-familial relationships, statutory rape, molestation, prostitution, or other form of sexual exploitation of children, or incest with children."
    b. Incest. The occurrence of sexual contacts or interaction between, or sexual exploitation of, close relatives, or between participants who are related to each other by a kinship bond that is regarded as a prohibition to sexual relations (e.g., caretakers, stepparents, stepsiblings).
    c. Indicators of Sexual Abuse.
        (1) Physical indicators.
        (2) Behavioral indicators.
5. Characteristics of the Abuser
    a. Parents who abuse their children were likely abused as children themselves.
    b. Retarded ego development, lack of knowledge of adequate child-rearing practices, lack of empathy, and low self-esteem.
    c. Certain environmental influences, such as numerous stresses, poverty, social isolation, and an absence of adequate support systems, may predispose to child abuse.
6. The Incestual Relationship
    a. Often there is an impaired spousal relationship.
    b. Father is often domineering, impulsive, and physically abusing.
    c Mother is commonly passive, submissive, and denigrates her role of wife and mother. She is often aware of, or at least suspects, the incestuous relationship, but uses denial or keeps quiet out of fear of being abused by her husband.
7. The Adult Survivor of Incest
    a. Common characteristics.
        (1) A fundamental lack of trust that arises out of an unsatisfactory mother-child relationship.
        (2) Low self-esteem and a poor sense of identity.
        (3) Absence of pleasure with sexual activity.
        (4) Promiscuity
C. Sexual assault
    1. Rape is an act of aggression, not passion. It is identified by the use of force and executed "against the person's will."
        a. Date Rape. Applied to sexual assault in which the rapist is known to the victim.
        b. Marital Rape. Sexual violence directed at a marital partner against that person's will.
        c. Statutory Rape. Unlawful intercourse between a male over age 16 and a female under the age of consent.
    2. Profile of the Victimizer
        a. The mother of the rapist has been described as "seductive but rejecting" toward her child. She is overbearing, with seductive undertones, but is quick to withdraw her "love" and attention when he goes against her wishes. Her dominance over her son often continues into his adult life.

265

    b.   Many rapists report growing up in abusive homes. Even when the abuse was discharged by the father, the rapist's anger is directed toward the mother for not providing adequate protection from the father's abuse.

   3. The Victim

      a.   Rape can occur at any age. The highest risk group appears to be between 16 and 24 years.

      b.   Most victims are single women, and the attack often occurs near their own neighborhood.

      c.   When the attack is a "stranger rape," victims are not chosen for any reason having to do with their appearance or behavior, but simply because they happened to be in that place at that particular time.

      d.   The presence of a weapon (real or perceived) appears to be the principal measure of the degree to which a woman resists her attacker.

      e.   Victim responses:

          (1)   Expressed response pattern--the victim expresses feelings of fear, anger, and anxiety through such behaviors as crying, sobbing, smiling, restlessness, and tension.

          (2)   Controlled response pattern--feelings of the victim are masked or hidden, and a calm, composed, or subdued affect is seen.

          (3)   Compounded rape reaction--additional symptoms such as depression and suicide, substance abuse, and even psychotic behaviors may be noted in the victim.

          (4)   Silent rape reaction--the victim tells no one about the assault. Anxiety is suppressed and the emotional burden may become overwhelming.

V.   Diagnoses/Outcome Identification

   A. Nursing diagnoses for the client who has been abused may include:

      1. Rape-trauma syndrome

      2. Powerlessness

      3. Altered growth and development

   B. Outcome criteria are identified for measuring the effectiveness of nursing care.

VI.   Planning/Implementation

   A. Nursing intervention for the victim of abuse or neglect is to provide shelter and promote reassurance of his or her safety.

   B. Other nursing concerns include:

      1. Tending to physical injuries

      2. Staying with the client to provide security

      3. Assisting the client to recognize options

      4. Promoting trust

      5. Reporting to authorities when there is "reason to suspect" child abuse or neglect

VII. Evaluation is based on accomplishment of previously established outcome criteria.

VIII. Treatment Modalities

   A. Crisis Intervention

   B. Safe House or Shelter

   C. Family Therapy

IX.   Summary

X.   Critical Thinking Exercise

XI.   Review Questions

ANSWERS TO CRITICAL THINKING EXERCISE

1.   "He doesn't act this way because of anything you do."

2.   Powerlessness related to cycle of battering.

3.   The nurse must help Lisa understand that alternatives to her current situation do exist, and it is her decision to choose one of the alternatives or return to her current living situation. Either way, she will be supported in her decision.

CASE STUDY FOR USE WITH STUDENT LEARNING

Case Study: Physical Neglect of a Child

Amy, age 5, started kindergarten this year. Her teacher noticed that she seems to spend a lot of time alone, standing on the sidelines during recess watching the other children play, but not entering into the interaction. She comes to school somewhat unkempt and with a noticeable body odor about her. She participates in the free school lunch program, and often gulps her food, appearing ravenous when the food is presented. As the weather turns cold, the teacher notices that Amy is coming to school without a coat. When questioned, she states, "I don't have a coat." The teacher reports Amy's case to the DHS and a home health nurse is sent to Amy's home to investigate. At Amy's home the nurse finds a teenager who identifies herself as Amy's sister, Carol. She is caring for three other children: an 8-year-old boy and a 3-year-old girl, whom she identifies are her siblings, and a 6-month-old girl, whom she identifies as her own child. There is no adult in the home. Carol tells the nurse that she is 16 years old and has full charge of these children most of the time. Carols' mother lives with her boyfriend most of the time, but comes to the house occasionally to bring a few groceries. Carol tells the nurse that she is worried because the electric company has threatened to turn off the electricity for lack of payment, and because there has been no food in the house for 2 days. She says she has talked to her mother several times, but her mother just responds that she doesn't have any money right now, and they must do the best that they can. DHS places all the children in foster care and tells the mother that she must undergo therapy in order to justify return of the children to her care. Devise a plan of care that the home health nurse might use to assist the mother in this effort.

LEARNING ACTIVITY

BEHAVIORS OF ABUSE OR NEGLECT

Match terms on the right to the situations they describe on the left.

_____ 1. John likes to brag of his sexual conquests to his friends.   a. Physical injury
          When Alice rejected his sexual advances on their first date,
          he became angry and forced intercourse with her.

_____ 2. Alice tells no one about the encounter with John. She   b. Compounded rape reaction
          suppresses her anxiety and tries to pretend it didn't happen.

_____ 3. Harry is 28 years old. He is very flattered when 15-year-old   c. Spouse abuse
          Lisa pays attention to him at a party. After the party, he takes
          her to his home, where she agrees to have sex with him.

_____ 4. At 9 p.m., Jack gets home from the bar where he had gone   d. Date rape
          after work with his friends. He is intoxicated, and when
          he finds his dinner cold, he slaps his wife across the face,
          knocks her down, and kicks her in the side.

_____ 5. Jack pulls his wife to their bed, and against her protests,   e. Expressed response pattern
          forces intercourse with her, yelling, "You can't say no
          to me! You're my wife!"

_____ 6. Janie is 16 years old. Her father left home a year ago and   f. Incest
          has never returned. Her mother frequently says to Janie,
          "See what you did?! If you had been a better little girl,
          Daddy wouldn't have left us!"

_____ 7. Janie attempts to establish a relationship with her mother,   g. Marital rape
          but whenever Janie approaches her mother for interaction,
          her mother yells, "Get away from me! I don't want to have
          anything to do with bad little girls!"

_____ 8. Janie has open sores on her buttocks. She tells the   h. Statutory rape
          babysitter, "My mommy made them with her cigarette."

_____ 9. Janie comes to school in the snow without a coat. When   i. Silent rape reaction
          the teacher asks her where her coat is, Janie replies, "I
          don't have one."

_____ 10. Scarlet is 15 years old. She is sent to the school nurse   j. Emotional injury
          by her homeroom teacher. She is obviously having
          symptoms of a panic attack. Upon becoming calmer,
          Scarlet explains to the nurse that Frank just asked her for
          her first date. With much encouragement, the nurse learns
          that Scarlet's father has been coming into her bed at night
          for 5 years now. At first he just touched her and fondled
          her, but last year he began having intercourse with her.

_____ 11. After being raped by a man in the deserted laundry room of her apartment building, Carol is taken to the hospital by her roommate. Carol is sobbing and yelling, "He had no right to do that to me!" She is tense, and is fearful of any man who comes near her.

k.   Emotional neglect

_____ 12. Carol's physical wounds heal, but in subsequent weeks, she becomes increasingly fearful. She is overcome with despair and talks of taking her life. She drinks a great deal of alcohol to help her get through each day.

l.   Physical neglect

CHAPTER 37. TEST QUESTIONS

Situation: Roberta is a 43-year-old married woman who has called in sick to work for 3 days. When she finally returns to work, her makeup cannot conceal bruises on her face. A coworker who is a good friend mentions the bruises, and says they look like the bruises she used to have after being beaten by her former husband. Roberta says, "It was an accident. He just had a terrible day at work. He's being so kind and gentle now. Yesterday he brought me flowers. He says he's going to get a new job, so it won't ever happen again."

1. Which phase of the cycle of battering does Roberta's response represent?
    a. Phase I. The Tension-Building Phase
    b. Phase II. The Acute Battering Incident
    •   c. Phase III. The Honeymoon Phase
    d. Phase IV. The Resolution Phase

2. Roberta's co-worker recommends that she seek assistance from her Employee Assistance Program. Roberta refuses because she believes her husband has reformed. What is the *best* alternative suggestion her co-worker can make at this point?
    a. Buy a gun.
    b. File for divorce.
    c. Press charges of assault and battery.
    •   d. Carry the number of the safe house for battered women.

Situation: Katie is a 9-year-old third grader. Her teacher, Mrs. Small, notices that Katie has had an open lesion on her left arm for a week. The lesion appears to have become infected, which is easy to see because Mrs. Small has never seen it covered with a bandage. Katie is often absent from school, and seems apathetic and tired when she attends. Other children in the classroom avoid her, and Mrs. Small has overheard them talking about Katie stealing food from them at lunch time.

3. Mrs. Small's observations are indications of which of the following?
    •   a. Physical neglect
    b. Emotional injury
    c. Physical abuse
    d. Sexual abuse

Situation: Teresa, an unmarried 37-year-old woman, has recently been referred from her family physician to the psychiatrist with the complaint of "anxiety attacks." These attacks occur in the evening before bedtime, and Teresa has also been experiencing insomnia. When she does get to sleep, she often has nightmares. She tells the psychiatrist that her father has recently been diagnosed with an inoperable brain tumor.

4. What might the psychiatrist suspect after making his initial assessment of Teresa?
    a. Possible depressive disorder.
    •   b. Possible history of childhood incest.
    c. Possible anticipatory grieving.
    d. Possible history of childhood physical abuse.

Situation: The police escort Zoe, a 29-year-old, married stock market analyst, to the emergency department of an inner-city hospital. She is sobbing, her clothing is torn and she has superficial cuts on her neck and chest. She was leaving her office after working late and was accosted from behind as she bent to unlock her car, which was parked at the periphery of the parking lot. Her assailant raped her and stole her purse and her car. She walked to a nearby telephone, dialed 911, and a police car was dispatched to assist her. Upon arrival at the ED, the triage nurse immediately calls a member of the Sexual Assault Crisis Team, who arrives within 20 minutes and remains with Zoe throughout her stay in the ED.

5. What is the most therapeutic thing for the nurse to say to Zoe when she arrives at the ED?
    - a. "You are safe now."
    b. "I'll call your husband."
    c. "The police will want to interview you."
    d. "We'll have to take photographs of those wounds."

6. Zoe is crying, pacing, and cursing her attacker. Which behavioral defense do these manifestations represent?
    a. Controlled response pattern
    b. Compounded rape reaction
    - c. Expressed response pattern
    d. Silent rape reaction

CHAPTER 38.   COMMUNITY MENTAL HEALTH NURSING

CHAPTER FOCUS

The focus of this chapter is on nursing care of psychiatric clients in the community setting, using the framework of the model of public health: primary, secondary, and tertiary prevention. Emphasis is given to the chronically mentally ill and the homeless mentally ill. Nursing care is presented in the context of the six steps of the nursing process. A discussion of rural mental health nursing is presented.

LEARNING OBJECTIVES

After reading this chapter, the student will be able to:

1.   Discuss the changing focus of care in the field of mental health.
2.   Define the concepts of care associated with the model of public health:
      a.   Primary prevention
      b.   Secondary prevention
      c.   Tertiary prevention
3.   Differentiate between the roles of basic level and advanced practice psychiatric/mental health registered nurses.
4.   Define the concepts of case management and identify the role of case management in community mental health nursing.
5.   Discuss primary prevention of mental illness within the community.
6.   Identify populations at risk for mental illness within the community.
7.   Discuss nursing intervention in primary prevention of mental illness within the community.
8.   Discuss secondary prevention of mental illness within the community.
9.   Describe treatment alternatives related to secondary prevention within the community.
10.   Discuss tertiary prevention of mental illness within the community as it relates to the chronically and homeless mentally ill.
11.   Relate historical and epidemiological factors associated with caring for the chronically and homeless mentally ill within the community.
12.   Identify treatment alternatives for care of the chronically and homeless mentally ill within the community.
13.   Apply steps of the nursing process to care of the chronically and homeless mentally ill within the community.
14.   Describe principal aspects of the role of the mental health nurse in rural settings.

KEY TERMS

deinstitutionalization
prospective payment
primary prevention
secondary prevention
tertiary prevention
community
store-front clinics

diagnostically related groups (DRGs)
managed care
case management
case manager
shelters
mobile outreach units

CHAPTER OUTLINE/LECTURE NOTES

I.   The Changing Focus of Care

A. before 1840, there was no known treatment for the mentally ill, who were removed from the community to a place where they could do no harm to themselves or others.
B. In 1841, Dorothea Dix, a former school teacher, started a campaign that resulted in the establishment of a number of hospitals for the mentally ill.
C. The mentally ill population grew faster than the number of hospitals, creating overcrowdedness and poor conditions.
D. In the 40s and 50s, a number of constitutional acts were passed, attempting to improve the quality of care for the mentally ill.
E. In 1963, the Community Mental Health Centers Act was passed. It called for the construction of community health centers.
F. Deinstitutionalization (the closing of state mental hospitals and discharging of mental ill individuals) had begun.
G. However, federal funding was reduced, and the number of community health centers was diminished.
H. Cost containment by prospective payment was initiated in 1983, drastically affecting the amount of reimbursement for health care services.
I. Clients are being discharged from the hospital with a greater need for aftercare than in the past, when hospital stays were longer. Outpatient services have become an essential part of the mental health care system.

II. The Public Health Model
A. Primary Prevention
1. Primary prevention is defined as reducing the incidence of mental disorders within the population.
2. Nursing in primary prevention is focused on targeting groups at risk and the provision of educational programs.
B. Secondary Prevention
1. Reducing the prevalence of psychiatric illness by shortening the course (duration) of the illness.
2. Accomplished through early identification of problems and prompt initiation of effective treatment.
C. Tertiary Prevention
1. Reducing the residual defects that are associated with severe or chronic mental illness.
2. Accomplished by preventing complications of the illness and promoting achievement of each individual's maximum level of functioning.

III. The Role of the Nurse
A. A way of coordinating health care services required to meet the needs of the client.
B. Managed care is a concept purposefully designed to control the balance between cost and quality of care. (HMOs and PPOs are examples of managed care.)
C. Case management is the method used to achieve managed care. Case management is especially beneficial for individuals who require long-term care (e.g., clients with chronic mental illness).
D. The case manager is responsible for negotiating with multiple health care providers to obtain a variety of services for the client.
E. The ANA suggests that nurses are particularly suited to provide case management for clients with multiple health problems that have a health-related component.

V. The Community as Client
A. Primary Prevention
1. To identify stressful life events that precipitate crises and target the relevant populations at risk.
2. To intervene with these high-risk populations to prevent or minimize harmful consequences.
3. Populations at Risk
a. Individuals experiencing maturational crises:
(1) Adolescence
(2) Marriage
(3) Parenthood
(4) Midlife
(5) Retirement
b. Individuals experiencing situational crises:
(1) Poverty
(2) High rate of life change events

        (3)   Environmental conditions

        (4)   Trauma

B. Secondary Prevention

    1. Early detection and prompt intervention with individuals experiencing mental illness symptoms

    2. Populations at Risk

        1. Individuals experiencing maturational crises:

           (1)   Adolescence

           (2)   Marriage

           (3)   Parenthood

           (4)   Midlife

           (5)   Retirement

        b. Individuals experiencing situational crises:

           (1)   Nursing care at the secondary level of prevention with clients undergoing situational crises occurs only if crisis intervention at the primary level failed and the individual is unable to function socially or occupationally.

C. Tertiary Prevention

    1. The Chronically Mentally Ill

        a. Historical and Epidemiological Aspects

           (1)   Approximately 120,000 mentally ill persons inhabit public mental hospitals.

           (2)   Deinstitutionalization occurred so rapidly that there was not sufficient time for planning for the needs of these individuals before they reentered the community.

           (3)   The Coalition of Psychiatric Nursing Organization (COPNO) has outlined the following essential services for mental health reform to assist the chronically mentally ill:

              (a)   Primary care mental health services

              (b)   Universal access to a basic mental health package

              (c)   Long-term care

              (d)   Managed care

        b. Treatment Alternatives

           (1)   Community Mental Health Centers

           (2)   Day-Evening Treatment/Partial Hospitalization Programs

           (3)   Community Residential Facilities

    2. The Homeless Mentally Ill

        a. Historical and Epidemiological Aspects

           (1)   The number of homeless in the U.S. has been estimated at somewhere between 250,000 and 4 million.

           (2)   It is thought that approximately 20 to 25 percent of the single adult homeless population suffers from some form of severe and persistent mental illness.

        b. Types of Mental Illness Among the Homeless

           (1)   Most common: schizophrenia

           (2)   Bipolar affective disorder

           (3)   Substance abuse and dependence

           (4)   Depression

           (5)   Personality disorders

           (6)   Organic mental disorders

        c. Contributing Factors to Homelessness Among the Mentally Ill

           (1)   Deinstitutionalization

           (2)   Poverty

           (3)   A scarcity of affordable housing

           (4)   Lack of affordable health care

           (5)   Domestic violence

           (6)   Addiction disorders

        d. Community Resources for the Homeless

           (1)   Interfering Factors

               (a)   Residential instability

          (b) Seasonal mobility

          (c) Migration

      (2) Health Issues

          (a) Alcoholism is common

          (b) Thermoregulation

          (c) Tuberculosis is on the rise

          (d) Dietary deficiencies are common

          (e) Sexually transmitted diseases

          (f) Special health needs of homeless children

      (3) Types of Resources Available

          (a) Homeless shelters

          (b) Health Care centers and Store-Front Clinics

          (c) Mobile Outreach Units

   e. The Homeless Client and the Nursing Process: A Case Study

      (1) Assessment

      (2) Diagnosis/Outcome Identification

      (3) Plan/Implementation

      (4) Evaluation

VI.   Rural Mental Health Nursing

   A. Approximately 25 percent of the U.S. population reside in rural areas.

   B. Mental health assistance is much less readily available to rural residents than it is to individuals in urban areas.

   C. Only about half of rural residents with emotional problems ever seek treatment, and those who do often receive it from a general practitioner, public health nurse, or social service worker.

   D. In comparison to the population in general, rural residents are commonly more religious, conservative, traditional, family-centered, clannish, inflexible, and work-oriented. They do not often establish trust easily.

   E. The rural mental health nurse must possess the ability to intervene with a variety of skills in a diversity of situations.

   F. The rural mental health nurse may serve in a community health center, make home visits, or even act as primary therapist in crisis intervention, and short-term and long-term individual counseling.

   G. The role of educator is most significant to the rural mental health nurse.

   H. Outreach programs, in which health care services are provided in the home, have been shown to be effective in providing care to underserved areas. For some chronically ill individuals, this home treatment may be the only alternative to institutionalization. These services have been shown to be very efficient and cost-effective, without diminishing quality of care.

VII. Summary

VIII. Review Questions

LEARNING ACTIVITY

CONCEPTS AND TERMS ASSOCIATED WITH COMMUNITY MENTAL HEALTH NURSING

Fill in the blanks of the statements below with the following terms and concepts associated with community mental health nursing.

deinstitutionalization
DRGs
primary prevention
secondary prevention
tertiary prevention

managed care
mobile outreach units
day treatment programs
health maintenance organization
homelessness

1. In _____, volunteers and paid professionals form teams to drive or walk around and seek out homeless persons who are in need of assistance.

2. _____ is a concept purposefully designed to control the balance between cost and quality of care.

3. A _____ is an example of the concept described in question #2.

4. Nurse Jones visits Sam, who has chronic schizophrenia, in his home to give him his monthly injection of antipsychotic medication. This is an example of _____.

5. The release of thousands of chronically mentally ill individuals from state hospitals into the community setting is called _____.

6. The concept defined in #5 has been identified as a contributing factor to _____ among the mentally ill.

7. _____ are designed to ease the transition from the hospitalization to community living.

8. _____, directed at control of Medicare costs, have reduced the length of hospital stays for psychiatric clients, and increased the importance of aftercare.

9. Teaching a class in prepared childbirth education is an example of _____.

10. Caring for a widow who has been hospitalized for major depression is an example of _____.

CHAPTER 38. TEST QUESTIONS

Situation: Victor is a 47-year-old man with schizophrenia. He lives with his 67-year-old mother, who has always managed his affairs. He has never been employed. Recently his mother had to have an emergency cholecystectomy, at which time Victor suffered an exacerbation of his psychosis and was hospitalized.

1. Victor's hospitalization represents an example of which of the following?
   - a. Primary prevention
   - • b. Secondary prevention
   - c. Tertiary prevention
   - d. None of the above

2. Upon discharge from the hospital, Victor's physician refers him for nursing case management. Which of the following statements *best* describes case management?
   - a. Reducing residual defects associated with chronic mental illness.
   - b. Provision of cost-effective care based on need.
   - • c. Long-term coordination of needed services by multiple providers.
   - d. Recognition of symptoms and provision of treatment.

3. Once a month, the home health nurse administers Victor's injection of haloperidol (Haldol) decanoate. This nursing intervention is an example of:
   - a. Primary prevention
   - b. Secondary prevention
   - • c. Tertiary prevention
   - d. None of the above.

4. One of the major problems in attempting to provide health care services to the homeless is:
   - a. Most of them don't want help.
   - b. They are suspicious of anyone who offers help.
   - c. Most are proud and will refuse charity.
   - • d. They have a penchant for mobility.

5. A recent increase in which of the following diseases has been noted among the homeless?
   - a. Meningitis
   - • b. Tuberculosis
   - c. Encephalopathy
   - d. Mononucleosis

6. Which of the following also are ongoing problems for many homeless individuals?
   - a. Alcoholism and thermoregulation
   - b. Sexually transmitted diseases, including HIV disease
   - c. Conditions related to dietary deficiencies
   - • d. All of the above

7. Which of the following interventions would be considered primary prevention for a homeless individual who lives at a shelter?
   - • a. Job training
   - b. A place to eat and sleep
   - c. Clean clothing
   - d. Nursing care

CHAPTER 39. CULTURAL CONCEPTS RELEVANT TO PSYCHIATRIC/MENTAL HEALTH NURSING

CHAPTER FOCUS

The focus of this chapter is the study of various sociocultural concepts that have an impact on the way individuals interact with each other. The nurse must have an understanding of these concepts and how they relate to various groups of people. Emphasis is given to Northern European Americans, African Americans, native Americans, Asian/Pacific Islander Americans, Latino Americans, and Western European Americans.

LEARNING OBJECTIVES

After reading this chapter, the student will be able to:

1. Define and differentiate between culture and ethnicity.
2. Describe six phenomena on which to identify cultural differences.
3. Identify cultural variances, based on the six phenomena, for:
   a. Northern European Americans
   b. African Americans
   c. Native Americans
   d. Asian/Pacific Islander Americans
   e. Latino Americans
   f. Western European Americans
4. Apply the nursing process in the care of individuals from various cultural groups.

KEY TERMS

culture
ethnicity
stereotyping
territoriality
density
distance
folk medicine
shaman
yin and yang
curandero
curandera

CHAPTER OUTLINE/LECTURE NOTES

I. Introduction
   A. Culture describes a particular society's entire way of living, encompassing shared patterns of belief, feeling, and knowledge that guide people's conduct and are passed down from generation to generation.
   B. Ethnicity relates to people who identify with each other because of a shared heritage.
   C. Nurses must understand these cultural concepts because cultural influences affect human behavior, the interpretation of human behavior, and the response to human behavior.

D. Caution must be taken not to assume that all individuals who share a culture or ethnic group are clones. This constitutes stereotyping, and must be avoided. All individuals must be appreciated for their uniqueness.

II. How Do Cultures Differ?
A. Communication
 1. Has its roots in culture
 2. Is expressed through language, paralanguage, and gestures
B. Space (the place where the communication occurs)
 1. Territoriality refers to the innate tendency to own space
 2. Density refers to the number of people within a given environmental space
 3. Distance is the means by which various cultures use space to communicate
  a. Intimate distance: 0 to 18 inches
  b. Personal distance: 18 inches to 3 feet
  c. Social distance: 3 to 6 feet
C. Social Organization
 1. Social organizations are the groups within which individuals are acculturated, acquiring knowledge and internalizing values.
 2. Examples of social organizations are families, religious groups, and ethnic groups.
D. Time
 1. Some cultures place great importance on values that are measured by time, whereas others are actually scornful of clock time.
 2. Whether individuals perceive time in the present orientation or future orientation influences many aspects of their lives.
E. Environmental Control
 1. Has to do with the degree to which individuals perceive that they have control over their environment.
 2. Cultural beliefs and practices influence how an individual responds to their environment during periods of wellness and illness.
F. Biological Variations
 1. Differences among people in various racial groups include body structure, skin color, physiological responses to medication, electrocardiographic patterns, susceptibility to disease, and nutritional preferences and deficiencies.

III. Application of the Nursing Process
A. Background Assessment Data
 1. Northern European Americans
  a. Language has roots in the first English settlers
  b. Descendants of these immigrants make up what is considered the dominant cultural group
  c. They value territory; personal space is about 18 inches to 3 feet
  d. Less value placed on marriage and religion as once was
  e. Punctuality and efficiency highly valued
  f. Future-oriented
  g. Most value a healthy lifestyle, but still enjoy fast food
  h. Medium body structure and fair skin
 2. African Americans
  a. Language dialect thought to be a combination of various African languages and the languages of other cultural groups present in the U.S. at the time of its settlement.
  b. Some African Americans are completely assimilated into the dominant culture while others find it too difficult and prefer to remain in their own social organization.
  c. About one-third of African American households are headed by a female.
  d. Large support groups of families and friends.
  e. Some African Americans (particularly from the deep South) practice folk medicine and receive their care from a "granny," "old lady," or "spiritualist."
  f. Body structure similar to dominant culture. Skin color varies from white to very dark brown.
  g.

g.   Hypertension and sickle cell anemia have genetic tendencies within the African American culture.

3. Native Americans

    a.   Less than half of Native Americans live on reservations.

    b.   Touch is not highly regarded by Native Americans and a handshake may be viewed as aggressive.

    c.   Sometimes appear silent and reserved.

    d.   Uncomfortable expressing emotions.

    e.   Primary social organization is the family and the tribe. Children are taught to respect tradition.

    f.   Native Americans are present-time oriented.

    g.   Medicine man is called a shaman, and uses a variety of methods in practice. May work closely with traditional medicine to heal the sick.

    h.   Average height with reddish-tinted skin that may be light to medium brown.

    i.   Health problems include tuberculosis, alcoholism, and nutritional deficiencies.

4. Asian/Pacific Islander Americans

    a.   Very large group in the U.S. today, with 11 million immigrants and their descendants from Japan, China, Vietnam, the Philippines, Thailand, Cambodia, Korea, Laos, and the Pacific Islands.

    b.   They are viewed as one (Asian) culture, but in fact constitute a multiplicity of differences regarding attitudes, beliefs, values, religious practices, and language.

    c.   Asian Americans are quiet spoken, for to raise the voice indicates a loss of control.

    d.   Many of the younger generation Asian Americans have become almost totally acculturated into the dominant cultural group.

    e.   Touching is not considered totally appropriate by some Asian Americans.

    f.   The family is the ultimate social organization in the Asian American culture, and loyalty to family is emphasized above all else.

    g.   Education is highly valued, although many remain undereducated.

    h.   Religious practices and beliefs are very diverse and exhibit influences of Taoism, Buddhism, Islam, and Christianity.

    i.   Time orientation is on both past and present.

    j.   Restoring the balance of yin and yang is the fundamental concept of Asian health practices.

    k.   Generally small of frame and build. Obesity is very uncommon. Skin color ranges from white to medium brown, with yellow tones.

    l.   Rice, vegetables, and fish are main staple foods.

    m.   Psychiatric illness is viewed as behavior that is out of control and brings great shame to the family.

    n.   Alcohol consumption is low due to a possible genetic intolerance of the substance.

5. Latino Americans

    a.   Ancestry traced to Mexico, Spain, Puerto Rico, Cuba, and other countries of Central and South America.

    b.   Common language is Spanish.

    c.   Touch is a common form of communication.

    d.   Latinos are very group oriented, and the primary social organization is a large extended family.

    e.   Latinos tend to be very present oriented.

    f.   Roman Catholicism is the predominant religion.

    g.   Folk medicine combines elements of Roman Catholicism and Indian and Spanish ancestries.

    h.   The folk healer is called a curandero (male) or curandera (female). Many still subscribe to the "hot and cold" theory of disease (a concept similar to the yin and yang beliefs of the Asian Americans).

    i.   Height tends to be somewhat shorter than those from the dominant cultural group. Skin color can vary from light tan to dark brown.

    j.   A strong cohesiveness within the family is thought to promote the fact that there is less mental illness among Latino Americans than in the general population.

6. Western European Americans
    a. Origin is from France, Italy and Greece.
    b. Each has unique language with unique dialects within each language.
    c. Warm and affectionate, very physically expressive, and use a lot of body language, including hugging and kissing.
    d. Very family oriented. Interact in large groups.
    e. A strong allegiance to the cultural heritage is common.
    f. Father is head of household. Women view their role as mother and homemaker. Children are prized and cherished, and elderly are respected for their age and wisdom.
    g. Roman Catholicism is the predominant religion for the French and Italians; Greek Orthodox for the Greeks.
    h. Western European Americans are present-oriented and view whatever happens in the future as God's will.
    i. Most follow health beliefs and practices of the dominant American culture, but some folk beliefs and superstitions still endure.
    j. Western Europeans are of average stature. Skin color ranges from fair to medium brown.
    k. Wine is the beverage of choice, but alcoholism rate is low.
B. Diagnosis/Outcome Identification
    1. Nursing diagnoses for individuals with varied cultural influences may include:
        a. Impaired verbal communication
        b. Anxiety (moderate to severe)
        c. Alteration in nutrition, less than body requirements
        d. Spiritual distress
C. Planning/Implementation
    1. Nursing intervention with clients whose beliefs are culturally influenced are aimed at insuring that those beliefs are not misunderstood and that nursing care includes elements that are important to the individual within his or her culture.
    2. Emphasis is also placed on developing a trusting relationship with the client and his or her family, and that any barriers to communication are eliminated.
D. Evaluation is based on accomplishment of previously established outcome criteria.
IV. Summary
V. Review Questions

LEARNING ACTIVITY

CONCEPTS AND TERMS RELATED TO CULTURE AND ETHNICITY

Match the terms on the left to the appropriate explanation on the right.

____ 1. Culture

____ 2. Ethnicity

____ 3. Stereotyping

____ 4. Folk medicine

____ 5. Shaman

____ 6. Yin and yang

____ 7. Curandero

____ 8. Acculturation

____ 9. Density and distance

____ 10. Social organization

a. Health care provided by a member of the cultural group.

b. Concepts of space that influence communication.

c. Internalizing the attitudes and beliefs of another cultural group.

d. A society's way of living that is passed down from generation to generation.

e. A folk healer in the Latino American culture.

f. The major groups in which an individual becomes acculturated.

g. Assuming that all individuals who share a culture or ethnic group are the same.

h. A concept of folk medicine beliefs in the Asian American culture.

i. Identification with a group because of a shared heritage.

j. The Native American "medicine man" or folk healer.

CHAPTER 39. TEST QUESTIONS

1. Asian Americans often view emotional illness as behavior that is out of control, and that which brings shame on the family. Which of the following responses to psychological distress is most likely to occur among this cultural group?
    - a. Obsessive-compulsive behavior
    - b. Depression
    - • c. Somatization disorder
    - d. Phobias

2. A common symptom of psychotic behavior is "flat" affect, or little change in facial expression that signals change in mood or feeling tone. Because of cultural differences, with which of the following cultural groups would care have to be taken in interpreting the affect as "flat?"
    - a. African Americans
    - • b. Native Americans
    - c. Latino Americans
    - d. Western European Americans

3. What is the *best* reason for including favorite or culturally required foods in the diets of clients from cultures other than the dominant culture?
    - a. It prevents malnutrition.
    - b. It prevents clients from becoming agitated.
    - c. It insures the client's cooperation with scientifically based treatment.
    - • d. It conveys acceptance of the client's beliefs and identity.

4. Albert, a homeless Native American, is taken to the emergency department (ED) by the shelter nurse. Albert has a known history of diabetes, and he presents with a sore on his foot that he says he has had for several weeks. He refuses to talk to the physician on call in the ED unless a shaman is present. Which of the following interventions would be most appropriate?
    - • a. Try to locate a shaman and ask him to come to the ED.
    - b. Explain to Albert that "voodoo" medicine will not heal the wound on his foot.
    - c. Ask Albert to explain what he thinks the shaman will do that would not be done by the ED physician.
    - d. Tell Albert that he has the right to refuse treatment by the ED physician; it is his choice.

5. Which of the following is associated with values of the Northern European American culture (dominant cultural group)?
    - a. They are present-oriented.
    - b. They are highly religious and church attendance is at an all time high.
    - • c. They value punctuality and efficiency.
    - d. With the advent of technology, increased emphasis is being placed on family cohesiveness.

6. Which of the following is typical of the African American culture?
    - • a. They often have a strong religious orientation.
    - b. Personal space tends to be larger than that of the dominant culture.
    - c. About one-half of all African American households are headed by a woman.
    - d. In the deep South, the African American folk practitioner is known as a shaman.

7. Which of the following relates to individuals of the Native American culture?
    - a. Most are warm and outgoing.
    - b. Touch is a common form of communication.
    - • c. Primary social organizations are family and tribe.
    - d. Most Native Americans are future-oriented.

8. Which of the following relates to individuals of the Asian American culture?
    - a. Obesity and alcoholism are common problems.
    - • b. The elderly maintain positions of authority within the culture.

     c.   "Hot" and "cold" are the fundamental concepts of Asian health practices.

     d.   Asian Americans willingly seek psychiatric assistance for emotional problems.

9.   Which of the following relates to individuals of the Latino American culture?

     a.   Latino Americans shy away from any form of touch.

     b.   Latino Americans tend to be future-oriented.

     c.   Roman Catholicism is the predominant religion, although the influence of the church is weak.

 •   d.   The first contact when illness is encountered is often with the curandero folk healer.

10.   Which of the following relates to individuals of the Western European American culture?

 •   a.   They are present-oriented; future is perceived as God's will.

     b.   Youth is valued; elderly are commonly placed in nursing homes.

     c.   Alcoholism is a major problem in the Western European American culture.

     d.   They have a large personal space.

CHAPTER 40. ETHICAL AND LEGAL ISSUES IN PSYCHIATRIC/MENTAL HEALTH NURSING

CHAPTER FOCUS

The focus of this chapter is on ethical and legal issues that affect psychiatric/mental health nursing. Ethical theories, dilemmas, and principles are explored as a foundation for decision-making. Various types of law are defined, and situation for which nurses may be held liable ar discussed.

LEARNING OBJECTIVES

After reading this chapter, the student will be able to:

1.   Differentiate among ethics, morals, values, and rights.
2.   Discuss ethical theories including utilitarianism, Kantianism, Christian ethics, natural law theories, and ethical egoism.
3.   Define *ethical dilemma.*
4.   Discuss the ethical principles of autonomy, beneficence, nonmaleficence, veracity and justice.
5.   Use an ethical decision-making model to make an ethical decision.
6.   Describe ethical issues relevant to psychiatric/mental health nursing.
7.   Define *statutory law* and *common law.*
8.   Differentiate between civil and criminal law.
9.   Discuss legal issues relevant to psychiatric/mental health nursing.
10.   Differentiate between *malpractice* and *negligence.*
11.   Identify behaviors relevant to the psychiatric/mental health setting for which specific malpractice action could be taken.

KEY TERMS

assault	libel
autonomy	Kantianism
battery	malpractice
beneficence	moral behavior
bioethics	natural law
Christian ethics	negligence
civil law	nonmaleficence
common law	privileged communication
defamation of character	right
ethical dilemma	slander
ethical egoism	statutory law
ethics	tort
false imprisonment	utilitarianism
informed consent	values
justice	values clarification
	veracity

CHAPTER OUTLINE/LECTURE NOTES

I. Introduction
    A. Nurses are constantly faced with the challenge of making difficult decisions regarding good and evil or life and death.
    B. Legislation determines what is "right" o "good" within our society.

II. Definitions
    A. Ethics: a branch of philosophy dealing with values related to human conduct, to the rightness and wrongness of certain actions, an to the goodness and badness of the motives and ends of such actions.
    B. Bioethics: applies to ethics when they refer to concepts within the scope of medicine, nursing and allied health.
    C. Moral Behavior: conduct that results from serious critical thinking about how individuals ought to treat others.
    D   Values: personal beliefs about the truth, beauty, or worth of thought, object, or behavior.
    E. Values clarification: a process of self-discovery by which people identify their personal values and their value rankings.
    F. Right: that to which an individual is entitled (by ethical or moral standards) to have, or to do, or to receive from within the limits of the law.
    G. Absolute right: when there is no restriction whatsoever upon the individual's entitlement.
    H. Legal right: a right upon which the society has agreed and formalized into law.

III. Ethical Considerations
    A. Theoretical Perspectives
        1   Utilitarianism. An ethical theory that promotes action based on the end results that produced the most good (happiness) for the most people.
        2. Kantianism. Suggests that decisions and actions are bound by a sense of duty. Also called deontology.
        3. Christian ethics. Do unto others as you would have them do unto you; and alteratively, do not do unto others what you would not have them do unto you.
        4. Natural Law Theories. Do good and avoid evil. Evil acts are never condoned, even if it is intended to advance the noblest of ends.
        5. Ethical Egoism. Decisions are based on what is best for the individual making the decision.
    B. Ethical Dilemmas
        1. Ethical dilemmas occur when moral appeals can be made for taking each of two opposing courses of action.
        2. Taking no action is considered an action taken.
    C. Ethical Principles
        1. Autonomy. This principle emphasizes the status of persons as autonomous moral agents whose right to determine their destinies should always be respected.
        2. Beneficence. Refers to one's duty to benefit or promote the good of others.
        3. Nonmaleficence. Abstaining from negative acts toward another, including acting carefully to avoid harm.
        4. Justice. Principle based upon the notion of a hypothetical social contract between free, equal, and rational persons. The concept of justice reflects a duty to treat all individuals equally and fairly.
        5. Veracity. Principle that refers to one's duty to always be truthful.
    D. A model for Making Ethical Decisions.
        1. Assessment
        2. Problem identification
        3. Plan
            a. Explore the benefits and consequences of each alternative
            b. Consider principles of ethical theories
            c. Select an alternative
        4. Implementation. Act upon the decision made and communicate decision to others
    E. Ethical Issues tin Psychiatric/Mental Health Nursing
        1. The right to refuse medication

      2. The right to the least restrictive treatment alternative

IV. Legal Considerations
- A. Nurse Practice Acts defines the legal parameters of professional and practical nursing
- B. Types of Law
  1. Statutory Law - those that have been enacted by legislative bodies, such as a county or city council, state legislature, or the Congress of the United States
  2. Common Law - derived from decisions mad in previous cases
- C. Classifications within Statutory and Common Law
  1. Civil Law - protects the private and property rights of individuals and businesses.
     - a. Tort - a violation of civil law in which an individual has been wronged. Torts may be intentional or unintentional.
     - b. Contracts - compensation or performance of the obligation set forth in the contract is sought.
  2. Criminal Law - provides protection from conduct deemed injurious to the public welfare.
- D. Legal Issues in Psychiatric/Mental Health Nursing
  1. Confidentiality and Right to Privacy
     - a. Doctrine of privileged communication
  2. Informed Consent
  3. Restraints and Seclusion
     - a. False Imprisonment
  4. Commitment Issues
     - a. Voluntary Admission
     - b. Involuntary Commitment
     - c. Emergency Commitments
     - d. The "Mentally Ill" Person in need of treatment
     - e. Involuntary Outpatient Commitment
     - f. The Gravely disabled client
- E. Nursing Liability
  1. Malpractice and Negligence
  2. Types of Lawsuits that occur in Psychiatric Nursing
     - a. Breach of confidentiality
     - b. Defamation of character
       - (1) libel
       - (2) slander
     - c. Invasion of privacy
     - d. Assault and battery
     - e. False imprisonment
- F. Avoiding Liability
  1. Practice within the scope of the nurse practice act.
  2. Observe the hospital's and department's policy manuals
  3. Measure up to established practice standards
  4. Always put the client's rights and welfare first
  5. Develop and maintain a good interpersonal relationship with each client and his or her family

V. Summary

VI. Review Questions

LEARNING ACTIVITY

ETHICAL AND LEGAL ISSUES IN PSYCHIATRIC/MENTAL HEALTH NURSING

Identify the following key terms associated with ethical and legal issues in psychiatric/mental health nursing with the descriptions/definitions listed below.

a. assault
b. battery
c. beneficence
d. Christian ethics
e. tort
f. common law
g. libel
h. ethical egoism
i. false imprisonment

j. Kantianism
k. malpractice
l. natural law
m. nonmaleficence
n. slander
o. statutory law
p. utilitarianism
q. civil law
r. criminal law
s. veracity

_____ 1. Ethical theory by which decisions are based on a sense of duty.
_____ 2. Writing false and malicious information about a person.
_____ 3. The unconsented touching of another person.
_____ 4. Provides protection from conduct deemed injurious to the public welfare.
_____ 5. Abstaining rom negative acts toward another, including acting carefully to avoid harm.
_____ 6. An act that results in a person's genuine fear and apprehension that he or she will be touched without consent.
_____ 7. The theory on which decisions are based in which evil acts are never condoned, even if they are intended to advance the noblest of ends.
_____ 8. A violation of a civil law in which an individual has been wronged.
_____ 9. The ethical theory on which decisions are based that ensure the greatest happiness to the greatest number of people.
_____ 10. The deliberate and unauthorized confinement of a person within fixed limits by the use of threat or force.
_____ 11. The failure of a professional to perform or to refrain from performing in a manner in which is reputable member within the profession would be expected to do so.
_____ 12. An ethical principle which refers to one's duty to benefit or promote the good of others.
_____ 13. Law that has been enacted by legislative bodies.
_____ 14. Verbalizing false and malicious information about a person
_____ 15. An ethical theory that espouses making decisions based on what is most advantageous for the person making the decision.
_____ 16. Law that is derived from decision mad in previous cases.
_____ 17. Law that protects the private and property rights of individuals and businesses.
_____ 18. The ethical theory that espouses "Do unto others as you would have others do unto you."
_____ 19. Ethical theory that refers to one's duty to always be truthful.

CHAPTER 40. TEST QUESTIONS

1. Raymond is a 54 year old man with chronic schizophrenia who is seen monthly by a community mental health nurse for administration of fluphenazine decanoate (Prolixin decanoate.) Raymond refuses his medication at one regularly scheduled monthly visit. Which of the following interventions by the nurse is considered to be ethically appropriate?
    - • a. Tell Raymond it is his right not to take the medication.
    - b. Tell Raymond that if he does not take his medication he will have to b hospitalized.
    - c. Arrange with a relative to add medication to Raymond's morning orange juice.
    - d. Call for help from Security to hold Raymond down while the shot is administered.

2. Raymond, a 54 year old man with chronic schizophrenia, is hospitalized when he becomes agitated, physically aggressive an unable to communicate cooperatively. With the help of hospital Security an the police, who brought him in, the ER nurse and resident apply leather restraints to Raymond's arms and legs against his very loud protests. Raymond yells that he is going to sue. Under which of the following conditions ar the staff protected?
    - a. Raymond is a voluntary commitment and poses no danger to self or others.
    - b. Raymond is a voluntary commitment, but poses a danger to self or others.
    - c. Raymond is an involuntary commitment, but poses no danger to self or others.
    - • d. Raymond is an involuntary commitment and poses a danger to self or others.

3. Raymond, an aggressive client who is placed in restraints, threatens to sue the physician and nurse who restrained him for assault an battery. Which of the following conditions identifies the criteria for this offense (outside of an emergency situation)?
    - a. The staff become angry at Raymond and call him offensive names.
    - • b. Raymond is touched (or fears being touched) without his consent.
    - c. The nurse hides Raymond's clothes so he cannot leave.
    - d. The nurse puts Raymond in restraints against his wishes.

4. The nurse states: "Well, I know Raymond is against us putting him in restraints, but if I ever get in this condition, I hope people would do the same for me." This is an example of which ethical philosophy?
    - a. Kantianism
    - b. Utilitarianism
    - • c. Christian ethics
    - d. Natural Law ethics

5. In an effort to adhere to the principle of least-restrictive alternative, instead of putting Raymond in leather restraints, the nurse might have (with physician's order):
    - • a. Given Raymond an injection of a major tranquilizer.
    - b. Put Raymond in a locked room by himself.
    - c. Told Raymond if he didn't calm down, he would be given an ECT treatment.
    - d. Put Raymond in soft, Posey restraints, rather than leather restraints.

CHAPTER 41. PSYCHIATRIC HOME NURSING CARE

CHAPTER FOCUS

The focus of this chapter is on care of clients with psychiatric problems in their home settings. Historical and cultural issues are described and the role of the nurse is presented in the context of the nursing process. Legal and ethical issues relating to psychiatric home nursing care are explored.

LEARNING OBJECTIVES

After reading this chapter, the student will be able to:

1. Define *home care* and *psychiatric home care.*
2. Discuss historical aspects related to the growth in the home health care movement.
3. Identify agencies that provide, and sources of reimbursement for, psychiatric home nursing care.
4. Identify client populations that benefit most from psychiatric home nursing care.
5. Describe advantages and disadvantages associated with psychiatric home nursing care.
6. Discuss cultural and boundary issues associated with psychiatric home nursing care.
7. Describe the role of the nurse in psychiatric home nursing care.
8. Apply steps of the nursing process to psychiatric home nursing care.
9. Discuss legal and ethical issues that relate to psychiatric home nursing care.

KEY TERMS

home care
psychiatric home care
Health Care Financing Administration (HCFA)
Medicare
informed consent
abandonment

CHAPTER OUTLINE/LECTURE NOTES

I.   Introduction
     A. Home care has created a way to provide quality, cost-effective care to psychiatric clients.
     B. Home care is defined as services that are delivered at home to recovering, disabled, chronically or terminally ill persons in need of medical, nursing, social, or therapeutic treatment and/or assistance with essential activities of daily living.
     C. Psychiatric home nursing care expounds upon the definition of home care to include the delivery of mental health services to clients in their home setting.
II. Historical Aspects
     A. Roots of home care lie in the practice of visiting nursing, which began in the U.S. in the late 1800s.
     B. Nursing home care increased dramatically beginning in 1965 with the passage of Medicare legislation, which included home care as one of its benefits.
     C. Psychiatric home nursing care was not included as a reimbursable service until 1979.
     D. Psychiatric home nursing care is a rapidly growing part of the home care industry today.
III. General Information Related to Psychiatric Home Nursing Care
     A. In 1996, 3.4 percent of all clients receiving home care services had a primary psychiatric diagnosis.
     B. Payment for Home Care

1. The majority of home health care is paid for by Medicare.
2. Medicaid
3. Private insurance
4. Self-pay
5. Others
   C. Requirements for Medicare Reimbursement
      1. Certification of homebound status
      2. Diagnosis of an acute psychiatric illness
      3. Client's requirement of specialized knowledge, skills, and abilities of a psychiatric registered nurse
   D. Types of Diagnoses
      1. Most common diagnoses include schizophrenia, major depression, bipolar disorder, substance abuse, agoraphobia, paranoia, and generalized anxiety disorder.
      2. Three predominant client populations that benefit from psychiatric home health nursing:
         a. The elderly
         b. The chronically mentally ill
         c. Those with acute mental health problems
   E. Advantages and Disadvantages of Home Care
      1. Advantages
         a. Cost-effective
         b. Being able to observe the client within the context of family and home environment allows for the most comprehensive biopsychosocial assessment.
         c. Psychiatric care in the home often perceived by the client as less threatening.
      2. Disadvantages
         a. The nurse may not have back-up services of other professionals.
         b. Authority and autonomy of the nurse are constrained by being in the domain of the family.
         c. Nurse's safety may be an issue.
   F. Cultural and Boundary Issues
      1. Acceptance of token gifts from clients?
IV. Role of the Nurse
   A. ANA definition of home health nursing: the practice of nursing applied to a patient with a health deficit in the patient's place of residence.
   B. Medicare requires that psychiatric home nursing care be provided by "psychiatrically trained nurses," which they define as "...nurses who have special training and/or experience beyond the standard curriculum required for a registered nurse."
   C. Must be highly adept at performing biopsychosocial assessments.
   D. Must be able to recognize signals in behavior that the client is decompensating either psychiatrically or medically.
   E. Monitoring the client's compliance with the regimen of psychotropic medications.
   F. Collaborate with other members of the health team providing care to the client.
V. Application of the Nursing Process
   A. Assessment
      1. Biopsychosocial assessment
      2. Mental status examination
      3. Global Assessment of Functioning (GAF) scale rating
   B. Diagnosis/Outcome Identification
   C. Plan/Implementation
   D. Evaluation
VI. Care for the Caregivers
   A. Caregiver role strain is a problem for primary caregivers who are responsible for care of a family member on a 7-day-a-week, 24-hour-a-day schedule.
   B. The nurse can assist the caregiver to find ways to ease their burden with suggestions for referrals and participation in support groups.
VII. Legal and Ethical Issues

A. Legal Issues. Both national and state laws influence a number of issues that may arise within a home care setting.
   1. Confidentiality
      a. Client confidentiality is protected by both federal and state statutes.
      b. Confidentiality affects all aspects of information that become known as a direct result of the agency-client relationship.
      c. Permission must be granted by the client for the nurse to share information with other members of the health team.
      d. Written permission to share information should be granted by the client so that third-party payers may have access to the information in order to make payment for services.
      e. Clients have a legal right to the information contained in their medical record. The original record usually stays with the home health agency, but the client may request a copy.
      f. One issue of concern: Does the nurse breach confidentiality when he or she discusses the client's condition with family or significant other? The nurse should be aware of the agency's policy.
      g. Another issue of concern: Does the nurse breach confidentiality by documenting that a client is HIV positive, when there is a possibility that these records may be viewed by others, such as third-party payers? The nurse should be aware of the agency's policy.
      h. Some instances require reporting, regardless of confidentiality.
         (1) Child abuse
         (2) Adult abuse
         (3) Possession of illegal substances
         (4) Specific communicable diseases
         (5) Injuries that appear to have been caused by a dangerous weapon
         (6) Deaths of uncertain nature
         (7) Animal bites
   2. Informed Consent
      a. A process in which information from the physician assists the client to make decisions about health care or treatment.
      b. It must not be assumed that mental illness infers lack of capacity to make independent decisions about treatment.
      c. Information must be given to the client in language that he or she can understand.
      d. The client's level of competence can be assessed by asking the client to paraphrase the information or by questioning the client specifically about the information.
   3. Careful documentation is critical for reasons of legal consequence.
B. Ethical Issues
   1. Right to Refuse Treatment
      a. Clients have the right to make reasoned decisions regarding their treatment.
      b. Clients have the right to withdraw consent after it has been given.
      c. Verbal withdrawal of consent is adequate.
      d. Refusal of treatment should be based on informed consent.
      e. Careful documentation by the nurse is critical.
   2. Abandonment
      a. Defined: a unilateral severance of the professional relationship between a health care provider and a client without reasonable notice at a time when there is still a need for continuing health care.
      b. Severance of care may occur for several reason:
         (1) The client refuses to cooperate in the provision of home care.
         (2) Reimbursement for services has been denied, the agency has ceased to be a Medicaid or Medicare provider, and the client will not or cannot pay for the service.
         (3) The client is unruly, obnoxious, or difficult to treat to the point that it is in the best interests of all concerned that the agency discontinue service.
         (4) Certain environmental factors exist that endanger agency staff, such as physical threats, a dangerous dog, or sexual harassment.

3. It is best when a reasonable amount of notice can be given to the client that discontinuation of services will be occurring.
4. Ongoing communication with the physician and detailed documentation in the agency record is critical.

ANSWERS TO CRITICAL THINKING EXERCISE

1. The comprehensive assessment would include the following components:
   a. Client's perception of the problem and need for assistance
   b. Information regarding client's strengths and personal habits
   c. Health history
   d. Recent changes
   e. Support systems
   f. Vital signs
   g. Current medications
   h. Client's understanding and compliance with medications
   i. Nutritional and elimination assessment
   j. Activities of daily living (ADLs) assessment
   k. Substance use assessment
   l. Neurological assessment
   m. Mental status examination (see Appendix B)
   n. Comprehension of proverbs
   o. Global Assessment of Functioning (GAF) scale rating

   Other important assessments include information about acute or chronic medical conditions, patterns of sleep and rest, solitude and social interaction, use of leisure time, education and work history, issues related to religion or spirituality, and adequacy of the home environment.

2. a. Alteration in nutrition, less than body requirements, evidenced by weight loss.
   b. Dysfunctional grieving, evidenced by depressed mood.

3. Sarah will return to premorbid levels related to:
   a. nutritional status
   b. mood
   c. independence
   d. activity

4. Antidepressant medication. Trazadone (Desyrel) and sertraline (Zoloft) are commonly used with elderly individuals. Both are generally prescribed to be taken at bedtime for the elderly. The nurse would monitor for effectiveness and side effects. Electroconvulsive therapy may be risky for Sarah because of cardiac history.

CHAPTER 41. TEST QUESTIONS

1. Wally is a 35-year-old man who was diagnosed with paranoid schizophrenia when he was 23 years old. He is disabled because of his illness and receives Medicaid. He lives with his widowed mother. Susan, a home health psychiatric nurse, is referred to Wally's case after he has been hospitalized for the 3rd time in 6 months. His mother tells Susan, "I just can't get him to take his medicine. He thinks I'm trying to poison him." What is Susan's likely intervention in this case?
    a. Stop by Wally's house every morning to administer his oral medication.
    b. Suggest Wally's mother hide the concentrate form of his medication in his orange juice.
    • c. Suggest the physician order biweekly injections of the decanoate form of his medication.
    d. Tell Wally that if doesn't start taking his medication regularly, he will have to be institutionalized.

2. In visiting the client with paranoid schizophrenia in his or her home, the nurse must strive to establish trust in the relationship before proceeding with interventions generally accepted as appropriate in home health nursing. "Hands on" assessment may need to be delayed because:
    • a. Individuals with paranoid schizophrenia may perceive touch as threatening.
    b. Psychiatric nurses need to have a medical staff nurse available to assist with the physical assessment.
    c. It is more important to assess mental status of psychiatric clients before assessing their physical status.
    d. Consent by the client will need to be granted after he or she is less delusional.

3. Wally is a 35-year-old man with paranoid schizophrenia who lives with his widowed mother. He quits taking his medication and decompensates about every 3 months. His mother says to the home health psychiatric nurse, "Sometimes I just get so weary. Nothing I try to do ever helps out situation." How may the home health psychiatric nurse help Wally's mother?
    a. Show her how to organize her time better so that she may do everything for Wally.
    b. Help her problem-solve how she may draw monetary support from the state so that she can stay home and take care of Wally.
    c. Encourage her to tell Wally that if he doesn't "straighten up," he will have to leave her home.
    • d. Encourage participation in a support group of family members of individuals with mental illness.

4. Wally, a 35-year-old client with paranoid schizophrenia, says to the home health psychiatric nurse, "I know you write stuff about me in your notes. I want to know what you write. I read that those notes really belong to me." What is the appropriate response by the nurse?
    a. "The notes do not belong to you, Wally. They belong to the home health agency."
    • b. "The notes belong to the home health agency, Wally. But I can make a copy for you if you'd like."
    c. "I will have to talk to the physician before I can share any of the information with you, Wally."
    d. "Yes, you are right, Wally. The notes do belong to you. I will give them to you when I finish writing them."

5. The home health psychiatric nurse visits Twila, a client with agoraphobia, once a week to assist with activities of daily living. With knowledge about confidentiality related to home health care, which of the following would the home health psychiatric nurse report, regardless of confidentiality?
    a. Twila answers the door with a bruise on her forehead and explains that she ran into the bathroom door.
    b. Twila's little girl, age 3, has a large scrape on her leg, and Twila explains that she fell off her tricycle.
    • c. Twila's husband and two of his friends are sitting in the living room openly snorting cocaine.
    d. Twila's mother, who lives with them, has an intermittent, loud, productive cough.

CHAPTER 42. FORENSIC NURSING

CHAPTER FOCUS

The focus of this chapter is on defining forensic nursing within varied aspects of the role. A discussion of historical perspectives is included, and care of the client is presented within the context of the nursing process.

LEARNING OBJECTIVES

After reading this chapter, the student will be able to:

1. Define the terms *forensic* and *forensic nursing*.
2. Discuss historical perspectives of forensic nursing.
3. Identify areas of nursing within which forensic nurses may practice.
4. Describe forensic nursing specialties.
5. Apply the nursing process within the role of clinical forensic nursing in trauma care.
6. Apply the nursing process within the role of forensic psychiatric nursing in correctional facilities.

KEY TERMS

Forensic
forensic nursing
sexual assault nurse examiner (SANE)
colposcope

CHAPTER OUTLINE/LECTURE NOTES

I.   Introduction
     A. The many roles of nurses continue to increase with the ever-expanding health service delivery system.
     B. Forensic nursing is an example of a new concept of the nursing role that is rapidly increasing in its scope of practice.
II. What is Forensic Nursing?
     A. Forensic is defined as "pertaining to the law; legal."
     B. The International Association of Forensic Nurses (IAFN) and the American Nurses Association (ANA) define forensic nursing as follows:
         1. The application of forensic science combined with the biopsychological education of the registered nurse, in the scientific investigation, evidence collection and preservation, analysis, prevention and treatment of trauma and/or death related medical-legal issues.
III. Historical Perspectives
     A. The first forensic nurses served in Canada around 1975 as medical examiners' investigators in the field of death investigation.
     B. The role of forensic nursing has expanded from concerns solely with death investigation to include the living --the survivors of violent crime--as well as the perpetrators of criminal acts.
     C. The goals of forensic nursing have been cited as: "the empowerment of victims of all races and cultures, the treatment of perpetrators in preventive studies, and the protection of their human rights."
IV. The Context of Forensic Nursing Practice
     A. Areas within which a forensic nurse may intervene:
         1. Interpersonal violence
         2. Public health and safety

3. Emergency/trauma nursing
4. Patient care facilities
5. Police and corrections
V. Forensic Nursing Specialities
   A. Clinical Forensic Nursing Specialty
      1. Clinical forensic nursing is the management of crime victims from trauma to trial.
         a. Collection of evidence
         b. Assessment of victims
         c. Investigation of death that occurs in the clinical setting
   B. The Sexual Assault Nurse Examiner (SANE)
      1. A clinical forensic registered nurse who has received specialized training to provide care to the sexual assault victim.
         a. Physical and psychosocial examination of victims
         b. Collection of physical evidence
         c. Therapeutic interactions to minimize the trauma and initiate healing.
         d. Coordination of referral and collaboration with community-based agencies involved in the rehabilitation of victims
      3. Judicial processing of sexual assault
   C. Forensic Psychiatric Nursing Specialty
      1. Registered nurses who integrate psychiatric/mental health nursing philosophy and practice with knowledge of the criminal justice system.
         a. Assessment of sociocultural influences on the individual clients, their families, and the community.
         b. Work with mentally ill offenders in their assessment and care, to identify and change behaviors that link criminal offenses to them.
         c. Work with victims of crime to cope with their emotional wounds.
         d. Help perpetrators and victims of crime deal with the criminal justice system.
         e. Assessment of inmates for fitness, criminal responsibility, disposition, and early release.
         f. Provide mental health treatment for convicted offenders and those who are not found criminally responsible.
   D. Correctional/Institutional Nursing Specialty
      1. Work in secure settings, such as jails, state and federal prisons, and halfway houses.
         a. Provides treatment, rehabilitation, and health promotions to clients who have been charged with or convicted of crimes.
   E. Nurses in General Practice
      1. Forensic applications in the acute care setting, particularly in emergency rooms and in critical care units.
         a. Assessment, documentation of care, and reporting of information to police or other law enforcement agencies.
         b. Collection and preservation of evidence.
VI. Application of the Nursing Process in Clinical Forensic Nursing in Trauma Care
   A. Assessment
      1. Victims of rape, drug and alcohol addiction, domestic violence, assaults, automobile/pedestrian accidents, suicide attempts, occupational related injuries, incest, medical malpractice and the injuries sustained therefrom, and food and drug tampering.
   B. Preservation of Evidence
      1. Crime related evidence must be safeguarded in a manner consistent with the investigation. May include:
         a. Clothing, bullets, blood stains, hairs, fibers, and small pieces of material such as fragments of metal, glass, paint, and wood.
   C. Investigation of Wound Characteristics
      1. The nurse should be able to identify types of undiagnosed trauma injuries and possible weapon involved.
         a. Sharp injuries

b. Blunt-force injuries
c. Dicing injuries
d. Patterned injuries
e. Bite mark injuries
f. Defense wounds
g. Hesitation wounds
h. Fast-force injuries
D. Deaths in the Emergency Department
1. Documentation of the appearance, condition, and behavior of the victim upon arrival at the hospital is critical.
2. In the emergency department, a determination must be made if the cause of death was natural or unnatural.
E. Nursing Diagnosis
1. Risk for posttrauma syndrome
2. Fear
3. Anxiety
4. Risk for self-mutilation
5. Risk for self-directed violence
6. Risk for dysfunctional grieving
F. Planning/Implementation
1. Preservation of Evidence
a. Medical stabilization
b. Examination of wounds
c. Careful preservation of clothing
d. SANE may be called in the event of a sexual assault
(1) Treatment and documentation of injuries
(2) Maintaining the proper chain of evidence
(3) Treatment and evaluation of sexually transmitted diseases
(4) Pregnancy risk evaluation and prevention
(5) Crisis management and arrangement for follow-up counseling
2. Deaths in the Emergency Department
a. Preservation of evidence
b. Protection of the body
c. Anatomical gifts
G. Evaluation
VII. Application of the Nursing Process in Forensic Psychiatric Nursing in Correctional Facilities
A. Assessment. Care of the mentally ill offender population is a highly specialized area of nursing practice.
1. Assessing Mental Health Needs of the Incarcerated
a. Three groups of psychiatric clients may be identified in the forensic population:
(1) Those who are mentally ill at the time of incarceration
(2) Those who become mentally ill while incarcerated
(3) Those with antisocial personality disorder
b. Psychiatric diagnoses commonly identified at the time of incarceration:
(1) Schizophrenia
(2) Affective psychoses
(3) Personality disorders
(4) Substance disorders
c. Common behaviors observed among the mentally ill incarcerated:
(1) Hallucinations
(2) Suspiciousness
(3) Thought disorders
(4) Anger/agitation
(5) Impulsivity

(6) Denial of problems
    d. Detoxification frequently occurs in jails and prisons
  2. Special Concerns
    a. Overcrowding and violence
    b. Sexual assault
    c. HIV infection in the prison population
    d. Female offenders
B. Nursing Diagnosis
  1. Defensive coping
  2. Dysfunctional grieving
  3. Anxiety/fear
  4. Altered thought processes
  5. Powerlessness
  6. Self-esteem disturbance
  7. Risk for self-mutilation
  8. Risk for violence, directed at self or others
  9. Ineffective individual coping
  10. Altered sexuality patterns
  11. Risk for infection
C. Planning/Implementation
  1. Development of a Therapeutic Relationship
    a. Preinteraction Phase
      (1) The nurse must examine his or her feelings, fears, and anxieties about working with prisoners-- violent offenders--perhaps murders, rapists, or pedophiles.
    b. Orientation (Introductory) Phase
      (1) The nurse works to establish trust with the client.
      (2) Set limits on manipulative behavior.
      (3) Touch and self-disclosure most commonly unacceptable with the prisoner population.
    c. Working Phase
      (1) Promoting behavioral change is the primary goal of the working phase.
      (2) Counseling and supportive psychotherapy.
      (3) Crisis intervention.
      (4) Education
        (a) Health teaching
        (b) HIV/AIDS education
        (c) Stress management
        (d) Substance abuse
    d. Termination Phase
      (1) Closure is difficult in a setting where prisoners may be transferred from one institution to another on short notice.
      (2) When possible, nurses may institute assistance for transition to the community setting.
D. Evaluation
VIII. Summary
IX. Critical Thinking Exercise
X. Review Questions

ANSWERS TO CRITICAL THINKING EXERCISE

1. First: Take care of life-threatening injuries (medical stabilization).
   Second: Protect physical evidence: blood, semen, hair, fibers, clothing.
           Take photographs or written descriptions of wounds.
           Careful documentation.
           Lock up evidence or keep under personal observation.

2. Prophylactic antibiotics for sexually transmitted diseases (STDs).
   Prophylaxis with Hepatitis B immunoglobulin.
   Prophylactic regimen for possible pregnancy.

3. Risk for posttrauma syndrome.

CHAPTER 42. TEST QUESTIONS

1. Karen, an 18-year-old college freshman, is brought to the emergency department by her roommate. She tells the admitting nurse that she was raped by her date when she refused to consent to his sexual advances. A sexual assault nurse examiner (SANE) is called in to assist with Karen's case. What is the priority intervention with Karen?
    -   a. Help her to bathe and clean up.
    -   • b. Ensure medical stabilization.
    -   c. Take pictures of the wounds.
    -   d. Call law enforcement officials to report the rape.

2. For the purpose of collecting evidence, the rape victim is asked to remove her clothing. The sexual assault nurse examiner (SANE) will preserve the clothing in which of the following ways?
    -   a. Shake the clothing so that any possible evidence that may be adhering to it is not missed.
    -   b. Place all items of clothing together in a plastic bag for protection.
    -   c. Store the clothing in the police department's evidence collection division.
    -   • d. Seal each item of clothing separately in a dated paper bag.

3. The nurse may advise the sexual assault victim that there are interventions which may be undertaken to prevent all of the following *except:*
    -   a. Pregnancy
    -   b. Gonorrhea
    -   • c. HIV
    -   d. Chlamydia

4. Which of the following behaviors has been identified as most common among the mentally ill incarcerated?
    -   • a. Denial of problems
    -   b. Thought disorders
    -   c. Hallucinations
    -   d. Delusions

5. Which of the following nursing interventions is *not* appropriate in the correctional setting?
    -   a. Encouragement of feelings.
    -   b. Guidance through the mourning process.
    -   c. Setting of personal boundaries.
    -   • d. Touch and self-disclosure.

APPENDIX: ANSWERS TO LEARNING ACTIVITIES

CHAPTER 1. An Introduction to the Concept of Stress

Exercise 1. "Fight or flight" response

When the body encounters a stressor, it prepares itself for "fight or flight." Identify the adaptation responses that occur in the initial stress response in each of the physical components listed.

Physical Component	Adaptation Response
Adrenal Medulla	Releases norepinephrine and epinephrine
Eye	Pupils dilate Secretion is increased from lacrimal glands
Respiratory System	Bronchioles dilate Respiration rate is increased
Cardiovascular System	Increased force of cardiac contraction Increased cardiac output Increased heart rate Increased blood pressure
Gastrointestinal System	Decreased gastric and intestinal motility Decreased secretions Sphincters contract
Liver	Increased glycogenolysis and gluconeogenesis Decreased glycogen synthesis
Urinary System	Increased ureter motility Bladder muscle contracts Bladder sphincter relaxes
Sweat Glands	Increased secretion
Fat Cells	Lipolysis

Exercise 2. Hormonal response to stress.

1. c
2. e
3. a
4. d
5. b

Exercise 3. Holmes and Rahe Social Readjustment Rating Scale

Each student self-administers the evaluation form to determine risk of physical illness due to stress. Method of scoring is included at the bottom of the form.

Exercise 4. Case Study

A. Precipitating Factors:

1. Genetic influences:
   a. Father and brother both alcoholics
   b. Mother, heavy smoker, died of lung cancer

2. Past experiences:
   a. First drink at age 12
   b. Increased amount and frequency since that time
   c. Hospitalized three months ago. Diagnosis: ulcer
   d. Erratic work history related to drinking
   e. Fired from his most recent job yesterday

3. Existing conditions:
   a. Smokes three packages of cigarettes per day
   b. Severe financial difficulties
   c. Supportive wife
   d. No insight into his drinking behavior (blames his boss each time he is fired)

B. Precipitating Stressor: drank two fifths of bourbon

CHAPTER 2:   Mental Health and Mental Illness

Exercise 1.   Please see Figure 2.3 in the text for an explanation of this activity.

Exercise 2.   Ego Defense Mechanisms - Definitions

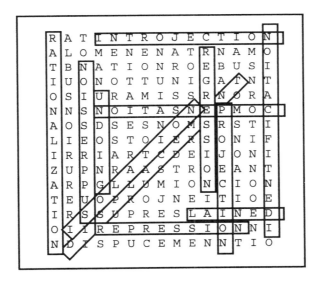

Exercise 3.   The Grief Response

1. Anger
2. Denial
3. Acceptance
4. Bargaining
5. Depression
6. Anger
7. Denial
8. Depression
9. Bargaining
10. Acceptance

CHAPTER 3:   Theories of Personality Development

Exercise 1.   Three Components of the Personality

1. id
2. superego
3. ego
4. id
5. id
6. ego
7. superego
8. id
9. ego
10. superego

Exercise 2.   Behaviors Identified by Erikson's Stages of Development

1. e
2. b
3. l
4. h
5. o
6. d
7. g
8. n
9. i
10. f
11. j
12. a
13. p
14. k
15. c
16. m

Exercise 3.   Stages of Moral Development

1. b
2. f
3. e
4. c

5. a
6. d

CHAPTER 4:   Concepts of Psychobiology

Exercise 1.   Label the parts of the brain.

<u>1</u> Frontal lobe   <u>4</u> Medulla
<u>5</u> Parietal lobe   <u>7</u> Cerebellum
<u>2</u> Temporal lobe   <u>3</u> Pons
<u>6</u> Occipital lobe

Exercise 2.   Crossword

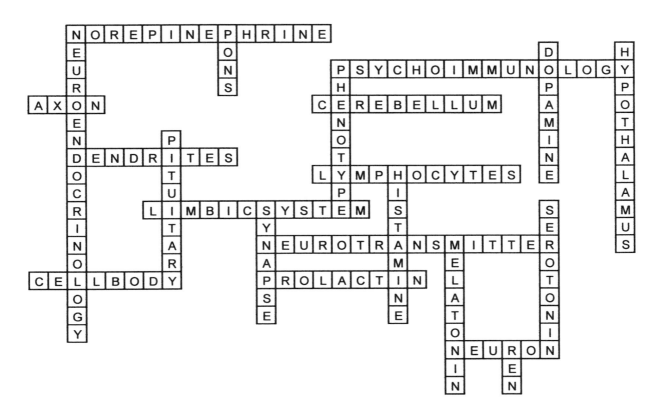

CHAPTER 5:   Relationship Development

Exercise 1.   Essential Conditions for Therapeutic Relationship Development

1.   b
2.   d
3.   a
4.   c
5.   e

Exercise 2. Phases of Relationship Development

1. b
2. a
3. c
4. b
5. d
6. a
7. c
8. d
9. d
10. c

CHAPTER 6: **Therapeutic Communication**

Exercise: Interpersonal Communication Techniques

1. Voicing doubt (T)
2. Belittling feelings (N)
3. Focusing (T)
4. Giving recognition (T)
5. Indicating an external source of power (N)
6. Reflecting (T)
7. Defending (N)
8. Exploring (T)
9. Verbalizing the implied (T)
10. Giving reassurance (N)
11. Restating (T)
12. Giving advice (N)
13. Giving broad openings (T)
14. Rejecting (N)
15. Requesting an explanation (N)

CHAPTER 7: **The Nursing Process in Psychiatric/Mental Health Nursing**

Exercise: Case Study

1. Assessment data
    a. Picks up a chair, as if to use it for protection. Threatened to harm anyone who came close to him in the department store.
    b. Talks and laughs to himself, and tilts his head to the side.
    c. Keeps to himself, and walks away when anyone approaches him.
    d. Appearance is unkempt. Clothes are dirty and wrinkled, hair is oily and uncombed, and there is obvious body odor about him.

2. Nursing diagnoses
    a. Risk for violence: directed toward others
    b. Sensory-perceptual alteration (hallucinations)
    c. Social isolation
    d. Self-care deficit

3. Outcome criteria

a. Sam has not harmed self or others.
b. Sam is able to define and test reality.
c. Sam approaches others in an appropriate manner for 1:1 interaction. Attends group activities voluntarily.
d. Sam carries out personal care independently and willingly.

4. Some appropriate nursing interventions include:
   a. Remove dangerous objects from client's environment.
   b. Redirect violent behavior with physical outlets.
   c. Have sufficient staff available to indicate show of strength.
   d. Administer antipsychotic medication, as ordered (scheduled and prn).
   e. Encourage client to share content of hallucination.
   f. Attend groups with client until he feels comfortable attending alone.
   g. Give positive feedback for voluntary interactions with others.
   h. Encourage client to be as independent with self-care activities as possible.
   i. Give positive feedback for self-care activities performed independently.

CHAPTER 8:   Therapeutic Groups

Group Attendance

Students should prepare a written report of their attendance in a group describing:
a. type of group attended
b. type of leadership identified
c. member roles identified
d. description of group dynamics

CHAPTER 9:   Intervention with Families

Exercise 1.   Family Developmental Stages

1. d
2. f
3. a
4. c
5. e
6. b

Exercise 2.   Personal Family Genogram

CHAPTER 10: Milieu Therapy -- The Therapeutic Community

Exercise 1.   The Interdisciplinary Team

1. recreational therapist
2. art therapist
3. clinical psychologist
4. chaplain
5. dietitian
6. music therapist

7. psychiatric clinical nurse specialist
8. psychiatrist
9. psychiatric staff nurse
10. psychiatric social worker
11. occupational therapist
12. psychodramatist
13. mental health technician

Exercise 2. Basic Assumptions of Milieu Therapy

1. e
2. a
3. g
4. f
5. b
6. d
7. c

CHAPTER 11: Crisis Intervention

Exercise 1. Types of Crisis

1. f
2. b
3. a
4. e
5. d
6. c

Exercise 2. Problem-solving a Crisis

1. Unresolved separation-individuation tasks:
    Unmet dependency needs
    Dysfunctional grieving

2. To develop a realistic and positive self-perception independent from parents.

    Relinquishing need to secure personal identity through interaction with others.

    To progress through the grief process triggered by loss of previous lifestyle and come to terms with acceptance of the change.

3. Explore with Jane those aspects which cannot be changed. For example:
    a. Ted's job requires that he live in the new town.
    b. Jane's family will continue to live in the town from which they moved.

4. Alternatives include:
    a. Stay with Ted and accept the move (an alternative that is developmentally appropriate for Jane, and that the nurse should encourage).
    b. Leave Ted and move back to home town where relatives live (a decision based on developmental regression).

5. Jane will need to weigh the personal benefits and consequences of staying with Ted in the new town and working to accept the move, or leaving him and moving back to live near her relatives.

6. Once Jane has made a decision, she may need assistance from the nurse to help her accept it and adapt to the change. Either decision will undoubtedly trigger a grief response, and assistance in progression to acceptance may be required. Jane must make the decision independently, based on knowledge and understanding of what each would mean for her. A decision to remain with Ted will require work on Jane's part to separate adaptively from her parents and form an independent identity (tasks which have gone unfulfilled by Jane). New coping strategies will have to be developed.

CHAPTER 12: Relaxation Therapy

Exercise 1. Inventory of vulnerability to stress.

Each student self-administers and scores own evaluation.
Explanation of the score is included.

Exercise 2. Stress diary.

Each student keeps a record of adaptation to stress.
Group discussion is encouraged.

CHAPTER 13: Assertiveness Training

Exercise: Assertive Techniques

1. d
2. f
3. j
4. h
5. a
6. c
7. e
8. i
9. g
10. b

CHAPTER 14: Promoting Self-Esteem

Exercise: Students perform self-evaluation.

CHAPTER 15: Anger/Aggression Management

Exercise: Students' personal experiences with anger.

CHAPTER 16: The Suicidal Client

Exercise: Facts and Fables About Suicide

1. F
2. T
3. T
4. F
5. F
6. F
7. T
8. T
9. F
10. F

CHAPTER 17: Behavior Therapy

Exercise: Techniques for Modifying Client Behavior

1. c
2. i
3. f
4. b
5. j
6. e
7. g
8. k
9. a
10. h
11. l
12. d

CHAPTER 18: Cognitive Therapy

Exercise 1.   Cognitive Distortions

1. f
2. c
3. j
4. a
5. i
6. b
7. g
8. d
9. e
10. h

Exercise 2.   Thought Recording

CHAPTER 19: Psychopharmacology

Exercise: Psychotropic Medication Quiz

1.   Increase levels of norepinephrine and serotonin

2. Sudden lifts in mood (may indicate suicidal intention)
3. Depending upon the medication, from 1 to 4 weeks
4. a. amitriptyline (Elavil)
   b. phenelzine (Nardil)
5. a. Dry mouth (offer sugarless candy, ice, frequent sips of water)
   b. Constipation (increase fluids and foods high in fiber)
   c. Sedation (request physician to order given at bedtime)
   d. Orthostatis hypotension (teach client to rise slowly from a sitting or lying position; take vital signs every shift)
   e. Lowers seizure threshold (closely observe client, especially those with history of seizures)
6. Hypertensive crisis; nurse should be on the alert for symptoms of severe occipital headache, palpitations, nausea and vomiting, muchal rigidity, fever, sweating, marked increase in blood pressure, chest pain, coma. Client must avoid foods high in tyramine, such as aged cheeses, pickled herring, preserved meats, beer, wine, chocolate, sour cream, yogurt, over-the-counter cold medications, diet pills.
7. Mania. Lithium has a lag time of 1 to 3 weeks. Antipsychotics are prescribed to decrease the hyperactivity on an immediate basis until the lithium can take effect.
8. Therapeutic range: 0.6 to 1.5 mEq/L. Initial signs and symptoms of lithium toxicity are blurred vision, ataxia, tinnitus, persistent nausea and vomiting, severe diarrhea.
9. a. Give with food.
   b. Ensure client gets adequate sodium in diet.
   c. Ensure client drinks 2500 to 3000 cc fluid per day.
   d. Check for lithium levels before administering dose.
   e. Monitor client's intake and output.
   f. May need to instruct client on diet to prevent weight gain.
10. CNS depression
11. Benzodiazepines: chlordiazepoxide (Librium) and diazepam (Valium)
12. Drowsiness, sedation, confusion, orthostatic hypotension
13. Client must be instructed not to stop taking the drugs abruptly
14. Decreases levels or activity of dopamine
15. Chlorpromazine (Thorazine) and fluphenazine (Prolixin)
16. Decreased libido; retrograde ejaculation; gynecomastia; amenorrhea; weight gain
17. sore throat, fever, malaise
18. Severe muscle rigidity, fever up to 107 degrees F, tachycardia, tachypnea, fluctuations in blood pressure, diaphoresis, and rapid deterioration of mental status to stupor and coma
19. a. pseudoparkinsonism (tremor, shuffling gait, drooling, rigidity)
    b. akinesia (muscular weakness)
    c. akathisia (continuous restlessness and fidgeting)
    d. dystonia (spasms of face, arms, legs, and neck)
    e. oculogyric crisis (uncontrolled rolling back of the eyes)
    f. sometimes tardive dyskinesia is considered as an extrapyramidal system (bizarre facial and tongue movements; stiff neck; and difficulty swallowing)
20. Antiparkinsonian agents: benztropine (Cogentin) and trihexyphenidyl (Artane)

CHAPTER 20: Electroconvulsive Therapy

Exercise: Electroconvulsive Therapy

1. c
2. j
3. f
4. b
5. h
6. a

7. d
8. i
9. g
10. e

CHAPTER 21: Complementary Therapies

CHAPTER 22: Disorders Usually First Diagnosed in Infancy, Childhood, or Adolescence

Exercise: Disorders of Infancy, Childhood, or Adolescence

1. h
2. e
3. j
4. b
5. d
6. g
7. f
8. i
9. c
10. a

CHAPTER 23: Delirium, Dementia, and Amnestic Disorders

Learning Activity:

	Delirium	Dementia	Amnestic Disorders
1.	x		
2.			x
3.		x	
4.		x	
5.	x		
6.			x
7.	x		
8.		x	
9.			x
10.		x	
11.	x		
12.	x		
13.	x		
14.		x	
15.			x

CHAPTER 24: Substance Related Disorders

Exercise: Symptoms Associated with Psychoactive Substances

Drugs	Symptoms of Use	Symptoms of Intoxication	Symptoms of Withdrawal

CNS Depressants
Examples:
  Anxiolytics
  Alcohol
  Sedatives
  Hypnotics
	Relaxation,
	loss of inhibitions,
	lack of concentration,
	drowsiness
	slurred speech
		Aggressiveness,
		disinhibition, impaired
		judgment,
		incoordination, unsteady
		gait, slurred speech,
		disorientation, confusion
			Tremors,
			nausea/vomiting,
			insomnia, seizures,
			hallucinations, irritability

CNS Stimulants
Examples:
  Amphetamines
  Caffeine
  Cocaine
  Nicotine
	Hyperactivity, agitation,
	euphoria, insomnia,
	anorexia, increased pulse
		Euphoria, grandiosity,
		fighting, elevates vital
		signs, nausea and
		vomiting, psychomotor
		agitation
			Anxiety, depressed
			mood, insomnia or
			hypersomnia, craving for
			the drug, suicidal ideas
			(with amphetamines and
			cocaine)

Opioids
Examples:
  Opium
  Morphine
  Codeine
  Heroin
  Meperidine
	Euphoria, lethargy,
	drowsiness, lack of
	motivation
		Euphoria, lethargy,
		somnolence, apathy,
		dysphoria, impaired
		judgment, slurred speech,
		constipation, decreased
		respiratory rate and blood
		pressure
			Craving for the drug,
			nausea/vomiting, muscle
			aches, lacrimation,
			rhinorrhea, piloerection
			or sweating, yawning,
			fever, insomnia

Hallucinogens
Examples:
  Mescaline
  LSD
  PCP
	Visual hallucinations,
	disorientation, confusion,
	paranoia, euphoria,
	anxiety, panic, increased
	pulse
		Belligerence,
		impulsiveness,
		psychomotor agitation,
		increased heart rate and
		blood pressure, ataxia,
		seizures, panic reaction,
		delirium
			The occurrence of a
			withdrawal syndrome
			with these substances has
			not been established.

Cannabinols
Examples:
  Marijuana
  Hashish
	Relaxation, talkativeness,
	lowered inhibitions,
	euphoria, mood swings
		Impaired judgment, loss
		of recent memory,
		tremors, muscle rigidity,
		conjunctival redness,
		panic, paranoia
			If high doses are used for
			a prolonged period,
			symptoms of
			nervousness, tremor,
			insomnia and
			restlessness may occur
			upon cessation of use.

CHAPTER 25: Schizophrenia and Other Psychotic Disorders

Exercise 1. Behaviors associated with Schizophrenia

1. g
2. d
3. o
4. n
5. m

6. a
7. h
8. k
9. b
10. i
11. c
12. j
13. e
14. l
15. f

Exercise 2.   Symptoms of Schizophrenia

1. paranoia
2. delusion of grandeur
3. echolalia
4. imitation
5. nihilistic delusion
6. anhedonia
7. body rocking
8. regression
9. anergia
10. apathy
11. autism
12. delusion of reference

a. Altered thought processes.
b. An antipsychotic medication.
c. (Refer to Chapter 18 for side effects of antipsychotic drugs)
d. Trust vs. Mistrust because of her extreme suspiciousness.
e. Generativity vs. Self-absorption

CHAPTER 26:   Mood Disorders

Exercise: Symptoms of Mood Disorders

1. c
2. f
3. a
4. d
5. b
6. b
7. e
8. a
9. e
10. a
11. b
12. e
13. f

CHAPTER 27: Anxiety Disorders

Exercise: Behaviors Associated with Anxiety Disorders

1. c
2. g
3. b
4. d
5. f
6. a
7. c
8. e
9. d
10. f
11. b
12. c
13. g
14. e
15. d

CHAPTER 28: Somatoform and Sleep Disorders

Exercise: Behaviors Associated with Somatoform Disorders

1. b; Chronic pain
2. e; Body image disturbance
3. d; Sensory-perceptual alteration
4. a; Ineffective individual coping
5. c; Fear

CHAPTER 29: Dissociative Disorders

Exercise: Behaviors Associated with Dissociative Disorders

1. c
2. e
3. a
4. g
5. b
6. f
7. d

CHAPTER 30: Sexual and Gender Identity Disorders

Values clarification.   Students provide their own answers.

CHAPTER 31: Eating Disorders

Exercise: Symptoms of Eating Disorders

	Anorexia Nervosa	Bulimia Nervosa	Obesity
1.	X	X	
2.	X		
3.			X
4.		X	
5.	X		
6.	X	X	
7.			X
8.	X		
9.		X	
10.			X
11.		X	
12.			X
13.	X	X	
14.	X	X	X
15.		X	

CHAPTER 32: Adjustment and Impulse Control Disorders

Exercise: Case Study

1. 30 years old
    never married
    successful
    active social life/many friends
    no significant other at this time
    recent mastectomy for malignancy
    physical condition good
    sad, tired
    trouble sleeping and concentrating
    unable to work
    personal statement of dissatisfaction with appearance
    personal statement of "My personal life is over."

2. a. Dysfunctional grieving related to loss of right breast evidenced by sadness, fatigue, difficulty sleeping and concentrating, inability to work.

    b. Impaired adjustment related to loss of right breast evidenced by, "No man will ever want to have anything to do with me because of the way I look. My personal life is over."

3. See Table 32.2 "Care Plan for the Client with Adjustment Disorder."

4. The client:
    a. is able to verbalize acceptable behaviors associated with each stage of the grief process.
    b. demonstrates a reinvestment in the environment.
    c. is able to accomplish activities of daily living independently.
    d. demonstrates ability for adequate occupational and social functioning.
    e. verbalizes awareness of change in body image and effect it will have on her life style.
    f. is able to problem solve and set realistic goals for the future.

g. demonstrates ability to cope effectively with change in body image.

CHAPTER 33: Psychological Factors Affecting Medical Condition

Exercise: Psychophysiological Disorders

Psychophysiological Disorders	Biological Influences	Psychosocial Influences
Asthma	Difficulty breathing, wheezing, productive cough. Bronchial constriction. Diaphoretic and anxious. May be hereditary. Allergies may also play a role.	Characterized by excessive dependency needs, particularly on the mother figure.
Cancer	A malignant neoplasm caused by changes in the DNA. Possible hereditary link; continuous irritation; exposure to carcinogens; viruses.	Type C personality; lack of a close relationship with one or both parents; lack of opportunity for self-gratification.
Coronary Heart Disease	Diminished coronary blood flow due to alteration in circulation in the coronary arteries. Discomfort ranges from feelings of indigestion to crushing pain. Hereditary and lifestyle factors are common.	Type A personality.
Peptic Ulcer	An erosion of the mucosal wall in the esophagus, stomach, duodenum, or jejunum. Pain is the characteristic symptom. Possible hereditary factor, as well as environmental lifestyle factors.	Unfulfilled dependency needs. Excessive worriers. Anxiety and depression common.
Essential Hypertension	Persistent elevated blood pressure (> 140/90) for which there is no apparent cause. Most often asymptomatic. Possible hereditary factors. Various physiological factors have been hypothesized.	Repressed anger.
Migraine Headache	Vascular headache where pain is experienced unilaterally behind the eye, top of the head, base of the skull. Hereditary, hormonal, and environmental factors are influential.	Migraine personality. Repressed or suppressed anger.
Rheumatoid Arthritis	Inflammatory disease of the joints and major organs of the body. Pain, fatigue, anorexia, fever, myalgia. Possible hereditary factors or dysfunctional immune mechanism.	Self-sacrificing, masochistic, with an inherent inability to express anger.
Ulcerative Colitis	Chronic mucosal inflammatory disease of the colon. Bloody diarrhea, fever, weight loss, nausea/vomiting. Possible hereditary factors or dysfunctional immune mechanism.	Obsessive-compulsive personality. Suppression of anger and hostility.

CHAPTER 34: Personality Disorders

1. d
2. j

3. f
4. a
5. e
6. i
7. c
8. h
9. g
10. k
11. b

CHAPTER 35:   The Aging Individual

Exercise: Case Study

1. 77 years old
   a widow for 20 years
   lives alone on small farm
   has always been very independent
   has become forgetful in last few years
   forgetfulness has become dangerous to self
   starting to wander
   has caring support system in son and daughter

2. a.   Risk for trauma related to confusion, disorientation, and wandering

   b.   Altered thought processes related to age-related changes that result in cerebral anoxia evidenced by memory loss, confusion, disorientation, and wandering

3. See Table 35.2, "Care Plan for the Elderly Client."

4. The client:
   a.   has not experienced injury.
   b.   maintains reality orientation consistent with cognitive level of functioning.
   c.   can distinguish between reality- and nonreality-based thinking.

   Caregivers and client:
   a.   verbalize understanding of possible need for long-term care placement.

CHAPTER 36:   The Individual with HIV Disease

Exercise: Terms Associated with HIV Disease

1. i
2. m
3. e
4. f
5. l
6. c
7. g
8. d
9. b
10. k

11. j
12. a
13. h

CHAPTER 37: Problems Related to Abuse or Neglect

Exercise: Behaviors of Abuse or Neglect

1. d
2. i
3. h
4. c
5. g
6. j
7. k
8. a
9. l
10. f
11. e
12. b

CHAPTER 38: Community Mental Health Nursing

Exercise: Concepts and Terms Associated with Community Mental Health Nursing

1. mobile outreach units
2. managed care
3. health maintenance organization
4. tertiary prevention
5. deinstitutionalization
6. homelessness
7. day treatment program
8. DRGs
9. primary prevention
10. secondary prevention

CHAPTER 39: Cultural Concepts to Psychiatric/Mental Health Nursing

Exercise: Concepts and Terms Related to Culture and Ethnicity

1. d
2. i
3. g
4. a
5. j
6. h
7. e
8. c
9. b
10. f

CHAPTER 40:   Ethical and Legal Issues in Psychiatric/Mental Health Nursing

1. j
2. g
3. b
4. r
5. m
6. a
7. l
8. e
9. p
10. i
11. k
12. c
13. o
14. n
15. h
16. f
17. q
18. d
19. s

Cybertest -- Psychiatric Mental Health Nursing: Concepts of Care
Mary C. Townsend

01   An Introduction to the Concept of Stress

01.   When an individual's stress response is sustained over a long time, the endocrine system involvement results in:
a.   Decreased resistance to disease
b.   Increased libido
c.   Decreased blood pressure
d.   Increased inflammatory response
Answer: a

2.   Which of the following symptoms would the nurse identify as typical of the "fight-or-flight" response?
a.   Pupillary constriction
b.   Increased heart rate
c.   Increased salivation
d.   Increased peristalsis
Answer: b

03.   Research undertaken by Holmes and Rahe in 1967 demonstrated a correlation between the effects of life change and illness. In the development of the Social Readjustment Rating Scale, which of the following concepts limits its effectiveness?
a.   Stress overload always precipitates illness.
b.   Individual abilities are activated.
c.   Stress is viewed as a physiological response.
d.   Personal perception of the event is excluded.
Answer: d

04.   In the transactional model of stress/adaptation, secondary appraisal takes place if the individual judges an event to be:
a.   Benign
b.   Irrelevant
c.   Challenging
d.   Pleasurable
Answer: c

05.   Diseases of adaptation occur when:
a.   Individuals have not had to face stress in the past
b.   Individuals inherit maladaptive genes
c.   Predisposing factors fail
d.   Physiological and psychological resources become depleted
Answer: d

06. Meditation has been shown to be an effective stress-management technique. Meditation works by:
   a. Producing a state of relaxation
   b. Providing insight into one's feelings
   c. Promoting more appropriate role behaviors
   d. Facilitating problem-solving ability
   Answer: a

02   Mental Health and Mental Illness

01. John, a 39-year-old Italian-American, lives in an ethnic community of Italian immigrants. He and most of his peers are of the lower socioeconomic class. Recently John was charged with an act of voyeurism. Which of the following individuals would be most likely to label John's behavior as mental illness?
   a. John's parents, who are ashamed of his behavior
   b. John's friends from his "Sons of Italy" social club
   c. John's employer who owns the company where he works
   d. John's wife, who feels she must protect their children
   Answer: c

02. Which of the following best describe the characteristics of panic-level anxiety?
   a. Decreased attention span, hypotension, mild muscle tension
   b. Frequent body changes, feeling of nervousness, enhanced learning
   c. Narrow perceptual field, problem solving, mild gastric upset
   d. Feeling of losing control, misperceptions of the environment
   Answer: d

03. Anne tends to use the defense mechanism of displacement. Her husband, whom she loves very much, yells at her for not having dinner ready when he comes home from work. She is most likely to react by:
   a. Telling her husband he has no right to yell at her.
   b. Yelling at their son for slouching in his chair.
   c. Burning dinner.
   d. Saying to her husband, "I'll try to do better tomorrow."
   Answer: b

04. Nancy hates her mother, who paid little attention to Nancy when she was growing up. Nancy uses the defense mechanism of reaction formation. Which of the following statements represents this defense mechanism?
   a. "I don't like to talk about my relationship with my mother."
   b. "It's my mother's fault that I feel this way."
   c. "I have a very wonderful mother whom I love very much."
   d. "My mom always loved my sister more than she loved me."
   Answer: a

05. Jack and Jill were recently divorced. Jill was devastated by the divorce and became very depressed. She sought counseling at the community mental health center. Which of the following statements by Jill would indicate that she has resolved the grief over loss of her marriage?
   a. "I know things would be different if we could only try again."
   b. "He will be back. I know he will."
   c. "I'm sure I did lots of things to provoke his anger."
   d. "Yes, it was a difficult relationship, and he abused the children and me."
   Answer: d

06. Sarah's husband Frank died 23 years ago. She has not changed a thing in their house since he died. She still has all of Frank's clothing in his closet, and his house slippers are still beside the bed where they were when he died. Sarah talks about Frank unceasingly to anyone who will listen. Which of the following pathological grief responses is Sarah exhibiting?
   a. Inhibited
   b. Prolonged
   c. Delayed
   d. Distorted
   Answer: b

07. The main difference between neurotic and psychotic behavior is that people experiencing neuroses
   a. Are unaware that they are experiencing distress
   b. Are unaware that their behaviors are maladaptive
   c. Are aware of possible psychological causes of their behavior
   d. Experience no loss of contact with reality
   Answer: d

03   Theories of Personality Development

01. Mrs. K. is 78 years old. She has been admitted to the psychiatric unit of a large hospital because she is depressed and told her daughter she no longer had anything to live for. She threatened to swallow her whole bottle of antihypertensive medication. Theoretically, in which level of psychosocial development (according to Erikson) would you place Mrs. K?
   a. Trust versus mistrust
   b. Industry versus inferiority
   c. Generativity versus stagnation
   d. Ego integrity versus despair
   Answer: d

02. Mrs. K. is 78 years old. She has been admitted to the psychiatric unit of a large hospital because she is depressed and told her daughter she no longer had anything to live for. She threatened to swallow her whole bottle of antihypertensive medication. Mrs. K. lives alone. She has been married and divorced five times. She told the nurse, "Every time I got married, I thought it was for the rest

of my life; but every time, we just couldn't get along. I like to be independent. I want to do what I want to do, when I want to do it, and I don't want some man getting in my way! Men are all alike. They think they own their wives. Well, not me!" According to Erikson's theory, where would you place Mrs. K. based on her behavior?

a. Trust versus mistrust, based on suspiciousness of others
b. Industry versus inferiority, based on difficulty in interpersonal relationships due to feelings of inadequacy
c. Generativity versus stagnation, based on lack of concern for the welfare of others
d. Ego integrity versus despair, based on sense of self-contempt and disgust with how life has progressed

Answer: b

03. Mrs. K. is 78 years old. She has been admitted to the psychiatric unit of a large hospital because she is depressed and told her daughter she no longer had anything to live for. She threatened to swallow her whole bottle of antihypertensive medication. On the unit, she is quarrelsome with the other clients. She changes the TV channel to what she wants to watch without consulting the group; she interrupts in group therapy to discuss her own situation when the focus is on another person; and most of the time, she prefers to stay in her room alone, rather than interact with the other clients. In what stage of development is Mrs. K. fixed according to Sullivan's interpersonal theory?

a. Infancy: She relieves anxiety through oral gratification.
b. Childhood: She has not learned to delay gratification.
c. Early adolescence: She is struggling to form an identity.
d. Late adolescence: She is working to develop a lasting relationship.

Answer: b

04. Mrs. K. is 78 years old. She has been admitted to the psychiatric unit of a large hospital because she is depressed and told her daughter she no longer had anything to live for. She threatened to swallow her whole bottle of antihypertensive medication. On the unit, she is quarrelsome with the other clients. She changes the TV channel to what she wants to watch without consulting the group; she interrupts in group therapy to discuss her own situation when the focus is on another person; and most of the time, she prefers to stay in her room alone, rather than interact with the other clients. Which of the following describes the psychoanalytical structure of Mrs. K.'s personality?

a. Weak id, strong ego, weak superego
b. Strong id, weak ego, weak superego
c. Weak id, weak ego, punitive superego
d. Strong id, weak ego, punitive superego

Answer: d

05. Mrs. K. is 78 years old. She has been admitted to the psychiatric unit of a large hospital because she is depressed and told her daughter she no longer had anything to live for. She threatened to swallow her whole bottle of antihypertensive medication. On the unit, she is quarrelsome with the other clients. She changes the TV channel to what she wants to watch without consulting the group; she interrupts in group therapy to discuss her own situation when the focus is on another person;

and most of the time, she prefers to stay in her room alone, rather than interact with the other clients. In which of Peplau's stages of development would you assess Mrs. K.?

a. Learning to count on others
b. Learning to delay gratification
c. Identifying oneself
d. Developing skills in participation

Answer: b

04   Concepts of Psychobiology

01. Which of the following cerebral structures is sometimes referred to as the "emotional brain?"

a. The cerebellum
b. The limbic system
c. The cortex
d. The left temporal lobe

Answer: b

02. Carl's wife of 34 years died unexpectedly 2 months ago. He is very depressed and is visited at home weekly by a community mental health nurse. The nurse encourages Carl to talk about his wife, their life together, and what he's lost with her death. In addition, at each visit she strongly reinforces the need for Carl to eat properly and get daily exercise and adequate rest. She emphasizes these self-care activities primarily because:

a. The nurse is substituting for Carl's wife
b. Carl has developed bad habits since his wife's death
c. It is routine practice to remind patients about nutrition, exercise, and rest
d. Carl is more susceptible to illness because of his depression

Answer: d

03. Increased dopamine may play a significant role in which of the following illnesses?

a. Alzheimer's disease
b. Schizophrenia
c. Anxiety disorders
d. Depression

Answer: b

04. Decreased norepinephrine may play a significant role in which of the following illnesses?

a. Alzheimer's disease
b. Schizophrenia
c. Anxiety disorders
d. Depression

Answer: d

05. Decreased gamma-aminobutyric acid (GABA) may play a significant role in which of the following illnesses?
    a. Alzheimer's disease
    b. Schizophrenia
    c. Anxiety disorders
    d. Depression
    Answer: c

06. Decreased acetylcholine may play a significant role in which of the following illnesses?
    a. Alzheimer's disease
    b. Schizophrenia
    c. Anxiety disorders
    d. Depression
    Answer: a

07. Elevated levels of the cortisol may play a role in which of the following illnesses?
    a. Acute mania
    b. Schizophrenia
    c. Anorexia nervosa
    d. Alzheimer's disease
    Answer: c

08. Elevated levels of thyroid hormone may play a role in which of the following illnesses?
    a. Acute mania
    b. Depression
    c. Anorexia nervosa
    d. Alzheimer's disease
    Answer: a

09. Decreased levels of the hormone prolactin may play a role in which of the following illnesses?
    a. Acute mania
    b. Schizophrenia
    c. Anorexia nervosa
    d. Alzheimer's disease
    Answer: b

05   Relationship Development

01. When there is congruence between what the nurse is feeling and what is being expressed, the nurse is conveying
    a. Respect

b. Genuineness
c. Sympathy
d. Rapport
Answer: b

02. Sally has made the decision to leave her alcoholic husband. She is feeling very depressed right now. Which of the following statements by the nurse conveys empathy?
   a. "I know you are feeling very depressed right now. I felt the same way when I decided to leave my husband. But I can tell you from personal experience, you are doing the right thing."
   b. "I can understand that you are feeling depressed right now. It was a very difficult decision to make. I'll sit here with you for a while."

   Answer: b

03. Sally has made the decision to leave her alcoholic husband. She is feeling very depressed right now. Which of the following statements by the nurse conveys sympathy?
   a. "I know you are feeling very depressed right now. I felt the same way when I decided to leave my husband. But I can tell you from personal experience, you are doing the right thing."
   b. "I can understand that you are feeling depressed right now. It was a very difficult decision to make. I'll sit here with you for a while."

   Answer: a

04. Which of the following tasks takes place during the working phase of relationship development?
   a. Establishing a contract for intervention
   b. Examining feelings about working with a particular client
   c. Establishing a plan for continuing aftercare
   d. Promoting the client's insight and perception of reality

   Answer: d

05. The Johari Window is a representation of the self and a tool that can be used to increase self-awareness. Because Nurse J. suppresses painful memories of an abortion, she would prefer not to discuss these issues with anyone. However, she volunteers her time to counsel potential abortion clients at the women's clinic. In the Johari Window, this is an example of:
   a. The Open or Public Self
   b. The Unknowing Self
   c. The Private Self
   d. The Unknown Self

   Answer: c

06 Therapeutic Communication

01. Roy is a client on the psychiatric unit. He has a diagnosis of antisocial personality disorder. Jack is assigned as Roy's nurse. Occasionally, Roy loses his temper and expresses his anger inappropriately. Which of the following statements would be appropriate feedback for Roy's angry outbursts?
    a. "You were very rude to interrupt the group the way you did."
    b. "You accomplish nothing when you lose your temper like that."
    c. "Showing your anger in that manner is very childish and insensitive."
    d. "You became angry in group, raised your voice, stomped out, and slammed the door."
    Answer: d

02. Roy is a client on the psychiatric unit. He has a diagnosis of antisocial personality disorder. Jack is assigned as Roy's nurse. Roy says to Jack, "I don't belong in this place with all these loonies. My doctor must be crazy!" Which of the following responses by Jack is most appropriate?
    a. "You are here for a psychological evaluation."
    b. "I'm sure your doctor has your best interests in mind."
    c. "Why do you think you don't belong here?"
    d. "Just bide your time. You'll be out of here soon."
    Answer: a

03. Nancy, a pregnant adolescent, asks the nurse on the psychiatric unit, "Do you think I should give my baby up for adoption?" Which of the following statements by the nurse is most appropriate?
    a. "It would probably be best for you and the baby."
    b. "Why would you want to give it up for adoption?"
    c. "What do you think would be the best thing for you to do?"
    d. "I'm afraid you would feel very guilty afterward if you gave your baby away."
    Answer: c

04. The purpose of providing feedback is to:
    a. Give the patient good advice
    b. Tell the patient how to behave
    c. Evaluate the patient's behavior
    d. Give the patient information
    Answer: d

05. When interviewing a psychiatric client, which of the following nonverbal behaviors should the nurse be careful to avoid?
    a. Maintaining eye contact
    b. Leaning back with arms crossed
    c. Sitting directly facing the client
    d. Smiling
    Answer: b

329

07   The Nursing Process in Psychiatric Nursing

01.   Laura is a nurse on an inpatient psychiatric unit. Much of her time is spent observing client activity, talking with clients, and striving to maintain a therapeutic environment in collaboration with other health care providers. This specific example of the implementation step of the nursing process is called:
a.   Health teaching
b.   Case management
c.   Milieu therapy
d.   Self-care activities
Answer: c

02.   Which of the following statements about nursing diagnosis is true?
a.   Nursing diagnosis is a brand new concept.
b.   All nurses are required by law to write nursing diagnoses.
c.   All nursing diagnoses must be approved by the North American Nursing Diagnosis Association.
d.   Nursing diagnoses are client responses to actual or potential health problems.
Answer: d

03.   Which of the following statements is not true about outcomes?
a.   Expected outcomes are specifically formulated by the nurse.
b.   Expected outcomes are derived from the nursing diagnosis.
c.   Expected outcomes must be measurable and estimate a time for attainment.
d.   Expected outcomes must be realistic for the client's capabilities.
Answer: a

04.   Nursing diagnoses are prioritized according to:
a.   The established goal of care
b.   The life-threatening potential
c.   The nurse's priority of care
d.   The specific focus of problem resolution
Answer: b

05.   The purpose of case management is to attempt to:
a.   Improve the medical welfare system
b.   Ensure that all individuals have medical coverage
c.   Maintain a balance between costs and quality of care
d.   Increase hospital lengths of stay for chronically ill individuals
Answer: c

08 Therapeutic Groups

01. Jane, a psychiatric nurse, leads a supportive-therapeutic group on the psychiatric unit. It is an open group, and clients come and go within the group as they are admitted to and discharged from the unit. Members discuss unresolved issues and ways to cope with stress in their lives. One evening when the group was breaking up, Jane heard one client say to another, "I never thought that other people had the same problems that I have." This statement represents which of Yalom's curative factors?
    a. Catharsis
    b. Group cohesiveness
    c. Universality
    d. Imitative behavior
    Answer: c

02. Meredith has been in a supportive-therapeutic group on the psychiatric unit for 2 weeks now. She dominates the conversation and does not permit others to participate. Meredith is assuming which of the following roles within the group?
    a. Aggressor
    b. Dominator
    c. Recognition seeker
    d. Monopolizer
    Answer: d

03. Jane, a psychiatric nurse, leads a supportive-therapeutic group on the psychiatric unit. One evening, several of the group members spoke up in group and expressed their dissatisfaction that Meredith, a group member, had been dominating the conversation and not permitting others to participate. They encouraged others in the group to express their feelings as well. Together, they decided that from then on all members who wished to do so would get a turn to talk in group, and time would be monitored so that everyone would get their turn. Jane remained silent during this group interaction. Which type of leadership style does Jane demonstrate?
    a. Autocratic
    b. Democratic
    c. Laissez-faire
    Answer: c

04. Jane, a psychiatric nurse, leads a supportive-therapeutic group on the psychiatric unit. Although Meredith, a client on the psychiatric unit, talks a lot in group, Jane, the psychiatric nurse group leader, notices that much of her expressions are kept on a superficial level. Jane decides that Meredith might benefit from psychodrama. She makes a referral for Meredith to the psychodramatist. Which of the following statements is not true about psychodrama?
    a. It provides a safe setting in which to discuss painful issues.
    b. Peers will act out roles that represent individuals with whom Meredith has unresolved conflicts.
    c. Meredith can choose who will play the role of her, while she observes the interaction from the audience.
    d. After the drama has been completed, a discussion will be held with members of the audience.
    Answer: c

05. Michael, a registered nurse with 3 years' experience on a psychiatric inpatient unit, has taken a position in a day treatment program, where he will be leading some groups. Which of the following groups is Michael qualified to lead?
    a. A parenting group
    b. A psychotherapy group
    c. A psychodrama group
    d. A family therapy group
    Answer: a

09   Intervention with Families

01. Sam and Carla have been married for 18 years. They have two children: a boy, Franklin, age 17, and a girl, Natalie, age 15. Natalie recently took an overdose of alprazolam that she found in her parents' medicine cabinet. She was in the hospital for a week and diagnosed with depression. This family seeks counseling at the community mental health center. Natalie says to the nurse, "I just want to go out and do things like all the rest of the kids. Mom says it's okay, but Dad says I'm too young." In the structural model of family therapy, which of the following has occurred?
    a. Multigenerational transmission
    b. Disengagement
    c. Mother-daughter subsystem
    d. Emotional cutoff
    Answer: c

02. Sam and Carla have been married for 18 years. They have two children: a boy, Franklin, age 17, and a girl, Natalie, age 15. Natalie recently took an overdose of alprazolam that she found in her parents' medicine cabinet. She was in the hospital for a week and diagnosed with depression. This family seeks counseling at the community mental health center. Sam and Natalie start to argue, and Sam states, "Your brother never gave us this kind of trouble. Why can't you be more like him?" This is an example of:
    a. Triangulation
    b. Pseudohostility
    c. Double-bind communication
    d. Pseudomutuality
    Answer: a

03. Sam and Carla have been married for 18 years. They have two children: a boy, Franklin, age 17, and a girl, Natalie, age 15. Natalie recently took an overdose of alprazolam that she found in her parents' medicine cabinet. She was in the hospital for a week and diagnosed with depression. This family seeks counseling at the community mental health center. As the nurse continues to take notes of the initial family visit, she writes, "marital schism." What does this mean?
    a. Sam and Carla have a compatible marriage relationship.
    b. Sam has a dominant relationship over Carla.
    c. Sam and Carla have an enmeshed relationship.
    d. Sam and Carla have an incompatible marriage relationship.
    Answer: d

04. Sam and Carla have been married for 18 years. They have two children: a boy, Franklin, age 17, and a girl, Natalie, age 15. Natalie recently took an overdose of alprazolam that she found in her parents' medicine cabinet. She was in the hospital for a week and diagnosed with depression. This family seeks counseling at the community mental health center. Sam says to Carla, "What you need to do is spend more time with your family!" Carla responds, "Okay, I'll turn in my resignation at the office tomorrow." To this Sam replies, "Just as I thought! You've always been a quitter!" This is an example of:
a. Emotional cutoff
b. Double-bind communication
c. Indirect messages
d. Avoidance
Answer: b

05. Sam and Carla have been married for 18 years. They have two children: a boy, Franklin, age 17, and a girl, Natalie, age 15. Natalie recently took an overdose of alprazolam that she found in her parents' medicine cabinet. She was in the hospital for a week and diagnosed with depression. This family seeks counseling at the community mental health center. Carla says to the nurse, "Every time we start to discuss rules for the children, we get into shouting matches. We can't ever settle on anything. We just shout at each other." The nurse instructs Sam and Carla to shout at each other for the next 2 weeks on Tuesdays and Thursdays from 6:30 to 7 <sc>PM This intervention is called:
a. Reframing
b. Restructuring the family
c. Expressive psychotherapy
d. Paradoxical intervention
Answer: d

10   Milieu: The Therapeutic Community

01. Which of the following statements is true about milieu therapy?
a. Punishments are used to eliminate negative behaviors.
b. Interpersonal therapy is the foundation for the program of treatment.
c. Staff performs all activities of care for the clients.
d. The environment is structured so that stresses are used as opportunities for learning.
Answer: d

02. To reinforce the democratic form of self-government on a milieu unit,
a. Clients are allowed to set forth the type of punishment for a peer who violates the rules.
b. Clients may choose whether or not to attend daily community meetings
c. Clients participate in decision making that affects management of the unit
d. Professional staff does not attend community meetings
Answer: c

03. Jack is a client on the psychiatric unit. At community meeting, Jack expressed which movie he wanted to see that night. His choice was denied due to majority rule. At movie time that evening, Jack put the tape he wanted to view into the VCR. He was reprimanded by his peers, who removed the tape and put in the one voted on by the majority. This is an example of which basic assumption of milieu therapy?
    a. Every interaction is an opportunity for therapeutic intervention.
    b. Peer pressure is a useful and powerful tool.
    c. Restrictions and punishment are to be avoided.
    d. The client owns his or her own environment.
    Answer: b

04. Jack is a client on the psychiatric unit. At community meeting, Jack expressed which movie he wanted to see that night. His choice was denied due to majority rule. At movie time that evening, Jack put the tape he wanted to view into the VCR. He was reprimanded by his peers, who removed the tape and put in the one voted on by the majority. The psychiatrist decides to have Jack undergo psychological testing. Which of the following members of the interdisciplinary team would Jack's psychiatrist consult for this purpose?
    a. The occupational therapist
    b. The psychiatric social worker
    c. The clinical psychologist
    d. The clinical nurse specialist
    Answer: c

05. Which of the following best describes the role of the nurse in the therapeutic milieu of a psychiatric unit?
    a. The treatment team member who is responsible for management of the therapeutic milieu
    b. The treatment team member who develops the medical diagnosis for all clients on the unit
    c. The treatment team member who provides for the spiritual and comfort needs of the client and his or her family
    d. The treatment team member who conducts individual, group, and family therapy after an in-depth psychosocial history
    Answer: a

11   Crisis Intervention

01. On Thursday, Camille, a college junior, is accompanied to the student health center by her roommate, Nancy. Nancy explains to the nurse that for 3 days Camille has been unable to attend her classes, has cried constantly, and has become panicky whenever Nancy leaves to go to classes and meals. The nurse performs an assessment and finds that Camille does not know the date and has difficulty with short-term memory. Nancy is not aware that Camille has received any bad news recently, but she offers that Camille is a good student and has been spending long hours at the computer center for nearly 2 weeks working on a major class project, usually returning to the dorm after Nancy is asleep. This is the strategy she has successfully used when working on projects in

the past and was the strategy employed through Monday of this week. What crucial information is missing that will most assist the nurse to plan interventions that will be helpful for Camille?

a. The precipitating stressor
b. Camille's usual ability to cope with stress
c. How far away Camille's home and parents are
d. The due date of Camille's project.

Answer: a

02. On Thursday, Camille, a college junior, is accompanied to the student health center by her roommate, Nancy. Nancy explains to the nurse that for 3 days Camille has been unable to attend her classes, has cried constantly, and has become panicky whenever Nancy leaves to go to classes and meals. The nurse performs an assessment and finds that Camille does not know the date and has difficulty with short-term memory. Nancy is not aware that Camille has received any bad news recently, but she offers that Camille is a good student and has been spending long hours at the computer center for nearly 2 weeks working on a major class project, usually returning to the dorm after Nancy is asleep. This is the strategy she has successfully used when working on projects in the past and was the strategy employed through Monday of this week. Camille reports to the student health nurse that she was nearly raped on Monday night when she took a shortcut on her way from the computer center to her dorm. She is referred to a nurse who is trained as a rape crisis counselor, who schedules appointments three times a week for 3 weeks. At the first session, Camille announces that she has decided to quit school and return home. What is the most therapeutic response for the counselor to make?

a. "I'm confident you know what's best for you."
b. "This is not a good time for you to make such an important decision."
c. "Your mother and father will be terribly disappointed."
d. "What will you do if you go home?"

Answer: b

2. On Thursday, Camille, a college junior, is accompanied to the student health center by her roommate, Nancy. Nancy explains to the nurse that for 3 days Camille has been unable to attend her classes, has cried constantly, and has become panicky whenever Nancy leaves to go to classes and meals. The nurse performs an assessment and finds that Camille does not know the date and has difficulty with short-term memory. Nancy is not aware that Camille has received any bad news recently, but she offers that Camille is a good student and has been spending long hours at the computer center for nearly 2 weeks working on a major class project, usually returning to the dorm after Nancy is asleep. This is the strategy she has successfully used when working on projects in the past and was the strategy employed through Monday of this week. Camille reports to the student health nurse that she was nearly raped on her way from the computer center to her dorm. This is an example of which of the following types of crises?

a. A psychiatric emergency
b. A crisis of anticipated life transition
c. A crisis reflecting psychopathology
d. A crisis resulting from traumatic stress

Answer: d

04. On Thursday, Camille, a college junior, is accompanied to the student health center by her roommate, Nancy. Nancy explains to the nurse that for 3 days Camille has been unable to attend her classes, has cried constantly, and has become panicky whenever Nancy leaves to go to classes and meals. The nurse performs an assessment and finds that Camille does not know the date and has difficulty with short-term memory. Nancy is not aware that Camille has received any bad news recently, but she offers that Camille is a good student and has been spending long hours at the computer center for nearly 2 weeks working on a major class project, usually returning to the dorm after Nancy is asleep. This is the strategy she has successfully used when working on projects in the past and was the strategy employed through Monday of this week. Camille reports to the student health nurse that she was nearly raped on Monday night when she took a shortcut on her way from the computer center to her dorm. She is referred to a nurse who is trained as a rape crisis counselor, who schedules appointments three times a week for 3 weeks. In her interventions with Camille, which of the following therapeutic approaches would best be implemented by the nurse?

a. A psychoanalytical approach.
b. A psychodynamic approach.
c. A reality-oriented approach
d. A family-oriented approach

Answer: c

05. On Thursday, Camille, a college junior, is accompanied to the student health center by her roommate, Nancy. Nancy explains to the nurse that for 3 days Camille has been unable to attend her classes, has cried constantly, and has become panicky whenever Nancy leaves to go to classes and meals. The nurse performs an assessment and finds that Camille does not know the date and has difficulty with short-term memory. Nancy is not aware that Camille has received any bad news recently, but she offers that Camille is a good student and has been spending long hours at the computer center for nearly 2 weeks working on a major class project, usually returning to the dorm after Nancy is asleep. This is the strategy she has successfully used when working on projects in the past and was the strategy employed through Monday of this week. Camille reports to the student health nurse that she was nearly raped on Monday night when she took a shortcut on her way from the computer center to her dorm. She is referred to a nurse who is trained as a rape crisis counselor, who schedules appointments three times a week for 3 weeks. During the final two sessions, Camille and the counselor review the work they have done together. Which of the following statements by Camille would most clearly suggest that the goals of crisis intervention have been met?

a. "Thanks a lot. You've really been helpful. I'll miss working with you."
b. "My instructor gave me a 3-week extension on my project."
c. "I'm really glad I didn't go home. It would have been hard to come back."
d. "I'm wearing the whistle my dad gave me when I go out walking. I've practiced using it, too."

Answer: d

12 Relaxation Therapy

01. Which of the following is known to be a physiological manifestation of relaxation?
a. Increased levels of norepinephrine

336

b. Pupil dilation
c. Reduced metabolic rate
d. Increased blood sugar level
Answer: c

02. Ellen is a registered nurse who works in an employee health facility for a large corporation. She teaches many kinds of preventive health care strategies to the employees, among them relaxation therapy. Which of the following is Ellen likely to teach as a beginning technique and is useful in conjunction with many other forms of relaxation therapy?
a. Deep-breathing exercise
b. Mental imagery
c. Biofeedback
d. Meditation
Answer: a

03. Physical exercise is an effective relaxation technique because it
a. Stresses and strengthens the cardiovascular system
b. Decreases the metabolic rate
c. Decreases levels of norepinephrine into the brain
d. Provides a natural outlet for release of muscle tension
Answer: d

04. Which of the following relaxation techniques is thought to improve concentration and attention?
a. Biofeedback
b. Physical exercise
c. Meditation
d. Mental imagery
Answer: c

13 Assertiveness Training

01. Tracy, a registered nurse and new graduate from the local university, is beginning her first position in a medical-surgical unit where clients from the psychiatric unit often receive care. Which of the following best describes Tracy's use of assertive behavior?
a. Tracy attempts to please others and apologizes for her awkwardness in her new role.
b. Tracy frequently stands up for herself by defending her behavior to the nurse manager.
c. Tracy has some problems making decisions and has a tendency to procrastinate with he work.
d. Tracy is open and direct with the nurse manager when asked to complete her assignments.
Answer: d

02. Tracy, a registered nurse and new graduate from the local university, is beginning her first position in a medical-surgical unit where clients from the psychiatric unit often receive care. Tracy is working with a male client who is complaining about the attention he is receiving. She responds to him calmly and nondefensively, "You are very angry right now. I don't want to discuss this with you while you are so upset. I will be back in 1 hour to meet with you, and we will talk about it then." This is an example of which of the following assertive techniques?
   a. Defusing
   b. Clouding or fogging
   c. Responding as a broken record
   d. Shifting from content to process
   Answer: a

03. Tracy, a registered nurse and new graduate from the local university, is beginning her first position in a medical-surgical unit where clients from the psychiatric unit often receive care. Tracy works with her clients to teach assertiveness and ways in which they can improve their communication. Which of the following nursing diagnoses is selected for clients needing assistance with assertiveness?
   a. Impaired adjustment
   b. Altered thought processes
   c. Defensive coping
   d. Impaired verbal communication
   Answer: c

04. The goal of assertive skills training is to:
   a. Help clients explain themselves and their life-cycle events, and to assist them in resolving problems
   b. Give reliable, expert information so that clients may correct faulty behaviors
   c. Clarify misconceptions and misperceptions that have caused clients to distort reality
   d. Improve communication skills in an effort to improve interpersonal relationships
   Answer: d

05. Tracy, a registered nurse and new graduate from the local university, is beginning her first position in a medical-surgical unit where clients from the psychiatric unit often receive care. Tracy has worked 10 days straight when her nurse manager approaches her with a request to stay on the 3 to 11 shift and work a double shift. Which of the following represents a passive-aggressive response on Tracy's part?
   a. "Get someone else to work 3 to 11! I've been working 10 days straight and I need a break!"
   b. "Okay. I'll do it," then purposefully leaving tasks undone when she leaves the unit at 11 <sc>PM
   c. "I have worked 10 days straight and I cannot work tonight. I will work for you tomorrow if you need me."
   d. "Yes, I'll do it. Anything to keep peace with the staff is a good thing, I guess."
   Answer: b

14 Promoting Self-Esteem

01. Allen is a 37-year-old man who has never married and has remained at home with his aging mother. He has not worked since he had a paper route as a teenager so that he can remain at home to care for his mother. She gives him a weekly allowance out of an estate left to her by her late husband, who died when Allen was 15 years old. A community health nurse visits the family once a month to administer vitamin B_{12} injections to the mother. On one of these visits, Allen confides to the nurse that he is terrified of what will happen to him should his mother die. The nurse recognizes that Allen has low self-esteem related to failure at which of Erikson's developmental tasks?
    a. Trust versus mistrust
    b. Initiative versus guilt
    c. Identity versus role confusion
    d. Ego integrity versus despair
    Answer: c

02. Allen is a 37-year-old man who has never married and has remained at home with his aging mother. He has not worked since he had a paper route as a teenager so that he can remain at home to care for his mother. She gives him a weekly allowance out of an estate left to her by her late husband, who died when Allen was 15 years old. A community health nurse visits the family once a month to administer vitamin B_{12} injections to the mother. On one of these visits, Allen confides to the nurse that he is terrified of what will happen to him should his mother die. She notices that Allen demonstrates certain behaviors consistent with low self-esteem. Which of the following behaviors is Allen not likely to exhibit?
    a. Hostility
    b. Meticulous grooming
    c. Rumination about his situation
    d. Complaints of various aches and pains
    Answer: b

03. Allen is a 37-year-old man who has never married and has remained at home with his aging mother. He has not worked since he had a paper route as a teenager so that he can remain at home to care for his mother. She gives him a weekly allowance out of an estate left to her by her late husband, who died when Allen was 15 years old. A community health nurse visits the family once a month to administer vitamin B_{12} injections to the mother. On one of these visits, Allen confides to the nurse that he is terrified of what will happen to him should his mother die. What kind of boundaries does Allen appear to have relative to his mother?
    a. Loose
    b. Rigid
    c. Flexible
    d. Enmeshed
    Answer: d

04. Allen is a 37-year-old man who has never married and has remained at home with his aging mother. He has not worked since he had a paper route as a teenager so that he can remain at home to care for his mother. She gives him a weekly allowance out of an estate left to her by her late husband, who died when Allen was 15 years old. A community health nurse visits the family once a month to administer vitamin B_{12} injections to the mother. On one of these visits, Allen confides to the nurse that he is terrified of what will happen to him should his mother die. Although Allen's mother is the community health nurse's primary client, the nurse identifies Allen's need for intervention regarding his low self-esteem. The nursing diagnosis she selects from which to identify goals and interventions is:
   a. Self-esteem disturbance
   b. Chronic low self-esteem
   c. Situational low self-esteem
   d. Social isolation
   Answer: b

05. Allen is a 37-year-old man who has never married and has remained at home with his aging mother. He has not worked since he had a paper route as a teenager so that he can remain at home to care for his mother. She gives him a weekly allowance out of an estate left to her by her late husband, who died when Allen was 15 years old. A community health nurse visits the family once a month to administer vitamin B_{12} injections to the mother. On one of these visits, Allen confides to the nurse that he is terrified of what will happen to him should his mother die. Allen has been diagnosed with chronic low self-esteem and is seeing a psychotherapist. After several months, the community health nurse who had made the referral notices some changes in Allen's behavior. Which of the following behaviors most clearly indicates improvement in Allen's self-esteem?
   a. He decides to save his money to buy a dog.
   b. He asks his mother for permission to buy a dog.
   c. He tells his mother he plans to buy a dog.
   d. He buys a dog and hides it in the garage.
   Answer: c

15   Anger and Aggression Management

01. Anna is the charge nurse on a psychiatric unit in a large inner-city hospital. She carefully reviews clients' histories when making assignments so that the most experienced staff is assigned to clients who may become violent. Which of the following risk factors does Anna recognize as the most reliable indicator for a client becoming violent?
   a. Diagnosis of schizophrenia
   b. Past history of violence
   c. Family history of violence
   d. Tense posture and agitation
   Answer: b

02. John, who has a diagnosis of paranoid schizophrenia, is admitted to Anna's unit after attempting to injure his father with a butcher knife. The nurse who writes John's care plan gives him the priority nursing diagnosis of Risk for violence toward others. Which of the following is the priority goal for John during his hospitalization?
   a. The client will not verbalize anger or hit anyone
   b. The client will verbalize anger rather than hit others.
   c. The client will not harm self or others.
   d. The client will be restrained if he becomes verbally or physically abusive.
   Answer: c

03. Because of the frequency with which they deal with violent clients, nurses on psychiatric units commonly have violence intervention protocols. Which of the following interventions would be contraindicated as part of such a protocol?
   a. Administration of psychotropic medication
   b. Soothing the client by stroking an arm or shoulder
   c. Application of leather restraints
   d. Observation for symptoms of the preassaultive tension state
   Answer: b

04. A client with a history of violence begins to lose control of his anger, and the nurse decides intervention must occur. The client cannot be "talked down," and he refuses medication. The nurse should then:
   a. Call for assistance from the assault team
   b. Ask the ward clerk to put in a call for the physician
   c. Make the client go to his room
   d. Tell the client if he doesn't calm down, he will be placed in restraints
   Answer: a

05. A client who becomes violent is placed in restraints, after which the nurse administers the p.r.n. dose of neuroleptic medication that the client had previously refused. Which of the following statements is true regarding this intervention?
   a. The physician must leave a standing order for this intervention to be appropriate.
   b. The nurse who intervenes in this manner is setting himself or herself up for a lawsuit, because the client always has a right to refuse medication.
   c. The physician must write an order to cover the nurse's actions after the intervention has taken place.
   d. Most states consider this intervention appropriate in emergency situations or if a client would likely harm self or others.
   Answer: d

16   The Suicidal Client

01. Edward is a 67-year-old white lawyer who has been diagnosed with major depression. He was widowed 3 years ago and has had no interest in attending synagogue services since that time. He has taken fluoxetine (Prozac) for several years. He made a suicide attempt 45 years ago during his first year in law school. He has been transported to the emergency department by ambulance after telling his son he was thinking of swallowing his whole bottle of fluoxetine. How many risk factors for suicide will the triage nurse document?
    a. Three
    b. Five
    c. Seven
    d. Nine
    Answer: c

02. Edward is a 67-year-old white lawyer who has been diagnosed with major depression. He was widowed 3 years ago and has had no interest in attending synagogue services since that time. He has taken fluoxetine (Prozac) for several years. He made a suicide attempt 45 years ago during his first year in law school. He has been transported to the emergency department by ambulance after telling his son he was thinking of swallowing his whole bottle of fluoxetine. The nurse initiates suicidal precautions for Edward. She understands that which of the following statements regarding suicide is correct?
    a. The more specific the plan is, the more likely the client will attempt suicide.
    b. Clients who talk about suicide never actually commit it.
    c. The client who fails to complete a suicide attempt will not try again.
    d. The nurse should refrain from actually saying the word "suicide," because this may give the client ideas.
    Answer: a

03. Edward is a 67-year-old white lawyer who has been diagnosed with major depression. He was widowed 3 years ago and has had no interest in attending synagogue services since that time. He has taken fluoxetine (Prozac) for several years. He made a suicide attempt 45 years ago during his first year in law school. He has been transported to the emergency department by ambulance after telling his son he was thinking of swallowing his whole bottle of fluoxetine. In creating the care plan for Edward, which of the following would be the priority nursing diagnosis?
    a. Risk for self-mutilation related to low self-esteem
    b. Risk for self-directed violence related to depressed mood
    c. Dysfunctional grieving related to unresolved loss
    d. Powerlessness related to dysfunctional grieving process
    Answer: b

04. What is the most immediate outcome criterion for a suicidal client?
    a. The client will not physically harm himself.
    b. The client will express hope for the future.
    c. The client will reveal his suicide plan.
    d. The client will establish a trusting relationship with the nurse.
    Answer: a

05. Which of the following interventions is not consistent with the outcome criteria for a suicidal client?
    a. Accept the client with unconditional positive regard.
    b. Encourage the client to talk about his or her pain.
    c. Provide the client with tasks to occupy himself or herself.
    d. Provide the client with ample privacy.
    Answer: d

06. Edward is a 67-year-old white lawyer who has been diagnosed with major depression. He was widowed 3 years ago and has had no interest in attending synagogue services since that time. He has taken fluoxetine (Prozac) for several years. He made a suicide attempt 45 years ago during his first year in law school. He has been transported to the emergency department by ambulance after telling his son he was thinking of swallowing his whole bottle of fluoxetine. Edward says to the nurse, "There's nothing to live for anymore." What is the nurse's most therapeutic response?
    a. "Now, Edward, you know that isn't true."
    b. "In your situation, I might feel the same way."
    c. "Things will look better in the morning."
    d. "It sounds like you are feeling pretty hopeless."
    Answer: d

17   Behavior Therapy

01. Gloria, a single mother, has been attending parenting classes with her 9-year-old son, Phil. She wants him to begin doing some chores and asks him to clean his room. When she checks on him, she discovers he has picked up everything on the floor and tossed it on to a chair. She says, "You've done a nice job of picking up things off the floor." This is consistent with which technique of behavior modification?
    a. Shaping
    b. Modeling
    c. Contracting
    d. Premack principle
    Answer: a

02. Gloria responds to an advertisement in the local newspaper soliciting subjects for a research program to investigate effective ways to stop smoking. She is told that she will be assigned to a group that will use a reciprocal inhibition technique. Which of the following exercises is based on reciprocal inhibition?
    a. Before she can smoke, she must first take a half-hour walk.
    b. When she has the urge to smoke, she is to imagine herself as short of breath.
    c. She will be paid $1 for each cigarette she does not smoke and must forfeit $2 for each cigarette that she does smoke.
    d. When she has the urge to smoke, she must first hold her breath to a count of 30, then perform a rhythmic breathing exercise to a count of 100.
    Answer: d

03. Claudia has been seeing a psychotherapist for treatment of a phobia for spiders. Her therapist has begun a program of systematic desensitization. Which of the following interventions would not be a part of this behavior modification technique?
    a. Breathing exercises
    b. One-hour audiotape describing being in a room full of spiders
    c. A visit to an insect zoo with the psychotherapist
    d. Self-paced computer program presenting progressively more anxiety-producing scenarios regarding spiders

    Answer: b

04. Claudia has been seeing a psychotherapist for treatment of a phobia for spiders. Her therapist decides to use the technique of "flooding." Which of the following interventions describes use of this technique?
    a. A system of rewards for demonstrating decrease in fear of spiders
    b. Use of a 1-hour audiotape describing being in a room full of spiders
    c. A visit to an insect zoo with the psychotherapist
    d. Self-paced computer program presenting progressively more anxiety-producing scenarios regarding spiders

    Answer: b

05. Tony is a 20-year-old man with a history of suicide attempts of low-to-moderate lethality. He has been seeing Norman, a nurse psychotherapist, for 4 years. Late one Friday evening Norman receives a telephone call from Tony, who informs Norman that he has ingested half a bottle of aspirin. Norman advises Tony to call 911 for emergency assistance and says that he (Norman) will be available to reschedule a psychotherapy appointment when Tony has recovered. What is the explanation for Norman's behavior?
    a. Norman is using an aversive stimulus in response to Tony's suicide attempt.
    b. Norman is using negative reinforcement in response to Tony's suicide attempt.
    c. Norman is minimizing reinforcement of Tony's suicidal behavior with the goal of extinction.
    d. Norman lacks empathy for Tony's recurring suicidal behavior.

    Answer: c

18   Cognitive Therapy

01. Nancy is an 18-year-old high school senior. She has dreamed of attending a large Ivy League college when she graduates. She has received rejection letters from all such colleges to which she has applied because of inadequate GPA and SAT scores. She is devastated and becomes depressed. She is referred to Carol, a nurse psychotherapist. Nancy says to Carol, "I guess I'll just have to forget about going to college. I'm just not good enough." This is an example of:
    a. Arbitrary inference
    b. Overgeneralization
    c. Dichotomous thinking
    d. Personalization

    Answer: b

02. Nancy is an 18-year-old high school senior. She has dreamed of attending a large Ivy League college when she graduates. She has received rejection letters from all such colleges to which she has applied because of inadequate GPA and SAT scores. She is devastated and becomes depressed. She is referred to Carol, a nurse psychotherapist. Nancy says to Carol, "I guess I'll just have to forget about going to college. I'm just not good enough." Carol responds to Nancy's statement, "I thought you had received a scholarship to the local university." To this, Nancy replies, "Oh, that doesn't count." This is an example of:
   a. Magnification
   b. Minimization
   c. Selective abstraction
   d. Catastrophic thinking
   Answer: c

03. Nancy is an 18-year-old high school senior. She has dreamed of attending a large Ivy League college when she graduates. She has received rejection letters from all such colleges to which she has applied because of inadequate GPA and SAT scores. She is devastated and becomes depressed. She is referred to Carol, a nurse psychotherapist. Nancy says to Carol, "I guess I'll just have to forget about going to college. I'm just not good enough." Carol wants to help Nancy by using problem solving. Which of the following represents intervention with this technique?
   a. "Let's look at what your alternatives are."
   b. "I know you are feeling unhappy now, but things will get better."
   c. "Tell me what you are thinking now."
   d. "When you start to think about the rejections, I want you to switch to thinking about something else."
   Answer: a

04. Carol, a nurse psychotherapist, uses cognitive therapy with her depressed clients. She asks them to keep a daily record of dysfunctional thoughts. The purpose of this tool in cognitive therapy is to:
   a. Identify automatic thoughts
   b. Modify automatic thoughts
   c. Identify rational alternatives
   d. All of the above
   Answer: b

05. Nancy is an 18-year-old high school senior. She has dreamed of attending a large Ivy League college when she graduates. She has received rejection letters from all such colleges to which she has applied because of inadequate GPA and SAT scores. She is devastated and becomes depressed. She is referred to Carol, a nurse psychotherapist. Nancy says to Carol, "I guess I'll just have to forget about going to college. I'm just not good enough." The nursing diagnosis that Carol would most likely choose to work with Nancy during this period would be:
   a. Chronic low self-esteem
   b. Risk for self-directed violence
   c. Powerlessness
   d. Situational low self-esteem
   Answer: d

01.   Carol has made an appointment to see her primary care provider because of increased anxiety. She sees a nurse practitioner who does a physical examination and takes a detailed history. The psychiatrist diagnoses Carol with anxiety disorder. Which of the following medications is prescribed for anxiety?
a.   Chlorpromazine (Thorazine)
b.   Imipramine (Elavil)
c.   Diazepam (Valium)
d.   Methylphenidate (Ritalin)
Answer: c

02.   Which of the following data would suggest that caution is necessary in prescribing a benzodiazepine to an anxious client?
a.   The client has a history of alcohol dependence.
b.   The client has a history of diabetes mellitus.
c.   The client has a history of schizophrenia.
d.   The client has a history of hypertension.
Answer: a

03.   Peter has been diagnosed with major depression. His psychiatrist prescribes imipramine (Tofranil). What information is specifically related to this class of antidepressants and should be included in client and family education?
a.   The medication may cause dry mouth.
b.   The medication may cause constipation.
c.   The medication should not be discontinued abruptly.
d.   The medication may cause photosensitivity.
Answer: d

04.   A psychiatrist prescribes a monoamine oxidase inhibitor for a client. When teaching the client about the effects of tyramine, which of the following foods and/or medications will the nurse caution the client not to consume?
a.   Pepperoni pizza and red wine
b.   Bagels with cream cheese and tea
c.   Apple pie and coffee
d.   Potato chips and diet coke
Answer: a

05.   Alex, a 24-year-old graduate student, is taken to the ED by one of his classmates because of increased suspiciousness and auditory hallucinations. He keeps asking others what they are whispering about him. The nurse who takes his history discovers that he has a history of depression and has been taking desipramine (Norpramine) for 3 years. He is in good physical health but has allergies to penicillin, prochlorperazine (Compazine), and beestings. Although a definitive

diagnosis is not made, it is clear that Alex is experiencing a psychotic episode. Using the assessment data gathered on admission, which of the following antipsychotic medications would be contraindicated for Alex?

a. Haloperidol, because it is intended for use only with elderly patients and would not be effective for Alex
b. Clozapine, because it is incompatible with desipramine
c. Risperidone, because it exacerbates symptoms of depression
d. Thioridazine, because of cross-sensitivity among phenothiazines

Answer: d

06. The physician prescribes an additional medication for a client on antipsychotic medication, with the order for it to be administered "p.r.n. for EPS." When should the nurse give this medication?

a. When the client's white cell count falls below 3000 mm^3
b. When the client exhibits tremors and shuffling gait
c. When the client complains of dry mouth
d. When the client experiences a seizure

Answer: b

07. Which of the following medications would most likely be prescribed for extrapyramidal side effects of antipsychotic medications?

a. Diazepam
b. Amitriptyline (Elavil)
c. Benztropine (Cogentin)
d. Methylphenidate

Answer: c

08. Nancy takes a maintenance dosage of lithium carbonate for a history of bipolar disorder. She has come to the community health clinic stating that she "has had the flu for over a week." She describes her symptoms as coughing, runny nose, chest congestion, fever, and gastrointestinal upset. Her temperature is 100.9°F. She is complaining of blurred vision and "ringing in the ears." What might the nurse suspect in Nancy's case?

a. She has consumed some foods high in tyramine.
b. She has stopped taking her lithium carbonate.
c. She has probably developed a tolerance to the lithium.
d. She may have become toxic on the lithium carbonate.

Answer: d

09. Joey, age 8, takes methylphenidate for attention-deficit-hyperactivity disorder. His mother complains to the nurse that Joey has a very poor appetite, and she struggles to help him gain weight. Which of the following would be appropriate for the nurse to advise Joey's mother?

a. Administer Joey's medication immediately after meals.
b. Administer Joey's medication at bedtime.
c. Skip a dose of the medication when Joey doesn't eat anything.
d. Assure Joey's mother that Joey will eat when he is hungry.

Answer: a

20 Electroconvulsive Therapy

01. Sarah, age 70, is a client on the psychiatric unit with a diagnosis of major depression. She has been seeing her psychiatrist on an outpatient basis for several months and has been taking an antidepressant medication, with no improvement in her symptoms. Her physician has suggested hospitalization for a series of electroconvulsive therapy (ECT) treatments. The nurse is doing some pretreatment teaching with Sarah and her family. Sarah's daughter asks, "Isn't this treatment dangerous?" Which is the most appropriate response by the nurse?
    a. "No, this treatment is absolutely safe."
    b. "There are some risks involved, but in your mother's case, the benefits outweigh the risks."
    c. "There are some risks involved, but your mother will have a thorough examination in advance to ensure that she is a good candidate for the treatment."
    d. "There are some side effects to the treatment, but they are not life-threatening."
    Answer: c

02. Which of the following statements is true regarding ECT?
    a. Electrical stimulation to the brain produces a grand mal seizure.
    b. Maximal muscle movement is required to ensure efficacy of the treatment.
    c. The client will sleep for about 12 hours following a treatment.
    d. The client will have full recall of what has occurred during the treatment.
    Answer: a

03. In explaining to the client and family what to expect immediately following an ECT treatment, which of the following statements is true?
    a. The client will most likely wake up right away and no longer be depressed.
    b. The client will likely be confused and somewhat disoriented.
    c. The client will be sleepy and very likely sleep for a number of hours.
    d. The client may experience some soreness in her muscles and joints
    Answer: b

04. The nurse tells the client that an injection of medication called atropine sulfate will be administered about 30 minutes prior to the ECT treatment. The nurse explains to the client that this is for:
    a. Alleviating her anxiety
    b. Relaxing her muscles
    c. Decreasing secretions
    d. Putting her to sleep
    Answer: c

05. The nurse constructs a plan of care for the hospital stay of a client receiving a series of ECT treatments, and it includes the following nursing diagnoses. Which must receive priority attention?
    a. Anxiety related to receiving ECT
    b. Knowledge deficit related to ECT
    c. Confusion related to side effects of ECT
    d. Risk for injury related to risks and side effects of ECT
    Answer: d

21 Complementary Therapies

01. Carol went to the community mental health clinic because she was feeling depressed. She told the therapist that she had broken up with her boyfriend 6 weeks ago, and she has been feeling depressed since that time. She wants to feel better, but she does not want to take medication. She told the therapist she would be willing to take an herbal medication if there was something that might help her feel better. The therapist may suggest which of the following for Carol?
    a. Chamomile
    b. Echinacea
    c. St. John's wort
    d. Feverfew
    Answer: c

02. Carol went to the community mental health clinic because she was feeling depressed. She told the therapist that she had broken up with her boyfriend 6 weeks ago, and she has been feeling depressed since that time. Carol decided to see a chiropractor for a recurring pain in her lower back. The chiropractor took x-rays and told Carol that he saw some displacement of vertebrae in her spine. In chiropractic medicine, these displacements are called:
    a. Maladjustments
    b. Manipulations
    c. Meridians
    d. Subluxations
    Answers: d

03. Carol went to the community mental health clinic because she was feeling depressed. She told the therapist that she had broken up with her boyfriend 6 weeks ago, and she has been feeling depressed since that time. The therapist suggested that Carol see a physician for a complete physical examination. Part of the examination included a health risk assessment. Carol's medical history revealed that her father had died of colon cancer and that her mother has had surgery for breast cancer, both of which may have a link to high-fat diet. The nurse does health teaching about diet with Carol. In terms of her risk factors, which of the following food groups should Carol modify her intake of?
    a. Fruit and grain
    b. Meat and cheese
    c. Meat and starches
    d. Milk and cereal
    Answer: b

04. Which of the following herbal remedies is thought to improve memory and blood circulation?
    a. Ginkgo
    b. Ginseng
    c. Kava kava
    d. St. John's wort
    Answer: a

05. The technique of yoga uses which of the following?
   a. Deep breathing
   b. Meditation
   c. Balanced body postures
   d. All of the above
   e. C only
   Answer: d

22 Disorders Diagnosed in Infancy, Childhood, or Adolescence

01. Glenda, diagnosed as mentally retarded, scored 47 on recent IQ testing. Her parents have called a local agency that serves the developmentally disabled and asked for advice regarding Glenda's potential. Which of the following statements from the nurse who counsels them is the best estimate of Glenda's eventual level of development?
   a. "Glenda may develop minimal verbal skills."
   b. "Glenda may be able to work at an unskilled job."
   c. "Glenda may eventually function at about a sixth-grade level."
   d. "Glenda will require constant supervision and care."
   Answer: b

02. Tommy, age 9, has been diagnosed with autistic disorder. The cause of this disorder is thought to be:
   a. Refrigerator parents
   b. Fragile X syndrome
   c. Increased glucose metabolism
   d. Unknown
   Answer: d

03. Tommy, age 9, has been diagnosed with autistic disorder. A psychiatric nurse frequently visits Tommy and his family, who also has a second son, Ronnie, age 3. Which of the following behaviors would the nurse regard as age-appropriate and not indicative of autistic disorder?
   a. Intense fascination with fans
   b. Parallel play
   c. Lack of eye contact
   d. Drinking large quantities of fluid
   Answer: b

04. Mrs. Smith tells the psychiatric nurse that her son, Ronnie, age 3, is in constant motion and is unable to sit still long enough to listen to a story or even to watch TV. She asks the nurse if she thinks he could be "hyperactive." The nurse's best response is:
   a. "I wouldn't worry about it."
   b. "It's certainly possible."

c. "It's hard to tell with a 3-year-old."

d. "Why would you think that?"

Answer: c

05. Mrs. Smith tells the psychiatric nurse that her son, Ronnie, age 3, is in constant motion and is unable to sit still long enough to listen to a story or even to watch TV. She asks the nurse if she thinks he could be "hyperactive." Which of the following factors would prompt the nurse to continue to evaluate Ronnie for ADHD?

a. Ronnie's father smokes.

b. Ronnie was born 7 weeks prematurely.

c. Ronnie develops hives when he eats foods with red food coloring added.

d. Ronnie has a cousin on his father's side who has ADHD.

Answer: b

06. Calming effects on hyperactive children have been found to occur with the administration of which of the following classifications of medications?

a. Central nervous system (CNS) stimulants

b. CNS Depressants

c. Nonsteroidal anti-inflammatory drugs

d. Antimanic drugs, such as lithium

Answer: a

07. A potential side effect from prolonged use of methylphenidate (Ritalin) is which of the following?

a. Psychosis

b. Decreased intelligence

c. Dry mouth and sore throat

d. Decrease in rate of growth and development

Answer: d

08. The primary nursing intervention in working with a child with a conduct disorder is to:

a. Plan activities that provide opportunities for success

b. Give the child unconditional acceptance for good behaviors that occur

c. Recognize behaviors that precede the onset of aggression and intervene before violence occurs

d. Provide immediate positive feedback for acceptable and unacceptable behaviors

Answer: c

09. Which of the following classes of medications is effective in the treatment of Tourette's syndrome?

a. Neuroleptics

b. Antimanics

c. Tricyclic antidepressants

d. MAOIs

Answer: a

10. In providing care for the adolescent with an overanxious disorder, the primary goal of the nurse is:
   a. To set very strict limits on what behavior can be tolerated
   b. To make the adolescent aware of the outcome of his or her desire to excel
   c. To establish an atmosphere of calm, trust, and unconditional acceptance
   d. To accept all "nervous habit" behavior and extinguish somatic symptoms
   Answer: c

11. The essential feature that distinguishes oppositional defiant disorder from other disorders is:
   a. Gender ratio
   b. Passive-aggressiveness
   c. Violence toward others
   d. Role of genetic predisposition
   Answer: b

23 Delirium, Dementia, and Amnestic Disorders

01. Gloria visits her Aunt Naomi about twice a year. Naomi is 74 years old and lives in a city about 300 miles away from Gloria. During her most recent visit, Gloria notices that her aunt has become quite forgetful. Two days' worth of mail is still in the mailbox, and Naomi has forgotten to have her prescription for her antihypertensive medication refilled. There is very little food in the house, and Naomi is unable to tell Gloria when or what she last ate. Gloria calls Naomi's physician, who has Naomi hospitalized for evaluation. The physician diagnoses Naomi with dementia. From the information given, which of the following types of dementia does Naomi probably have?
   a. Dementia of the Alzheimer's type
   b. Vascular dementia
   c. Dementia due to head trauma
   d. Dementia due to Parkinson's disease
   Answer: b

02. Which of the following statements is true about vascular dementia?
   a. It is reversible.
   b. It is characterized by plaques and tangles in the brain.
   c. It exhibits a gradual, progressive deterioration.
   d. It exhibits a fluctuating pattern of deterioration.
   Answer: d

03. The physician orders cyclandelate (Cyclan) for a client with dementia. The rationale for this order is:
   a. To enhance circulation to the brain
   b. To elevate levels of acetylcholine in the brain
   c. To control aggressive behavior
   d. To prevent depression
   Answer: a

04. Which of the following nursing diagnoses would be a priority for the nurse caring of the client with dementia?
   a. Altered thought processes
   b. Self-care deficit
   c. Risk for trauma
   d. Risk for violence toward others
   Answer: c

05. Gloria visits her Aunt Naomi about twice a year. Naomi is 74 years old and lives in a city about 300 miles away from Gloria. During her most recent visit, Gloria notices that her aunt has become quite forgetful. Two days' worth of mail is still in the mailbox, and Naomi has forgotten to have her prescription for her antihypertensive medication refilled. There is very little food in the house, and Naomi is unable to tell Gloria when or what she last ate. Gloria calls Naomi's physician, who has Naomi hospitalized for evaluation. The physician diagnoses Naomi with vascular dementia. Naomi can no longer live alone. Arrangements are made for her to move into a nursing home, where she becomes very depressed and withdrawn. The physician believes Naomi would benefit from an antidepressant medication. Which of the following is an example of an antidepressant that the physician may prescribe for Naomi?
   a. Haloperidol (Haldol)
   b. Tacrine (Cognex)
   c. Amitriptyline (Elavil)
   d. Diazepam (Valium)
   Answer: c

24 Substance-Related Disorders

01. Michael, a 47-year-old salesman, is brought to the emergency department at midnight by the police because of aggressive, uninhibited behavior; slurred speech; and impaired motor coordination. His blood alcohol level is 347 mg/dl. He is admitted to the alcohol and drug treatment unit for detoxification. At what minimum blood alcohol level blood is an individual considered to be intoxicated?
   a. 50 mg/dl
   b. 100 mg/dl
   c. 200 mg/dl
   d. 300 mg/dl
   Answer: b

02. Michael, a 47-year-old salesman, is brought to the emergency department at midnight by the police because of aggressive, uninhibited behavior; slurred speech; and impaired motor coordination. His blood alcohol level is 347 mg/dl. Michael's wife reports to the admitting nurse that Michael's drinking has increased over the last several years. Lately, Michael has been drinking a pint of bourbon a day, mostly in the evening but sometimes also during the day. "He usually just comes home from work and drinks until he passes out." She stated that yesterday Michael's boss told him

if he didn't increase his sales, he would be fired. Michael started drinking in the early afternoon and drank continuously into the night. She didn't know what time he left the house. It is now 2 <sc>AM When might the nurse expect withdrawal symptoms to begin?

    a. Around 4 to 6 <sc>AM
    b. Around 10 <sc>AM
    c. In 2 to 3 days
    d. Around 4 to 6 <sc>PM

Answer: a

03.   For what initial symptoms should the nurse be alert with a client who is withdrawing from alcohol?

    a. Suicidal ideation, increased appetite
    b. Lacrimation, rhinorrhea, piloerection
    c. Tremors, tachycardia, sweating
    d. Belligerence, assaultiveness

Answer: c

04.   What would be the expected treatment for a client who is withdrawing from alcohol?

    a. Tricyclic antidepressants
    b. A long-acting barbiturate, such as phenobarbital
    c. Alcohol deterrent therapy, such as disulfiram
    d. Substitution therapy with chlordiazepoxide

Answer: d

05.   Michael, a 47-year-old salesman, is brought to the emergency department at midnight by the police because of aggressive, uninhibited behavior; slurred speech; and impaired motor coordination. His blood alcohol level is 347 mg/dl. The physician orders daily administration of thiamine for Michael, a chronic alcoholic who has been hospitalized for alcohol withdrawal. What is the rationale behind this order?

    a. To restore nutritional balance
    b. To prevent pancreatitis
    c. To prevent alcoholic hepatitis
    d. To prevent Wernicke's encephalopathy

Answer: d

06.   Which of the following describes symptoms of Wernicke's encephalopathy?

    a. Peripheral neuropathy and pain
    b. Epigastric pain and nausea and/or vomiting
    c. Diplopia, ataxia, somnolence
    d. Inflammation and necrosis of the liver

Answer: c

07. Michael, a 47-year-old salesman, is brought to the emergency department at midnight by the police because of aggressive, uninhibited behavior; slurred speech; and impaired motor coordination. His blood alcohol level is 347 mg/dl. Although Michael denies that he is an alcoholic, the nurse encourages him to seek rehabilitative treatment. The nurse understands that for Michael to be successful in treatment, he must first:
   a. Identify someone to whom he can go for support
   b. Give up all his old drinking buddies
   c. Understand the dynamics of alcohol on the body
   d. Correlate life problems to his drinking of alcohol
   Answer: d

25   Schizophrenia and Other Psychotic Disorders

01. Frankie, a 20-year-old college student, has become increasingly suspicious and isolated over the last few months. He has begun accusing his roommate and other students of conspiring against him. Last night, he charged after his roommate with a knife in his hands. He was taken to the local hospital by police, where he was admitted to the psychiatric unit. The psychiatrist diagnosed Frankie with paranoid schizophrenia. Based on the this information, what initial nursing diagnosis would the nurse make?
   a. Risk for self-directed violence
   b. Sensory-perceptual alteration
   c. Risk for violence directed toward others
   d. Altered thought processes
   Answer: c

02. Frankie, a 20-year-old college student, has become increasingly suspicious and isolated over the last few months. He has begun accusing his roommate and other students of conspiring against him. Last night, he charged after his roommate with a knife in his hands. He was taken to the local hospital by police, where he was admitted to the psychiatric unit. The psychiatrist diagnosed Frankie with paranoid schizophrenia. Based on background knowledge, in what stage of development would the nurse place her new client Frankie?
   a. Trust versus mistrust
   b. Autonomy versus shame and doubt
   c. Identity versus role confusion
   d. Intimacy versus isolation
   Answer: a

03. Because of the developmental level, what must be an initial intervention for the nurse who is working with a paranoid schizophrenic client?
   a. Allowing the client to take charge of his self-care independently
   b. Putting the client in the first group therapy session with an opening
   c. Helping the client decide where he wants to go in his life from here
   d. Helping the client to decrease his anxiety and establish trust
   Answer: d

04. Frankie, a 20-year-old college student, has become increasingly suspicious and isolated over the last few months. He has begun accusing his roommate and other students of conspiring against him. Last night, he charged after his roommate with a knife in his hands. He was taken to the local hospital by police, where he was admitted to the psychiatric unit. The psychiatrist diagnosed Frankie with paranoid schizophrenia. The physician orders 100 mg chlorpromazine (Thorazine) bid and 2 mg benztropine (Cogentin) bid p.r.n. The rationale for the chlorpromazine order is:
   a. To ensure that Frankie can get enough sleep
   b. To reduce psychotic symptoms
   c. To decrease Frankie's aggressiveness
   d. To prevent tardive dyskinesia
   Answer: b

05. Frankie, a 20-year-old college student, has become increasingly suspicious and isolated over the last few months. He has begun accusing his roommate and other students of conspiring against him. Last night, he charged after his roommate with a knife in his hands. He was taken to the local hospital by police, where he was admitted to the psychiatric unit. The psychiatrist diagnosed Frankie with paranoid schizophrenia. The physician orders 100 mg chlorpromazine (Thorazine) bid and 2 mg benztropine (Cogentin) bid p.r.n. Under what circumstances would the nurse administer a p.r.n. dose of Cogentin?
   a. When Frankie becomes aggressive
   b. When Frankie needs to be calmed down before bedtime
   c. When Frankie exhibits tremors and shuffling gait
   d. When Frankie complains of constipation
   Answer: c

06. Frankie, a 20-year-old college student, has become increasingly suspicious and isolated over the last few months. He has begun accusing his roommate and other students of conspiring against him. Last night, he charged after his roommate with a knife in his hands. He was taken to the local hospital by police, where he was admitted to the psychiatric unit. The psychiatrist diagnosed Frankie with paranoid schizophrenia. Frankie says to the nurse, "My roommate was plotting with others to have me killed!" The most appropriate response by the nurse would be:
   a. "I find that hard to believe, Frankie."
   b. "What would make you think such a thing?"
   c. "No one was trying to kill you, Frankie."
   d. "I might feel the same way if you came after me with a knife!
   Answer: a

07. Frankie, a 20-year-old college student, has become increasingly suspicious and isolated over the last few months. He has begun accusing his roommate and other students of conspiring against him. Last night, he charged after his roommate with a knife in his hands. He was taken to the local hospital by police, where he was admitted to the psychiatric unit. The psychiatrist diagnosed Frankie with paranoid schizophrenia. The nurse notices that Frankie is stopping in midsentence when they are talking. He tilts his head to the side as if listening to something. The most appropriate intervention by the nurse would be:

a. Call and report the behavior to the physician.
b. Give Frankie a p.r.n. dose of benztropine.
c. Say to Frankie, "What are the voices saying to you, Frankie?"
d. Say to Frankie, "Well, I see you are distracted right now. We'll talk more later."
Answer: c

26 Mood Disorders

01. Janet, age 28, was diagnosed at age 24 with bipolar I disorder. She had been taking lithium carbonate 300 mg tid for maintenance therapy. Today she was brought to the emergency department (ED) by police called to a local department store when she became belligerent and aggressive after being confronted for shoplifting. Janet lives with her mother, who is summoned to the hospital, and who reports that Janet quit taking her lithium about 3 months ago because it caused her to gain weight. On the psychiatric unit, Janet is agitated, pacing, talking loudly and abusively as if in response to an unseen person, and flailing her arms in exaggerated gestures. She is begun on lithium carbonate and haloperidol (Haldol) immediately. What is the rationale for the haloperidol order?
a. Haloperidol cures manic symptoms.
b. Haloperidol prevents extrapyramidal side effects.
c. Haloperidol will ensure that she gets a good night's sleep.
d. Haloperidol will calm hyperactivity until the lithium takes effect.
Answer: d

02. In the initial stages of caring for a client experiencing an acute manic episode, what must the nurse consider to be the priority nursing diagnosis?
a. Risk for injury related to excessive hyperactivity
b. Sleep pattern disturbance related to manic hyperactivity
c. Alteration in nutrition, less than body requirements related to inadequate intake
d. Self-esteem disturbance related to embarrassment from being arrested for shoplifting
Answer: a

03. Janet, age 28, was diagnosed at age 24 with bipolar I disorder. She had been taking lithium carbonate 300 mg tid for maintenance therapy. Today she was brought to the emergency department (ED) by police called to a local department store when she became belligerent and aggressive after being confronted for shoplifting. Janet lives with her mother, who is summoned to the hospital, and who reports that Janet quit taking her lithium about 3 months ago because it caused her to gain weight. On the psychiatric unit, Janet is agitated, pacing, talking loudly and abusively as if in response to an unseen person, and flailing her arms in exaggerated gestures. She is begun on lithium carbonate and haloperidol (Haldol) immediately. Janet, whose diagnosis is bipolar I disorder, current episode manic, tells the physician that she does not want to take lithium carbonate because she has gained a lot of weight on this medication. She says that if he sends her home on this drug, she will just stop taking it. The physician decides to change her medication in

hopes that she will be more compliant. Which of the following medications might the physician choose to prescribe for Janet?
a. Sertraline (Zoloft)
b. Valproic acid (Depakote)
c. Trazodone (Desyrel)
d. Paroxetine (Paxil)
Answer: b

04. Janet, who has been hospitalized for mania in the past, maintains stability with medication. Because of cutbacks and downsizing, Janet is laid off from her job. She becomes very depressed, refuses to look for another job, stays in her room, eats very little, and neglects her personal hygiene. She tells her mother, "What's the use of trying? I fail at everything I do, anyway. Nothing ever works out for me." The next morning, Janet's mother went in to check on her and found Janet unconscious, but still breathing, with an empty bottle of sertraline beside her. She called an ambulance and had Janet transported to the hospital ED. Janet was stabilized in the ED and admitted to the psychiatric unit. Her diagnosis is bipolar I disorder, current episode depressed. Why does the physician give Janet this diagnosis rather than Major Depression?
a. Because he does not feel she is that severely depressed
b. Because she has experienced a manic episode in the past
c. Because he needs to make a more extensive assessment before he decides
d. Because she has no history of major depression in her family
Answer: b

05. Janet, who has been hospitalized for mania in the past, maintains stability with medication. Because of cutbacks and downsizing, Janet is laid off from her job. She becomes very depressed, refuses to look for another job, stays in her room, eats very little, and neglects her personal hygiene. She tells her mother, "What's the use of trying? I fail at everything I do, anyway. Nothing ever works out for me." The next morning, Janet's mother went in to check on her and found Janet unconscious, but still breathing, with an empty bottle of sertraline beside her. She called an ambulance and had Janet transported to the hospital ED. Janet was stabilized in the ED and admitted to the psychiatric unit. Her diagnosis is bipolar I disorder, current episode depressed. What would be the priority nursing diagnosis for Janet at this time?
a. Alteration in nutrition, less than body requirements related to refusal to eat
b. Anxiety (severe) related to threat to self-esteem
c. Risk for self-directed violence related to depressed mood
d. Dysfunctional grieving related to loss of employment
Answer: c

06. Janet, who has been hospitalized for mania in the past, maintains stability with medication. Because of cutbacks and downsizing, Janet is laid off from her job. She becomes very depressed, refuses to look for another job, stays in her room, eats very little, and neglects her personal hygiene. She tells her mother, "What's the use of trying? I fail at everything I do, anyway. Nothing ever works out for me." The next morning, Janet's mother went in to check on her and found Janet unconscious, but still breathing, with an empty bottle of sertraline beside her. She called an

ambulance and had Janet transported to the hospital ED. Janet was stabilized in the ED and admitted to the psychiatric unit. Her diagnosis is bipolar I disorder, current episode depressed. The physician prescribes paroxetine for Janet. She is encouraged to participate in unit activities and to talk about her feelings. Despite all efforts, her depression becomes profound. She is in total despair and in a vegetative state. The physician obtains consent to perform electroconvulsive therapy (ECT). What is the rationale behind this treatment for profound depression?

a. The client is made to forget painful memories from the past and go on with his or her life.
b. The treatment causes stimulation of the central nervous system (CNS) similar to CNS stimulant medication, thereby lifting mood.
c. The treatment satisfies the need for punishment that severely depressed clients sometimes think they deserve.
d. The treatment is thought to increase levels of norepinephrine and serotonin, resulting in mood elevation.

Answer: d

07. The physician orders a medication to be administered by the nurse 30 minutes prior to each ECT treatment that will decrease secretions and maintain heart rate during the convulsion. Which of the following medications would the physician prescribe for this purpose?

a. Thiopental sodium (Pentothal)
b. Atropine sulfate
c. Succinylcholine (Anectine)
d. Clonazepam (Klonopin)

Answer: b

08. Which of the following currently receives the most credibility as etiologically implicated in the development of bipolar disorder.

a. Genetics and biochemical alterations
b. Poor mother-child relationship
c. Evidence of lesion in temporal lobe
d. Learned helplessness within a dysfunctional family system

Answer: a

27 Anxiety Disorders

01. Sharon is a new client on the psychiatric unit with a diagnosis of obsessive-compulsive disorder. After her initial assessment and introduction to the unit, Sharon goes to her room to unpack her suitcase. She begins to arrange her belongings in the drawers and closet. Forty-five minutes later, when the nurse comes to check on her, Sharon is still folding and unfolding her clothes and arranging and rearranging them in the drawers. What is the appropriate nursing intervention at this time?

a. Explain to Sharon that she must come out of her room and join the others in the dayroom at this time.
b. Give Sharon a task to complete, to get her mind off the ritual.

c. Allow Sharon as much time as she wants to perform the ritual.
d. Take Sharon by the hand and state, "It's time to go to group therapy now.
Answer: c

02. Sharon is a new client on the psychiatric unit with a diagnosis of obsessive-compulsive disorder. After her initial assessment and introduction to the unit, Sharon goes to her room to unpack her suitcase. She begins to arrange her belongings in the drawers and closet. Forty-five minutes later, when the nurse comes to check on her, Sharon is still folding and unfolding her clothes and arranging and rearranging them in the drawers. The most likely reason for Sharon's behavior is:
a. It relieves her anxiety.
b. Her mother taught her to be very neat.
c. It provides her with a feeling of control over her life.
d. It makes her feel good about herself.
Answer: a

03. Which of the following is an appropriate prescription for a client with obsessive-compulsive disorder?
a. Diazepam (Valium)
b. Fluvoxamine (Luvox)
c. Propranolol (Inderal)
d. Alprazolam (Xanax)
Answer: b

04. Sharon is a new client on the psychiatric unit with a diagnosis of obsessive-compulsive disorder. After her initial assessment and introduction to the unit, Sharon goes to her room to unpack her suitcase. She begins to arrange her belongings in the drawers and closet. Forty-five minutes later, when the nurse comes to check on her, Sharon is still folding and unfolding her clothes and arranging and rearranging them in the drawers. Which of the following would be an appropriate nursing intervention with Sharon?
a. Distract Sharon with other activities whenever she tries to clean out her drawers.
b. Report the behavior to the physician each time she begins the ritual.
c. Lock Sharon's room so that she cannot engage in the ritualistic behavior.
d. Help Sharon to identify what is causing the anxiety that leads to the ritualistic behavior.
Answer: d

05. Sharon is a new client on the psychiatric unit with a diagnosis of obsessive-compulsive disorder. After her initial assessment and introduction to the unit, Sharon goes to her room to unpack her suitcase. She begins to arrange her belongings in the drawers and closet. Forty-five minutes later, when the nurse comes to check on her, Sharon is still folding and unfolding her clothes and arranging and rearranging them in the drawers. Sharon is becoming more comfortable on the unit and beginning to interact with others. What change, if any, should the nurse make in her initial plan of care?
a. Begin to set limits on the amount of time Sharon may engage in the ritual.

b. Give negative reinforcement to the behavior by pointing out its inappropriateness.

c. Establish firm consequences if Sharon performs the ritualistic behavior.

d. No change should be made in the plan of care.

Answer: a

06. Recently, the biochemical theory of the etiology of obsessive-compulsive disorder has been given an increasing amount of credibility. Which neurotransmitter has been associated with this disorder?

a. Norepinephrine

b. Dopamine

c. Serotonin

d. Acetylcholine

Answer: c

28 Somatoform and Sleep Disorders

01. Louise has just moved to a new city and sees her new primary care practitioner (PCP) for the first time because of gastrointestinal distress. When she takes Louise's history, the PCP suspects some type of somatoform disorder. What is the next step necessary to confirm a diagnosis in this category?

a. Gastrointestinal work-up

b. Thorough physical examination

c. Review of old medical records

d. Referral to a psychiatrist

Answer: b

02. Which of the following data enables a physician to distinguish between hypochondriasis and somatization disorder in arriving at a diagnosis for a client?

a. Pain

b. Gender distribution

c. Persistent fear

d. Impaired functioning

Answer: c

03. Tyler, a 25-year-old law school graduate who has worked in his first job with a private law firm for a year, makes an appointment with his PCP because of weakness in his right hand and arm that he discovered when he awoke yesterday morning. He delayed making the appointment because he thought he "slept on it wrong," but it has not improved. He is unable to hold a pen or use his computer. He plays racquetball twice a week and last played 4 days ago, but he denies recent injury. Other extremities are normal, and he shows no other evidence of neurological impairment. Tyler says he enjoys the challenge of his job and has gotten used to the hectic pace and stress. He is scheduled to take the bar examination, for the second time, in 10 days but seems philosophical

about his inability to use his hand. Which of these data, taken together, form the basis for a diagnosis of conversion disorder?

1. Sudden onset
2. The specific functional loss
3. Negative neurological findings
4. Upcoming bar examination
5. Philosophical attitude

a. 1 & 2
b. 3 only
c. 4 only
d. All of the above

Answer: d

04. The psychodynamic theory underlying symptoms of conversion disorder is:
a. Relief from despair
b. Repression of anger
c. Unconscious resolution of conflict
d. Cognitive deficit

Answer: c

05. Tommy, age 9, has begun sleepwalking, and his parents are afraid for his safety. He has begun getting up and wandering around outside their house in the middle of the night. Which of the following interventions might the practitioner prescribe for Tommy?
a. Low-dose alprazolam (Xanax) and bell on side of bed
b. Methylphenidate (Ritalin) and biofeedback
c. Temazepam (Restoril) and relaxation therapy
d. Sertraline (Zoloft) and phototherapy

Answer: a

06. Edith, a 69-year-old widow, is very troubled by increasing difficulty sleeping well at night. She wakes frequently during the night and feels tired when she wakes early in the morning. What is the outcome that best indicates that treatment of Edith's sleep disorder is successful?
a. Is compliant with medications
b. Has not experienced injury
c. Verbalizes understanding of the sleep disorder
d. Reports increased sense of well-being and feeling rested

Answer: d

29 Dissociative Disorders

01. Tracy is a 27-year-old woman who, after being diagnosed with major depression, borderline personality disorder, and antisocial personality disorder in previous contacts with the mental health system, has recently been diagnosed with dissociative identity disorder. She has been hospitalized because one of her personalities attempted suicide. What is the primary consideration in planning care for Tracy?
    a. Safety
    b. Establishing trust
    c. Awareness of all personalities
    d. Recognition of events that trigger transition between personalities
    Answer: a

02. Tracy is a 27-year-old woman who, after being diagnosed with major depression, borderline personality disorder, and antisocial personality disorder in previous contacts with the mental health system, has recently been diagnosed with dissociative identity disorder. She has been hospitalized because one of her personalities attempted suicide. The primary nursing diagnosis for Tracy during this hospitalization is:
    a. Personal identity disturbance
    b. Sensory-perceptual alteration
    c. Altered thought processes
    d. Risk for self-directed violence
    Answer: d

03. Anxiety is involved in understanding the problem of dissociative amnesia. The defense mechanism used in this psychogenic process is:
    a. Suppression
    b. Denial
    c. Repression
    d. Rationalization
    Answer: c

04. Bill C. has been diagnosed with a dissociative disorder that is identified as a fugue state. Which of the following behaviors best illustrates this diagnosis?
    a. Seeking privacy in his office
    b. Driving a long distance to visit a friend
    c. Sudden unexpected travel away from home
    d. Taking a vacation to a place he would not usually go
    Answer: c

05. Symptoms associated with a fugue state usually occur in response to which of the following?
    a. Severe psychological stress
    b. Excessive alcohol use

c.   Psychogenic amnesia

d.   a or b

Answer: d

06.   Which of the following is an example of systematized amnesia?

a.   George has no memory of his entire lifetime, including his personal identity.

b.   Ann Marie knows her mother beat her as a child, but she cannot remember the details of any of the beatings.

c.   Nancy, who was driving the car in which her best friend was killed, cannot recall the accident or events since the accident.

d.   Sarah, whose home was destroyed in a tornado, only remembers hearing the tornado hit, the ambulance siren, and waking up in the hospital.

Answer: b

30   Sexual and Gender Identity Disorders

01.   Tom and Susan are seeking treatment at the sex therapy clinic. They have been married for 3 years. Susan was a virgin when they married. She admits that she has never really enjoyed sex, but lately, she has developed an aversion to it. They have not had sexual intercourse for about 5 months. Sexual history reveals that Susan grew up in a family that was very closed about sexual issues, with the implication that sex was sinful and dirty. The physician would most likely assign which of the following diagnoses to Susan?

a.   Dyspareunia

b.   Vaginismus

c.   Anorgasmia

d.   Sexual aversion disorder

Answer: d

02.   Tom and Susan are seeking treatment at the sex therapy clinic. They have been married for 3 years. Susan was a virgin when they married. She admits that she has never really enjoyed sex, but lately, she has developed an aversion to it. They have not had sexual intercourse for about 5 months. Sexual history reveals that Susan grew up in a family that was very closed about sexual issues, with the implication that sex was sinful and dirty. The most appropriate nursing diagnosis for Susan would be:

a.   Pain related to vaginal constriction

b.   Sexual dysfunction related to negative teachings about sex

c.   Altered sexuality patterns related to lack of desire for sex

d.   Self-esteem disturbance related to inability to please her husband sexually

Answer: b

03.   Tom and Susan are seeking treatment at the sex therapy clinic. They have been married for 3 years. Susan was a virgin when they married. She admits that she has never really enjoyed sex, but lately,

she has developed an aversion to it. They have not had sexual intercourse for about 5 months. Sexual history reveals that Susan grew up in a family that was very closed about sexual issues, with the implication that sex was sinful and dirty. The physician has assigned a diagnosis of female sexual aversion disorder. Which of the following interventions by the nurse may initiate treatment for Tom and Susan?

a. An explanation of the diagnosis
b. Initiating sensate focus exercises
c. Initiating directed masturbation training
d. Teaching the "squeeze" technique

Answer: a

04. Tom and Susan are seeking treatment at the sex therapy clinic. They have been married for 3 years. Susan was a virgin when they married. She admits that she has never really enjoyed sex, but lately, she has developed an aversion to it. They have not had sexual intercourse for about 5 months. Sexual history reveals that Susan grew up in a family that was very closed about sexual issues, with the implication that sex was sinful and dirty. The physician has assigned a diagnosis of female sexual aversion disorder. The sex therapist assigned to the case would likely choose which of the following therapies for Susan?

a. Sensate focus exercises
b. Systematic desensitization
c. Hypnotherapy
d. Gradual dilation of the vagina

Answer: b

05. Tom and Susan are seeking treatment at the sex therapy clinic. They have been married for 3 years. Susan was a virgin when they married. She admits that she has never really enjoyed sex, but lately, she has developed an aversion to it. They have not had sexual intercourse for about 5 months. Sexual history reveals that Susan grew up in a family that was very closed about sexual issues, with the implication that sex was sinful and dirty. The physician has assigned a diagnosis of female sexual aversion disorder. The sex therapist assigned to the case initiates therapy with desensitization techniques. Additional therapy may include:

a. Minor tranquilizers
b. Group therapy
c. Tricyclic antidepressant
d. Injections of testosterone

Answer: c

31 Eating Disorders

01. Stephanie, age 23, calls the eating disorders clinic for an appointment. She tells the nurse who does the assessment interview that she was hospitalized and diagnosed with anorexia nervosa when she was 14 years old. Since that time, she has seen a therapist periodically when she feels her anxiety is increasing and the fear of eating starts to take hold. She recently graduated from college and moved

to this city, where she began a new job as a production assistant at a local TV station. She is nervous about starting the new job and wants to "do a perfect job, so I can move up quickly to a more challenging position." She tells the nurse that she has been taking laxatives every day, and some days after eating, she will self-induce vomiting. She knows this is not good but feels powerless to stop. She is 5'6" tall and weighs 105 lb. What other physical manifestations might the nurse expect to find upon assessment?

a. High blood pressure, fever.
b. Low blood pressure, low temperature
c. Slow heart rate, fever
d. Fast heart rate, low blood pressure

Answer: b

02. Stephanie, age 23, calls the eating disorders clinic for an appointment. She tells the nurse who does the assessment interview that she was hospitalized and diagnosed with anorexia nervosa when she was 14 years old. Since that time, she has seen a therapist periodically when she feels her anxiety is increasing and the fear of eating starts to take hold. She recently graduated from college and moved to this city, where she began a new job as a production assistant at a local TV station. She is nervous about starting the new job and wants to "do a perfect job, so I can move up quickly to a more challenging position." She tells the nurse that she has been taking laxatives every day, and some days after eating, she will self-induce vomiting. She knows this is not good but feels powerless to stop. She is 5'6" tall and weighs 105 lb. The primary nursing diagnosis on which the nurse will base her plan of care is:

a. Ineffective denial
b. Body image disturbance
c. Self-esteem disturbance
d. Altered nutrition, less than body requirements

Answer: d

03. What pharmacotherapy might the physician prescribe for the client with anorexia nervosa?

a. Fluoxetine (Prozac)
b. Diazepam (Valium)
c. Fenfluramine (Pondimin)
d. Meprobamate (Equanil)

Answer: a

04. Betty, a 38-year-old woman, is followed up in the eating disorders clinic. Betty is 5'4" and weighs 250 lb. When she first came to the clinic 2 years ago, she weighed 347 lb. Her diagnosis at that time was morbid obesity. The dietitian put her on a 1500-calorie per-day diet and the physician at the clinic prescribed fenfluramine and phentermine, the "fen-phen" drugs that were so popular at that time. Since then, fenfluramine has been taken off the market because it caused pulmonary hypertension in a number of individuals. Betty says to the nurse, "I don't know what to do! I know I can't lose weight without those drugs. That's the only reason I lost any at all. And I've already gained some back since I quit taking them!" Fenfluramine and phentermine are part of which of the following classifications of drugs?

a. Antidepressants
b. Anorexigenics
c. Antianxiety
d. Anticonvulsants
Answer: b

05. Betty, a 38-year-old woman, is followed up in the eating disorders clinic. Betty is 5'4" and weighs 250 lb. When she first came to the clinic 2 years ago, she weighed 347 lb. Her diagnosis at that time was morbid obesity. The dietitian put her on a 1500-calorie per-day diet and the physician at the clinic prescribed fenfluramine and phentermine, the "fen-phen" drugs that were so popular at that time. Since then, fenfluramine has been taken off the market because it caused pulmonary hypertension in a number of individuals. Betty says to the nurse, "I don't know what to do! I know I can't lose weight without those drugs. That's the only reason I lost any at all. And I've already gained some back since I quit taking them!" The nurse explains to Betty that the physician may be able to prescribe another medication to help her lose weight. Which of the following might the nurse expect the physician to prescribe?
a. Diazepam (Valium)
b. Dexfenfluramine (Redux)
c. Sibutramine (Meridia)
d. Pemoline (Cylert)
Answer: c

06. Betty, a 38-year-old woman, is followed up in the eating disorders clinic. Betty is 5'6" tall and weighs 250 lb. When she first came to the clinic 2 years ago, she weighed 347 lb. Her diagnosis at that time was morbid obesity. The dietitian put her on a 1500-calorie per-day diet and the physician at the clinic prescribed fenfluramine and phentermine, the "fen-phen" drugs that were so popular at that time. Since then, fenfluramine has been taken off the market because it caused pulmonary hypertension in a number of individuals. Betty says to the nurse, "I don't know what to do! I know I can't lose weight without those drugs. That's the only reason I lost any at all. And I've already gained some back since I quit taking them!" The nurse tells Betty that she will lose weight even without medication if she just sticks to her diet and adds some exercise to her routine. What would be the most appropriate exercise for the nurse to suggest for Betty?
a. Low-impact aerobics 3 times a week
b. Jogging ½ mile twice a week
c. Swimming at the YWCA 30 minutes per day
d. Walking around her neighborhood for 20 minutes per day (weather permitting)
Answer: d

32   Adjustment and Impulse Control Disorders

01. Tommy, age 6, has just been admitted to the child psychiatric unit. His parents report that until the last 6 months Tommy has never presented a problem for them. However, since his baby sister was born 6 months ago, they have been unable to control his behavior. He bullies the other students at

school and has temper tantrums when he cannot have his way at home. Today his parents became fearful when they heard the baby screaming and coughing and found Tommy flinging baby powder all over the baby and the nursery. Tommy is admitted with a diagnosis of adjustment disorder with mixed disturbance of emotions and conduct. The primary nursing diagnosis for Tommy would be:

a. Dysfunctional grieving related to perceived loss of parental love
b. Impaired adjustment related to birth of baby sister
c. Ineffective individual coping related to loss of only-child status
d. Risk for violence directed at others related to anger at birth of sister

Answer: a

02. The category of adjustment disorder with mixed disturbance of emotions and conduct identifies the individual who:

a. Expresses symptoms that reveal a panic level of anxiety
b. Expresses feelings of suicidal ideation
c. Violates the rights of others to feel better
d. Exhibits severe social isolation and withdrawal

Answer: c

03. Tommy, age 6, has just been admitted to the child psychiatric unit. His parents report that until the last 6 months Tommy has never presented a problem for them. However, since his baby sister was born 6 months ago, they have been unable to control his behavior. He bullies the other students at school and has temper tantrums when he cannot have his way at home. Today his parents became fearful when they heard the baby screaming and coughing and found Tommy flinging baby powder all over the baby and the nursery. Tommy is admitted with a diagnosis of adjustment disorder with mixed disturbance of emotions and conduct. The most likely treatment modality for Tommy would be:

a. Family therapy
b. Group therapy
c. Behavior therapy
d. Individual psychotherapy

Answer: d

04. Tommy, age 6, has just been admitted to the child psychiatric unit. His parents report that until the last 6 months Tommy has never presented a problem for them. However, since his baby sister was born 6 months ago, they have been unable to control his behavior. He bullies the other students at school and has temper tantrums when he cannot have his way at home. Today his parents became fearful when they heard the baby screaming and coughing and found Tommy flinging baby powder all over the baby and the nursery. Tommy is admitted with a diagnosis of adjustment disorder with mixed disturbance of emotions and conduct. The focus of therapy with Tommy would most likely be:

a. To treat the dysfunctional family system
b. To allow input from his peer group in an effort to gain insight
c. To keep him from hurting others
d. To focus on his anger at the baby's birth and his fear of parental abandonment

Answer: d

05. The predisposition to adjustment disorder is most likely related to which of the following?
    a. Mental retardation
    b. Temperamental characteristics at birth that promote vulnerability
    c. Retarded superego development
    d. Presence of psychiatric illness
    Answer: b

06. What is the identifying dysfunction in all impulse control disorders?
    a. Disinhibition
    b. Thought disorder
    c. Mood disorder
    d. Loss of memory
    Answer: a

07. Which of the following impulse control disorders has the strongest genetic predisposing factor?
    a. Kleptomania
    b. Pyromania
    c. Pathological gambling
    d. Trichotillomania
    Answer: c

08. Psychosocial factors that are observed in many kleptomaniacs include which of the following?
    a. Stealing is due to a conduct disorder.
    b. Feelings of being neglected, injured, or unwanted occur.
    c. Intense pleasure, gratification, and relief occur during the event.
    d. The degree of aggressiveness in an episode is out of proportion to the stressor.
    Answer: b

33   Psychological Factors Affecting Medical Condition

01. Which of the following psychosocial influences has been correlated with the predisposition to asthma?
    a. Unresolved Oedipus complex
    b. Underdeveloped ego
    c. Punitive superego
    d. Unresolved dependence on the mother
    Answer: d

02. Type C personality characteristics include all of the following except:
    a. Exhibits a calm, placid exterior
    b. Puts others' needs before their own

c. Has a strong competitive drive

d. Holds resentment toward others for perceived "wrongs"

Answer: c

03. Friedman and Rosenman identified two major character traits common to individuals with type A personality. They are:

   a. Excessive competitive drive and chronic sense of time urgency

   b. Unmet dependency needs and low self-esteem

   c. Chronic depression and tendency toward self-pity

   d. Self-sacrificing and perfectionistic

   Answer: a

04. Which of the following statements is true about type B personality?

   a. Their personalities are the exact opposite of type As.

   b. They lack the need for competition and comparison as do type As.

   c. They are usually less successful than type As.

   d. They do not perform as well under pressure as type A's.

   Answer: b

05. Which of the following has not been implicated in the etiology of peptic ulcer disease?

   a. Genetics

   b. Cigarette smoking

   c. Allergies

   d. Unfulfilled dependency needs

   Answer: c

06. The individual with essential hypertension is thought to:

   a. Suppress anger and hostility

   b. Fear social interactions with others

   c. Project feelings onto the environment

   d. Deny responsibility for own behavior

   Answer: a

07. The "migraine personality" includes which of the following sets of characteristics?

   a. Compulsive, perfectionistic, and somewhat inflexible

   b. Excessively ambitious, easily aroused hostility, and highly competitive

   c. Highly extroverted, impulsive, and expresses anger inappropriately

   d. Chronic feelings of depression and despair and tendency toward self-pity

   Answer: a

08. The individual who suffers from migraine headaches is thought to have:

a. Repressed anger
b. Suppressed anxiety
c. Unresolved dependency needs
d. Displaced aggression
Answer: a

09. The individual with ulcerative colitis has been found to have which of the following types of personality characteristics?
a. Passive-aggressive
b. Obsessive-compulsive
c. Antisocial-suspicious
d. Hostile-aggressive
Answer: b

10. Individuals with ulcerative colitis and rheumatoid arthritis share which of the following personality characteristics?
a. Highly negativistic
b. Strongly independent
c. Excessively introverted
d. Inability to express anger directly
Answer: d

34   Personality Disorders

01. Claudia is a 27-year-old woman who has been married and divorced four times. She is admitted to the psychiatric unit with a diagnosis of borderline personality disorder. Which of the following behavior patterns best describes someone with borderline personality disorder?
a. Social isolation
b. Suspiciousness of others
c. Belligerent and argumentative
d. Emotional instability
Answer: d

02. Claudia is a 27-year-old woman who has been married and divorced four times. She is admitted to the psychiatric unit with a diagnosis of borderline personality disorder. As Nancy Nurse starts to leave the unit at the end of her shift, Claudia runs up to her, puts her arms around her, and yells, "Please don't go! You're the only one who understands me. If you go, I won't have anyone!" This is an example of what type of behavior common to individuals with borderline personality disorder?
a. Splitting
b. Manipulation
c. Clinging
d. Impulsivity
Answer: c

371

03. Which of the following nursing interventions is appropriate to help the client with borderline personality disorder extinguish clinging behaviors?
    a. Put the client on room restriction each time it happens.
    b. Ignore such behaviors so that they will be extinguished for lack of reinforcement.
    c. Secure a verbal contract with the client that he or she will discontinue this type of behavior.
    d. Ensure that various staff members are rotated to work with the client while he or she is in the hospital.
    Answer: d

04. Joe is a client of the psychiatric day treatment program. He has been referred by his probation officer for treatment after an arrest for driving under the influence of substances). Joe has a history of many arrests for assault, grand larceny, and other serious crimes and has served two prison sentences. His diagnosis is antisocial personality disorder. Which of the following quotes is Joe's most probable comment on his past behavior?
    a. "It's not my fault."
    b. "I'm too ashamed to talk about it."
    c. "I just don't remember doing it."
    d. "I'm really sorry about all the people I've hurt."
    Answer: a

05. Joe is a client of the psychiatric day treatment program. He has been referred by his probation officer for treatment after an arrest for driving under the influence of substances). Joe has a history of many arrests for assault, grand larceny, and other serious crimes and has served two prison sentences. His diagnosis is antisocial personality disorder. When he arrives at the day treatment unit for the day's activities, Joe says to the nurse, "Wow, you look great today! I'm so glad you're on duty today. You're the best nurse who works here, you know." This comment of Joe's is an example of what type of behavior commonly associated with antisocial personality disorder?
    a. Impulsivity
    b. Manipulation
    c. Exploitation of others
    d. Inability to delay gratification
    Answer b

06. Which of the following therapies is considered best for the client with antisocial personality disorder?
    a. Milieu therapy
    b. Family therapy
    c. Individual psychotherapy
    d. Pharmacological therapy
    Answer: a

07. Looking at the slightly bleeding paper cut she has just received, Linda screams, "Somebody help me, quick! I'm bleeding. Call 911! Hurry!" This response may reflect behavior associated with which personality disorder?
   a. Schizoid
   b. Obsessive-compulsive
   c. Histrionic
   d. Paranoid
   Answer: c

08 John had an extra calendar of the new year and left it on Andrew's desk as a gift. Andrew thinks, "I wonder what he wants from me?" This thought by Andrew may be associated with which personality disorder?
   a. Schizotypal
   b. Narcissistic
   c. Avoidant
   d. Paranoid
   Answer: d

09. Fred works long hours at his job as a research analyst. He then goes home where he lives alone. He has no friends and seldom speaks to others. This behavior is reflective of which personality disorder?
   a. Paranoid
   b. Schizoid
   c. Passive-Aggressive
   d. Avoidant
   Answer: b

10. When a new graduate nurse comes up with a plan and shows Thelma how everyone can be guaranteed every other weekend off, Thelma responds, "We can't makes these kinds of changes! Who do you think you are? We've always done it this way, and we will continue to do it this way!" Thelma's statement reflects behavior associated with which personality disorder?
   a. Dependent
   b. Histrionic
   c. Passive-aggressive
   d. Obsessive-compulsive
   Answer: d

35 The Aging Individual

01. As Eleanor, age 79, became increasingly unable to fulfill her self-care needs, her children, who lived in a distant city, agreed it would be best for her to move to a nursing home near them. Eleanor became depressed when she knew she would have to sell her home that she had lived in for more

than 50 years. The physician prescribed an antidepressant for Eleanor. Which of the following physiological changes in the elderly may require special consideration when prescribing psychotropic medications for them?

a. Changes in cortical and intellectual functioning
b. Changes in cardiac and respiratory functioning
c. Changes in liver and kidney functioning
d. Changes in endocrine and immune functioning

Answer: c

02. As Eleanor, age 79, became increasingly unable to fulfill her self-care needs, her children, who lived in a distant city, agreed it would be best for her to move to a nursing home near them. Eleanor became depressed when she knew she would have to sell her home that she had lived in for more than 50 years. The physician prescribed an antidepressant for Eleanor. However, she does not respond to the medication and becomes more depressed. She tells the nurse, "I don't want to live here. I would rather die than live here." After hearing Eleanor make this statement, the nurse would be expected to add which of the following nursing diagnoses to Eleanor's care plan?

a. Risk for self-mutilation
b. Risk for self-directed violence
c. Risk for violence toward others
d. Risk for injury

Answer: b

03. As Eleanor, age 79, became increasingly unable to fulfill her self-care needs, her children, who lived in a distant city, agreed it would be best for her to move to a nursing home near them. Eleanor became depressed when she knew she would have to sell her home that she had lived in for more than 50 years. The physician prescribed an antidepressant for Eleanor. However, she does not respond to the medication and becomes more depressed. She tells the nurse, "I don't want to live here. I would rather die than live here." When Eleanor does not respond to the antidepressant medication, the physician considers another therapy. Which of the following is he likely to choose?

a. Electroconvulsive therapy
b. Neuroleptic therapy
c. An antiparkinsonian agent
d. Anxiolytic therapy

Answer: a

04. Which of the following therapies is commonly used and has been found to be effective in decreasing depression in the elderly person?

a. Behavior therapy
b. Group therapy
c. Orientation therapy
d. Reminiscence therapy

Answer: d

05. As Eleanor, age 79, became increasingly unable to fulfill her self-care needs, her children, who lived in a distant city, agreed it would be best for her to move to a nursing home near them. Eleanor became depressed when she knew she would have to sell her home that she had lived in for more than 50 years. The physician prescribed an antidepressant for Eleanor. However, she does not respond to the medication and becomes more depressed. She tells the nurse, "I don't want to live here. I would rather die than live here." Which of the following nursing interventions would help Eleanor be as independent as possible in her self-care activities?
    a. Assign a variety of caregivers so that one person does not become used to doing everything for Eleanor.
    b. Allow Eleanor a specified amount of time to complete activities of daily living (ADLs), then finish them for her.
    c. Tell her at the beginning of each day what is expected of her that day.
    d. Allow ADLs to follow her home routine as closely as possible.
    Answer: d

36   The Individual with HIV Disease

01. Tessa, a 27-year-old mother of three children, is admitted to a dual-diagnosis program for clients with mental illness and substance abuse. Tessa has been HIV-positive for 5 years. She was infected with HIV by contaminated needles used to inject heroin IV. Her husband recently died from AIDS. Her diagnoses are major depression; alcohol dependence; and opioid dependence, in remission. Which of the following data is most useful to determine Tessa's stage of HIV disease?
    a. T4-cell count
    b. Hemoglobin and hematocrit
    c. Date of seroconversion
    d. Presence of opportunistic infection
    Answer: a

02. Tessa, a 27-year-old mother of three children, is admitted to a dual-diagnosis program for clients with mental illness and substance abuse. Tessa has been HIV-positive for 5 years. She was infected with HIV by contaminated needles used to inject heroin IV. Her husband recently died from AIDS. Her diagnoses are major depression; alcohol dependence; and opioid dependence, in remission. She is found to be in early-stage HIV disease. She states, "I don't need to be treated for AIDS. I've never had any symptoms." The nurse's response is based on the knowledge that:
    a. Tessa is most likely in denial about her illness
    b. Tessa is lying about having no symptoms
    c. The physician will likely prescribe an antiviral medication for her
    d. Individuals in early-stage disease may not have symptoms for many years
    Answer: d

03. Tessa, a 27-year-old mother of three children, is admitted to a dual-diagnosis program for clients with mental illness and substance abuse. Tessa has been HIV-positive for 5 years. She was infected with HIV by contaminated needles used to inject heroin IV. Her husband recently died from AIDS.

Her diagnoses are major depression; alcohol dependence; and opioid dependence, in remission. She is found to be in early-stage HIV disease. Tessa says to the nurse, "I'm so afraid my kids are going to get the disease from me." To help Tessa prevent this from happening, which of the following should she be instructed to do?

a. Wear a face mask when preparing their food.
b. When hands are chapped or cut, wear protective gloves when preparing their food.
c. Do not kiss them on the lips or face.
d. All family members should use disposable dishes and utensils from which to eat

Answer: b

04. Tessa, a 27-year-old mother of three children, is admitted to a dual-diagnosis program for clients with mental illness and substance abuse. Tessa has been HIV-positive for 5 years. She was infected with HIV by contaminated needles used to inject heroin IV. Her husband recently died from AIDS. Her diagnoses are major depression; alcohol dependence; and opioid dependence, in remission. She is found to be in early-stage HIV disease. She continues to be followed for her HIV disease by her family physician and remains symptom-free for 3 years. During one visit, her physician notices an enlarged lymph node in her armpit and one in the groin. Tessa's temperature is 100.9°F. The physician suspects that Tessa has progressed to middle-stage HIV disease. He orders a lymphocyte count. If his suspicion is correct, what would he expect the blood test to show?

a. A T4-cell count between 700 and 800 mm^3
b. A T4-cell count between 500 and 600 mm^3
c. A T4-cell count between 200 and 500 mm^3
d. A T4-cell count below 200 mm^3

Answer: c

05. Which of the following statements is true about hospice services?

a. Staff is on-call to families on a 24-hour basis.
b. Hospice services to the family will be discontinued upon a client's death.
c. The hospice will ensure that the client is hospitalized at the time of death.
d. The hospice is staffed solely with volunteers.

Answer: a

37 Problems Related to Abuse or Neglect

01. Roberta is a 43-year-old married woman who has called in sick to work for 3 days. When she finally returns to work, her makeup cannot conceal bruises on her face. A coworker who is a good friend mentions the bruises and says that they look like the bruises she used to have after being beaten by her former husband. Roberta says, "It was an accident. He just had a terrible day at work. He's being so kind and gentle now. Yesterday he brought me flowers. He says he's going to get a new job, so it won't ever happen again." Which phase of the cycle of battering does Roberta's response represent?

a. Phase I: The Tension-Building Phase
b. Phase II: The Acute Battering Incident

c. Phase III: The Honeymoon Phase
d. Phase IV: The Resolution Phase
Answer: c

02. Roberta is a 43-year-old married woman who has called in sick to work for 3 days. When she finally returns to work, her makeup cannot conceal bruises on her face. A coworker who is a good friend mentions the bruises and says that they look like the bruises she used to have after being beaten by her former husband. Roberta says, "It was an accident. He just had a terrible day at work. He's being so kind and gentle now. Yesterday he brought me flowers. He says he's going to get a new job, so it won't ever happen again." Roberta's co-worker recommends that Roberta seek assistance from her employee assistance program. Roberta refuses because she believes her husband has reformed. What is the best alternative suggestion her coworker can make at this point?
a. Buy a gun.
b. File for divorce.
c. Press charges of assault and battery.
d. Carry the number of the safe house for battered women.
Answer: d

03. Katie is a 9-year-old third grader. Her teacher, Mrs. Small, notices that Katie has had an open lesion on her left arm for a week. The lesion, which has never been covered with a bandage, appears to have become infected. Katie is often absent from school and seems apathetic and tired when she attends. Other children in the classroom avoid her, and Mrs. Small has overheard them talking about Katie stealing food from them at lunchtime. Mrs. Small's observations are indications of which of the following?
a. Physical neglect
b. Emotional injury
c. Physical abuse
d. Sexual abuse
Answer: a

04. Teresa, an unmarried 37-year-old woman, has recently been referred from her family physician to a psychiatrist with the complaint of "anxiety attacks." These attacks occur in the evening before bedtime, and Teresa has also been experiencing insomnia. When she does get to sleep, she often has nightmares. She tells the psychiatrist that her father has recently been diagnosed with an inoperable brain tumor. What might the psychiatrist suspect after making his initial assessment of Teresa?
a. Possible depressive disorder.
b. Possible history of childhood incest
c. Possible anticipatory grieving
d. Possible history of childhood physical abuse
Answer: b

05. The police escort Zoe, a 29-year-old married stock market analyst, to the emergency department (ED) of an inner-city hospital. She is sobbing, her clothing is torn, and she has superficial cuts on

her neck and chest. She was leaving her office after working late and was accosted from behind as she bent to unlock her car, which was parked at the periphery of the parking lot. Her assailant raped her and stole her purse and her car. She walked to a nearby telephone, dialed 911, and a police car was dispatched to assist her. Upon arrival at the ED, the triage nurse immediately calls a member of the sexual assault crisis team, who arrives within 20 minutes and remains with Zoe throughout her stay in the ED. What is the most therapeutic thing for the nurse to say to Zoe when she arrives at the ED?

a. "You are safe now."
b. "I'll call your husband."
c. "The police will want to interview you."
d. "We'll have to take photographs of those wounds."

Answer: a

06. The police escort Zoe, a 29-year-old married stock market analyst, to the emergency department (ED) of an inner-city hospital. She is sobbing, her clothing is torn, and she has superficial cuts on her neck and chest. She was leaving her office after working late and was accosted from behind as she bent to unlock her car, which was parked at the periphery of the parking lot. Her assailant raped her and stole her purse and her car. She walked to a nearby telephone, dialed 911, and a police car was dispatched to assist her. Upon arrival at the ED, the triage nurse immediately calls a member of the sexual assault crisis team, who arrives within 20 minutes and remains with Zoe throughout her stay in the ED. By now, Zoe is crying, pacing and cursing her attacker. Which behavioral defense do these manifestations represent?

a. Controlled response pattern
b. Compounded rape reaction
c. Expressed response pattern
d. Silent rape reaction

Answer: c

38   Community Mental Health Nursing

01. Victor is a 47-year-old man with schizophrenia. He lives with his 67-year-old mother, who has always managed his affairs. He has never been employed. Recently his mother had to have an emergency cholecystectomy, at which time Victor suffered an exacerbation of his psychosis and was hospitalized. Victor's hospitalization represents an example of which of the following?

a. Primary prevention
b. Secondary prevention
c. Tertiary prevention
d. None of the above

Answer: b

02. Victor is a 47-year-old man with schizophrenia. He lives with his 67-year-old mother, who has always managed his affairs. He has never been employed. Recently his mother had to have an emergency cholecystectomy, at which time Victor suffered an exacerbation of his psychosis and

was hospitalized. On discharge from the hospital, Victor's physician refers him for nursing case management. Which of the following statements best describes case management?
a. Reducing residual defects associated with chronic mental illness
b. Provision of cost-effective care based on need
c. Long-term coordination of needed services by multiple providers
d. Recognition of symptoms and provision of treatment

Answer: c

03. Victor is a 47-year-old man with schizophrenia. He lives with his 67-year-old mother, who has always managed his affairs. He has never been employed. Recently his mother had to have an emergency cholecystectomy, at which time Victor suffered an exacerbation of his psychosis and was hospitalized. On discharge from the hospital, Victor's physician refers him for nursing case management. Once a month, the home health nurse administers Victor's injection of haloperidol (Haldol). This nursing intervention is an example of:
a. Primary prevention
b. Secondary prevention
c. Tertiary prevention
d. None of the above

Answer: c

04. One of the major problems in attempting to provide health care services to the homeless is:
a. Most of them do not want help.
b. They are suspicious of anyone who offers help.
c. Most are proud and will refuse charity.
d. They have a penchant for mobility.

Answer: d

05. A recent increase in which of the following diseases has been noted among the homeless?
a. Meningitis
b. Tuberculosis
c. Encephalopathy
d. Mononucleosis

Answer: b

06. Which of the following are ongoing problems for many homeless individuals?
a. Alcoholism and thermoregulation
b. Sexually transmitted diseases, including HIV disease
c. Conditions related to dietary deficiencies
d. All of the above

Answer: d

07. Which of the following interventions would be considered primary prevention for a homeless individual who lives at a shelter?
    a. Job training
    b. A place to eat and sleep
    c. Clean clothing
    d. Nursing care
    Answer: a

39 Cultural Concepts Relevant to Psychiatric Nursing

01. Asian-Americans often view emotional illness as behavior that is out of control and that which brings shame on the family. Which of the following responses to psychological distress is most likely to occur among this cultural group?
    a. Obsessive-compulsive behavior
    b. Depression
    c. Somatization disorder
    d. Phobias
    Answer: c

02. A common symptom of psychotic disorders is "flat" affect, or little change in facial expression that signals change in mood or feeling tone. Because of cultural differences, with which of the following cultural groups would care have to be taken in interpreting the affect as "flat?"
    a. African-Americans
    b. Native-Americans
    c. Latino-Americans
    d. Western European-Americans
    Answer: b

03. What is the best reason for including favorite or culturally required foods in the diets of clients from other cultures?
    a. It prevents malnutrition.
    b. It prevents clients from becoming agitated.
    c. It ensures the client's cooperation with scientifically based treatment.
    d. It conveys acceptance of the client's beliefs and identity.
    Answer: d

04. Albert, a homeless Native-American, is taken to the emergency department (ED) by the shelter nurse. Albert has a known history of diabetes, and he has a sore on his foot that he says he has had for several weeks. He refuses to talk to the physician on-call in the ED unless a shaman is present. Which of the following interventions would be most appropriate?
    a. Try to locate a shaman and ask him to come to the ED.
    b. Explain to Albert that "voodoo" medicine will not heal the wound on his foot.

c. Ask Albert to explain what he thinks the shaman will do that would not be done by the ED physician.

d. Tell Albert that he has the right to refuse treatment by the ED physician—it is his choice.

Answer: a

05. Which of the following is associated with values of the Northern European-American culture (dominant cultural group)?

a. They are present oriented.

b. They are highly religious, and church attendance is at an all time high.

c. They value punctuality and efficiency.

d. With the advent of technology, increased emphasis is being placed on family cohesiveness.

Answer: c

06. Which of the following is typical of the African-American culture?

a. They often have a strong religious orientation.

b. Personal space tends to be larger than that of the dominant culture.

c. About one-half of all African American households are headed by a woman.

d. In the Deep South, the African-American folk practitioner is known as a shaman.

Answer: a

07. Which of the following relates to individuals of the Native-American culture?

a. Most are warm and outgoing.

b. Touch is a common form of communication.

c. Primary social organizations are family and tribe.

d. Most Native-Americans are future oriented.

Answer: c

08. Which of the following relates to individuals of the Asian-American culture?

a. Obesity and alcoholism are common problems.

b. The elderly maintain positions of authority within the culture.

c. "Hot" and "cold" are the fundamental concepts of Asian health practices.

d. Asian-Americans willingly seek psychiatric assistance for emotional problems.

Answer: b

09. Which of the following relates to individuals of the Latino-American culture?

a. Latino-Americans shy away from any form of touch.

b. Latino-Americans tend to be future-oriented.

c. Roman Catholicism is the predominant religion, although the influence of the church is weak.

d. When illness is encountered, the first contact is often with the curandero folk healer.

Answer: d

10. Which of the following relates to individuals of the Western European-American culture?
   a. They are present oriented; future is perceived as God's will.
   b. Youth is valued; elderly are commonly placed in nursing homes.
   c. Alcoholism is a major problem in the Western European-American culture.
   d. They have a large personal space.
   Answer: a

40 Ethical and Legal Issues in Psychiatric Nursing

01. Raymond is a 54-year-old man with chronic schizophrenia who is seen monthly by a community mental health nurse for administration of fluphenazine decanoate (Prolixin Decanoate). Raymond refuses his medication at one regularly scheduled monthly visit. Which of the following interventions by the nurse is considered to be ethically appropriate?
   a. Tell Raymond it is his right not to take the medication.
   b. Tell Raymond that if he does not take his medication he will have to be hospitalized.
   c. Arrange with a relative to add medication to Raymond's morning orange juice.
   d. Call for help to hold Raymond down while the shot is administered.
   Answer: a

02. Raymond is a 54-year-old man with chronic schizophrenia who is seen monthly by a community mental health nurse for administration of fluphenazine decanoate (Prolixin Decanoate). Raymond refuses his medication at one regularly scheduled monthly visit. He is hospitalized when he becomes agitated, physically aggressive and unable to communicate cooperatively. With the help of hospital security and the police who brought him to the emergency department, the nurse and resident apply leather restraints to Raymond's arms and legs against his very loud protests. Raymond yells that he is going to sue them for assault and battery. Under which of the following conditions is the staff protected?
   a. Raymond is a voluntary commitment and poses no danger to self or others.
   b. Raymond is a voluntary commitment but poses a danger to self or others.
   c. Raymond is an involuntary commitment but poses no danger to self or others.
   d. Raymond is an involuntary commitment and poses a danger to self or others.
   Answer: d

03. Raymond is a 54-year-old man with chronic schizophrenia who is seen monthly by a community mental health nurse for administration of fluphenazine decanoate (Prolixin Decanoate). Raymond refuses his medication at one regularly scheduled monthly visit. He is hospitalized when he becomes agitated, physically aggressive and unable to communicate cooperatively. With the help of hospital security and the police who brought him to the emergency department, the nurse and resident apply leather restraints to Raymond's arms and legs against his very loud protests. Raymond yells that he is going to sue them for assault and battery. Which of the following conditions identifies the criteria for this offense (outside an emergency situation)?
   a. The staff becomes angry with Raymond and calls him offensive names.
   b. Raymond is touched (or fears being touched) without his consent.

c. The nurse hides Raymond's clothes so he cannot leave.

d. The nurse puts Raymond in restraints against his wishes.

Answer: b

04. Raymond is a 54-year-old man with chronic schizophrenia who is seen monthly by a community mental health nurse for administration of fluphenazine decanoate (Prolixin Decanoate). Raymond refuses his medication at one regularly scheduled monthly visit. He is hospitalized when he becomes agitated, physically aggressive and unable to communicate cooperatively. With the help of hospital security and the police who brought him to the emergency department, the nurse and resident apply leather restraints to Raymond's arms and legs against his very loud protests. Raymond yells that he is going to sue them for assault and battery. The nurse states, "Well, I know Raymond is against us putting him in restraints, but if I ever get in this condition, I hope people would do the same for me." This is an example of which ethical philosophy?

a. Kantianism

b. Utilitarianism

c. Christian ethics

d. Natural Law ethics

Answer: c

05. Raymond is a 54-year-old man with chronic schizophrenia who is seen monthly by a community mental health nurse for administration of fluphenazine decanoate (Prolixin Decanoate). Raymond refuses his medication at one regularly scheduled monthly visit. He is hospitalized when he becomes agitated, physically aggressive and unable to communicate cooperatively. With the help of hospital security and the police who brought him to the emergency department, the nurse and resident apply leather restraints to Raymond's arms and legs against his very loud protests. Raymond yells that he is going to sue them for assault and battery. To adhere to the principle of least-restrictive alternative, instead of putting Raymond in leather restraints, the nurse might have (with physician's order):

a. Given Raymond an injection of a major tranquilizer

b. Put Raymond in a locked room by himself

c. Told Raymond if he did not calm down, he would be given an electroconvulsive therapy treatment.

d. Put Raymond in soft, Posey restraints, rather than in leather restraints.

Answer: a

41 Psychiatric Home Nursing Care

01. Wally is a 35-year-old man who was diagnosed with paranoid schizophrenia when he was 23 years old. He is disabled because of his illness and receives Medicaid. He lives with his widowed mother. Susan, a home health psychiatric nurse, is referred to Wally's case after he has been hospitalized for the third time in 6 months. His mother tells Susan, "I just can't get him to take his medicine. He thinks I'm trying to poison him." What is Susan's likely intervention in this case?

a. Stop by Wally's house every morning to administer his oral medication.

b. Suggest Wally's mother hide the concentrate form of his medication in his orange juice.

c. Suggest the physician order biweekly injections of the decanoate form of his medication.

d. Tell Wally that if he does not start taking his medication regularly, he will have to be institutionalized.

Answer: c

02. I n visiting the client with paranoid schizophrenia in his or her home, the nurse must strive to establish trust in the relationship before proceeding with interventions generally accepted as appropriate in home health nursing. "Hands-on" assessment may need to be delayed because:

a. Individuals with paranoid schizophrenia may perceive touch as threatening.

b. Psychiatric nurses need to have a medical staff nurse available to assist with the physical assessment.

c. It is more important to assess mental status of psychiatric clients before assessing their physical status.

d. Consent by the client will need to be granted after he or she is less delusional.

Answer: a

03. Wally is a 35-year-old man who was diagnosed with paranoid schizophrenia when he was 23 years old. He is disabled because of his illness and receives Medicaid. He lives with his widowed mother. Susan, a home health psychiatric nurse, is referred to Wally's case after he has been hospitalized for the third time in 6 months. He quits taking his medication and decompensates about every 3 months. His mother says to the home health psychiatric nurse, "Sometimes I just get so weary. Nothing I try to do ever helps our situation." How may the home health psychiatric nurse help Wally's mother?

a. Show her how to organize her time better so that she may do everything for Wally.

b. Help her to problem-solve how she may draw monetary support from the state so that she can stay home and take care of Wally.

c. Encourage her to tell Wally that if he doesn't "straighten up," he will have to leave her home.

d. Encourage participation in a support group of family members of individuals with mental illness.

Answer: d

04. Wally is a 35-year-old man who was diagnosed with paranoid schizophrenia when he was 23 years old. He is disabled because of his illness and receives Medicaid. He lives with his widowed mother. Susan, a home health psychiatric nurse, is referred to Wally's case after he has been hospitalized for the third time in 6 months. He quits taking his medication and decompensates about every 3 months. Wally, a 35-year-old client with paranoid schizophrenia, says to the home health psychiatric nurse, "I know you write stuff about me in your notes. I want to know what you write. I read that those notes really belong to me." What is the appropriate response by the nurse?

a. "The notes do not belong to you, Wally. They belong to the home health agency."

b. "The notes belong to the home health agency, Wally. But I can make a copy for you if you'd like."

c. "I will have to talk to the physician before I can share any of the information with you, Wally."

d. "Yes, you are right, Wally. The notes do belong to you. I will give them to you when I finish writing them."
Answer: b

05. The home health psychiatric nurse visits Twila, a client with agoraphobia, once a week to assist with activities of daily living. With knowledge about confidentiality in home health care, which of the following would the home health psychiatric nurse report, regardless of confidentiality?
a. Twila answers the door with a bruise on her forehead and explains that she ran into the bathroom door.
b. Twila's little girl, age 3, has a large scrape on her leg, and Twila explains that she fell off her tricycle.
c. Twila's husband and two of his friends are sitting in the living room openly snorting cocaine.
d. Twila's mother, who lives with them, has an intermittent, loud, productive cough.
Answer: c

42 Forensic Nursing

01. Karen, an 18-year-old college freshman, is brought to the emergency department by her roommate. She tells the admitting nurse that she was raped by her date when she refused to consent to his sexual advances. A sexual assault nurse examiner (SANE) is called in to assist with Karen's case. What is the priority intervention with Karen?
a. Help her to bathe and clean up.
b. Ensure medical stabilization.
c. Take pictures of the wounds.
d. Call law enforcement officials to report the rape.
Answer: b

02. For the purpose of collecting evidence, the rape victim is asked to remove her clothing. The SANE will preserve the clothing in which of the following ways?
a. Shake the clothing so that any possible evidence that may be adhering to it is not missed.
b. Place all items of clothing together in a plastic bag for protection.
c. Store the clothing in the police department's evidence collection division.
d. Seal each item of clothing separately in a dated paper bag.
Answer: d

03. The nurse may advise the sexual assault victim that there are interventions that may be undertaken to prevent all of the following except:
a. Pregnancy
b. Gonorrhea
c. HIV
d. Chlamydia
Answer: c

04. Which of the following behaviors has been identified as most common among the mentally ill incarcerated?
   a. Denial of problems
   b. Thought disorders
   c. Hallucinations
   d. Delusions
   Answer: a

05. Which of the following nursing interventions are not appropriate in the correctional setting?
   a. Encouragement of feelings
   b. Guidance through the mourning process
   c. Setting of personal boundaries
   d. Touch and self-disclosure
   Answer: d